INTERVIEWS FOR MEDICAL SCHOOL

Multiple Mini Interview (MMI) Practice

Thanthullu Vasu, Shreya Shyam &
the RISE Foundation Leicestershire

tfm Publishing Limited, Castle Hill Barns, Harley, Shrewsbury, SY5 6LX, UK
Tel: +44 (0)1952 510061; Fax: +44 (0)1952 510192
E-mail: info@tfmpublishing.com; Web site: www.tfmpublishing.com

Editing: Dr. Christine Graham PhD
Editing, design & typesetting: Nikki Bramhill BSc (Hons), Dip Law
Cover photo: © iStock.com
Credit: sdecoret; stock illustration ID: 1219662779

First edition:	© 2023
Paperback	ISBN: 978-1-913755-32-4
E-book editions:	© 2023
ePub	ISBN: 978-1-913755-33-1
Mobi	ISBN: 978-1-913755-34-8
Web pdf	ISBN: 978-1-913755-35-5

Printed by L&C PRINTING GROUP, Tadeusza Romanowicza 11, 30-702 Kraków, Poland
Tel: +48 690 565 600; E-mail: office@lcprinting.eu; Web site: www.lcprinting.eu

Contents

Section 2: General ethics

Section 4: Communication – general scenarios   281

Introduction to non-medical communication   282
Shreya Shyam

Section 9: Other topics

Preface

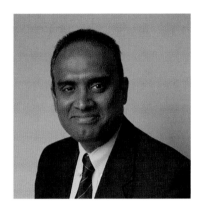 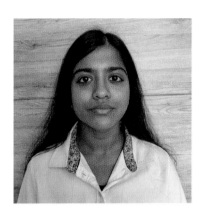

Dear Friends,

Securing a place in a medical school is becoming more competitive nowadays! Studying medicine is very satisfying as it leads to a fulfilling career that involves communicating, treating and caring for patients. In the aftermath of the COVID 19 pandemic, many have been motivated to take up a career path in healthcare, resulting in more medical school applicants than ever before. In turn, universities have a much more rigorous screening process. Medical schools seek out students with qualities including compassion, honesty, teamwork skills and many more, along with a baseline knowledge and skills.

The RISE Foundation Leicestershire is a charity based in the United Kingdom. We run regular interview courses to prepare candidates aspiring to become future doctors. Our team has a combined experience, expertise and motivation to teach, and our courses continually receive excellent feedback.

The money raised through these courses goes to charitable causes via the Foundation. We came up with the innovative idea of publishing a book after running these courses successfully and thus putting all the knowledge, experience and interview tips into a printed and ebook format. The book contains practice questions from a range of interview stations, as well as top tips and model answers to help the next generation of medical students to prepare for their interview. The author royalties from sales of the book will be donated to worthy causes through the RISE charity.

We thank Nikki Bramhill from tfm publishing Ltd, and her team, who have given us enthusiasm, energy and support round the clock to carry out this project successfully. Without the help of Nikki, this project would not have been possible.

Our team hopes that you find this book useful in your quest for medical placement and we wish you success in all your future efforts. We thank you for all your support for our RISE Foundation Leicestershire charity.

Dr Thanthullu Vasu
Consultant in Pain Medicine
University Hospitals of Leicester NHS Trust, Leicester, UK
Trustee, RISE Foundation Leicestershire Charity, UK

Ms Shreya Shyam
Medical Student
University of Birmingham, Birmingham, UK

Contributors

Ms Sheena Abraham
Medical Student
University of Manchester, Manchester, UK

Dr Shyam Sundar Balasubramanian MBBS MD FRCA FFPMRCA MSc (Medical Leadership)
Consultant Anaesthetist and Associate Medical Director
University Hospital Coventry & Warwickshire, Coventry, UK

Dr James Francis MBBS FRCP(UK)
Consultant Rheumatologist
University Hospitals of Leicester NHS Trust, Leicester, UK

Ms Roshni Francis
Medical Student
Barts and the London School of Medicine and Dentistry (QMUL), London, UK.

Dr Satya Francis MBBS FRCA
Consultant Anaesthetist & Honorary Senior Lecturer
University Hospitals of Leicester NHS Trust, Leicester, UK

Dr Prabhu Gandhimani MD FRCA FIPP FFPMRCA MA CMgr MCMI
Clinical Lead and Consultant in Pain Service
Kingston Hospital, Surrey, UK

Dr Subramanian Ganesan MBBS DCH MRCPCH FRCPCH Paed Epilepsy SPIN
Consultant Paediatric Neurodisability and Epilepsy
Leicestershire Partnership NHS Trust, Leicester, UK

Ms Shivani Ganesh iBSc
Medical Student
Barts and the London School of Medicine and Dentistry, London, UK

Dr Priya Gauthama MBBS MD FRCA
Consultant Anaesthetist
University Hospitals of Leicester NHS Trust, Leicester, UK

Dr Rupa Jayaraj MBBS DA FRCA PGCE
Consultant Anaesthetist
University Hospitals of Leicester NHS Trust, Leicester, UK

Ms Pritika Kandamaran
Medical Student
The University of the West Indies, Barbados

Dr Hema Kannappan MBBS MRCPCH FRCPCH
Clinical Lead for Paediatric Gastroenterology
University Hospital of Coventry & Warwickshire, Coventry, UK

Mr Kaviarasan Karunanidhi MSc (Computer Science)
Director, HealthyAA Ltd UK
Director, HealthyAA India Pvt Ltd
Leicester, UK

Dr Kodaganallur Parthasarathi Krishnan MBBS FRCA FCARCSI
Consultant Anaesthetist
Sandwell and West Birmingham Hospitals NHS Trust, Birmingham, UK

Mr Jatin Naidu
Medical Student
University College of London, UK

Dr Leena Naidu MBBS MRCP FRCR
Consultant Radiologist, University Hospitals of Northamptonshire, UK and
Clinical Director in Diagnostic Imaging
Honorary Lecturer
Leicester Medical School, UK

Dr Vijaianitha Nallendran MBBS MD MRCOG
Locum Consultant Gynaecologist
University Hospitals of Leciester NHS Trust, Leicester, UK

Dr Balamurugan Nambi MBBS MRCPsych CCT CAMHS
Consultant Child & Adolescent Psychiatrist
Derbyshire Healthcare NHS Foundation Trust, Derby, UK

Dr Selvakumar Panchatsharam MBBS DA FRCA FFICM EDIC
Consultant in Intensive Care and Anaesthesia & Clinical Lead for Intensive Care
Kettering General Hospital NHS Trust, Kettering, UK

Mr Gokul Parameswaran
Medical Student
University of Oxford, Oxford, UK

Mr Hari Adharsh Prabhu
Medical Student
Imperial College London, London, UK

Mr Gamma Manohara Prasad B Arch M Plan (Urban Planning) MSc (CPRED) CoA ITPI
Senior Procurement Manager, National Health Service
Leicester, UK

Mr Suresh Seetharaman BE DPSI (Law)
Director, Global Aspire
Director, HealthyAA Ltd
Leicester, UK.

Ms Shreya Shyam
Medical Student
University of Birmingham, Birmingham, UK

Dr Arani Sridhar MBBS DCH MD DNB MSc PG Cert Med Ed FRCPCH FRCP
Consultant Paediatrician/Rheumatologist
University Hospitals of Leicester NHS Trust, UK
Honorary Senior Lecturer, University of Leicester, Leicester, UK

Ms Swetha Sridhar BSc Hons Biological Sciences (Neuroscience)
London, UK

Dr Thiagarajan Sridhar MBBS MRCP FRCR PGdip in Clinical Oncology
Consultant Clinical Oncologist
University Hospitals of Leicester NHS Trust, Leicester, UK

Mr Paul Sanjay Sundaram BMedSc Clinical Cancer Sciences
Medical student
University of Birmingham, Birmingham, UK

Dr Premkumar Sundaram MBBS MD DCH DNB(Paeds) FRCPCH
Consultant Paediatrician and Paediatric Diabetologist
University Hospitals of Leicester NHS Trust, Leicester, UK

Mr Siva Thanthullu
Student
Leicester, UK

Dr Balaji Varadhan
Specialist Doctor Medical Oncology
University Hospitals of Leicester NHS Trust, Leicester, UK

Dr Thanthullu Vasu MBBS MD DNB FRCA FIPP FFPMRCA Dip Pain Mgt
Consultant in Pain Medicine
University Hospitals of Leicester NHS Trust, Leicester, UK

Section **1**

Medical ethics

Section editor: Thanthullu Vasu

Introduction to medical ethics

Questions on ethical scenarios or dilemmas are unavoidable in a multiple mini interview (MMI) or medical interview. However, most candidates appearing for the MMI find this problematic unless they are well prepared. For entrance to medical school, the candidate is not expected to solve complex ethical problems. Still, they should clearly understand the dilemma, and be able to explain the pros and cons of both sides of the dilemma, existing controversies, and possible solutions and their limitations.

If a candidate has a good approach to tackling the scenario and has a systematic way of explaining this, examiners will be satisfied to give good scores; it is the duty of the candidate to provide confidence to the examiners that they understand the problem and its complexity. Practising as many scenarios as possible helps face this MMI station.

Must do

To deal with an ethical scenario, a candidate should:

- Understand the ethical dilemma and make a structured plan before the discussion.
- Start explaining the extent or consequences of the problem or dilemma.
- Try to summarise both sides of the argument or dilemma in clear, simple language.
- If possible, present evidence for both sides.
- Conclude by explaining their position/stance in this dilemma.

Common mistakes

Common mistakes made by candidates include:

- Being anxious and thinking that they need to solve the problem.
- Not explaining what the problem or dilemma is.
- Staying on one side of a situation without explaining the other side.
- Being firm towards one side and not describing the limits of their preferred side.
- Not presenting in a balanced way.
- Not concluding clearly.
- Not helping the examiner to believe that they understand the problem.

Please remember that ethical problems are debatable and controversial and do not always have a simple solution.

Four pillars of medical ethics

If possible, always approach the medical ethics question based on the four pillars of medical ethics explained below; having this as a basic framework will guide the candidate to give more value to their answer:

1. Autonomy — giving respect to the patient and letting them decide.
2. Non-maleficence — not doing harm.
3. Beneficence — always act to benefit the patient.
4. Justice — consideration of the law and the overall benefit to society.

We strongly suggest that the candidate practises a few ethical dilemma questions with these four themes and clarifies their answers.

GMC ethical guidance

Always quote the ethical guidance published by the UK General Medical Council (GMC); this is available on their website: https://www.gmc-uk.org/ethical-guidance.

The GMC has published guidance for doctors on professional standards and medical ethics. The GMC provides 32 pieces of ethical guidance, set out in 11 categories. These include:

1. Good medical practice — core guidance for doctors; it is the foundation on which the rest of the guidance is built.

2. Confidentiality — includes guidance on disclosing patient information. Guidance includes handling patient information, disclosing information for training/education, disclosing information for employment/insurance, disclosing information about serious communicable diseases, fitness to drive and reporting to the Driver and Vehicle Licensing Agency (DVLA), reporting gunshot/knife wounds, and responding to criticism in the media.

3. Maintaining professionalism — includes advice on maintaining appropriate boundaries and guidance on social media. Guidance includes personal beliefs, conflicts of interest, social media, ending a professional relationship with the patient, chaperones/intimate examinations, maintaining the professional boundary between patient and doctor, and sexual behaviour and duty to report colleagues.

4. Children and young people — includes two documents on protecting children/young people and care for 0-18-year-olds.

5. Prescribing — guidance on good practice for prescribing and managing medicines and devices.

6. Decision making and consent — three guidances include shared decision making/consent, making and using audio-visual recordings of patients, and consent to research.

7. Care at the end of life — two guidances include treatment and care towards the end of life and assistance to die requests.

8. Leadership and management — guidance includes leadership and management, raising and acting on concerns about patient safety, a duty of candour (being open and honest if something goes wrong, apologising, and sharing mistakes with colleagues for learning purposes), delegation and referral, acting as a witness in legal proceedings, reporting criminal and regulatory proceedings, and writing references.

9. Candour and raising concerns — duty of candour (as mentioned above) and raising/acting on concerns about patient safety.
10. Cosmetic interventions — guidance on cosmetic interventions.
11. Research — two guidances, including good research practice and consent to research.

A candidate might not know all these guidances in full, but even if they quote these GMC documents/guidances, they can add value to their answer in an ethical scenario. It is worth reading the summary of the 'Good medical practice' guideline of the GMC.

Common scenarios

The candidate must practice common scenarios such as euthanasia, abortion, opt in/opt out of transplant, use of contraceptive pills, Jehovah's Witnesses and refusal of treatments. Complex arguments for and against each side should be practised before approaching the station. Always use the four pillars of medical ethics to justify the answer. Always recognise these are complex and sensitive problems and prove to the examiner that you understand this complexity.

Confidentiality

Confidentiality is an ethical and legal obligation for doctors; the GMC provides detailed guidance on confidentiality. In addition, it helps to build trust with the patient.

Informed consent

The clinician should explain in detail using understandable simple language about the intervention, the practicalities, the risks and the possible side effects. Next, the patient must be given enough time to think and decide. Finally, the patient must have the capacity to decide on their own.

Capacity

All adults aged 16 years or more are presumed to have capacity unless shown otherwise.

Mental Capacity Act 2005

When applicable, it is prudent to quote the Mental Capacity Act to provide more evidence or support to your answer.

Gillick competence

Children under 16 years of age may be able to make decisions after the informed consent process if they demonstrate the capacity for mature thinking.

Question 1

Patient confidentiality: disclosing personal information to close family members

Vijaianitha Nallendran

Question

A 23-year-old woman undergoes a termination of pregnancy under general anaesthesia. Unfortunately, the patient had a complication during surgery and her care needed to be transferred to the intensive care unit.

The patient's spouse/partner would like to know the nature of the procedure and the reason for the surgery. The patient has expressed her wishes preoperatively not to disclose her pregnancy and the procedure to her family members.

In the next station, you will discuss these issues with the examiner and explain your opinion regarding the scenario.

Themes for discussion (■ Table 1.1)

Table 1.1.	
Question themes	**What is expected from the candidate?**
1 The candidate greets the examiner and has good body language.	The candidate is presentable and uses good communication skills; always recommended in any station.
2 Is it right for doctors to disclose personal information to close family members?	The candidate gives a good opening statement showing that they understand the situation.
3 The candidate volunteers the cons for disclosing personal information in this scenario.	The candidate clearly understands the cons of disclosing personal information: • Trust is an essential part of the doctor-patient relationship and confidentiality is central to this. • The patient has explicitly expressed her wishes that the doctor must not disclose information regarding her medical condition to family members. • Women may avoid attending abortion clinics to receive safe care if confidentiality is not maintained; this can lead to unsafe procedures. • The overall public trust in doctors will be reduced if the confidentiality of the patient is breached.
4 The candidate also explains the pros of disclosing information in this scenario.	The candidate clearly understands the pros of disclosing information: • Close family members play a significant role in supporting or caring for the patient; they may want, insist or need information regarding the patient's diagnosis, treatment or care. • Discussions with those close to the patient might give information that might help the care given to the patient.

Table 1.1.

Question themes	What is expected from the candidate?
	• GMC advice is to be considerate to those close to the patient and be responsive in giving them information and support whilst maintaining patient confidentiality. • Family members can become upset, frustrated and angry because details are not given, leading to complaints and dissatisfaction.
5 What actions does the doctor need to take in this situation?	• The doctor needs to listen to the concerns and views of the spouse/partner. • Give the information regarding the general condition and prognosis of the patient. Explain the information empathetically and that we are doing everything in the patient's best interest, as per their wish. • Do not disclose confidential information regarding the termination of pregnancy.
6 What factors must be considered if disclosing personal information when a patient lacks capacity?	• The healthcare professional should work on the presumption that every adult patient has the capacity to consent regarding the disclosure of their personal information. • Assess the patient's mental capacity at the time when the decision needs to be taken. • If the capacity is lacking, consider whether their lack of capacity is permanent/temporary. • If temporary, consider whether it is reasonable to wait before disclosing information. • Disclose information if it is of overall benefit to the patient. This aspect should be carefully assessed and, if needed, always involve the multidisciplinary team. • Patient care should always be the priority. • Respect the patient's dignity and privacy. • Consider the patient's previously expressed views and feelings. • Consider the views of people with legal authority to make decisions on behalf of the patient. • Consider and listen to the opinions of people close to the patient regarding the patient's preferences, views and feelings.

Table 1.1.

Question themes	What is expected from the candidate?
7 Do you know the five statutory principles that underpin the Mental Capacity Act 2005?	• A person must be assumed to have capacity unless it is established that they lack capacity. • A person is not to be treated as unable to make a decision, unless all practicable steps to help him to do so have been taken without success. • A person is not to be treated as unable to make a decision merely because he makes an unwise decision. • An act done, or decision made, under this act for or on behalf of a person who lacks capacity must be done, or made, in their best interests. • Before the act is done, or the decision is made, regard must be made as to whether the purpose for which it is needed can be as effectively achieved in a way that is less restrictive of the person's rights and freedom of action.
8 Where can advice be obtained regarding these ethical dilemmas in the hospital/trust?	• Senior clinicians and multidisciplinary team. • Caldicott guardian of the trust. • Trust legal advisers. • Trust ethical committee.
9 Judgement and clarity.	The candidate has clarity in their answer and can explain the pros and cons, concluding clearly. A clear presentation, smiling throughout and avoiding repetition — these steps can increase the scores in this station.
10 Conclusion.	The candidate concludes the session and thanks the examiner at the end. This gains the candidate extra bonus points.

Discussion

Please make sure that you can explain the pros and cons in clear, simple language. It is key to ensure that the examiner has confidence in the candidate understanding the ethical dilemmas. The UK General Medical Council has clear guidance on what actions doctors should take when dealing with situations that carry ethical dilemmas. This guidance helps us to care for our patients in the best possible way without breaking their trust while protecting other individuals and society.

Key Points

- Any ethical dilemma has pros and cons; the candidate must be aware of both.
- The candidate should be able to come to a clear conclusion and explain the reasoning behind their decision.
- Quote the UK General Medical Council's code of ethics/'Good medical practice' document to show awareness of the ethics behind the scenario.

References

1. General Medical Council. Disclosures for the protection of patients and others. Available from: https://www.gmc-uk.org/ethical-guidance/ethical-guidance-for-doctors/confidentiality/disclosures-for-the-protection-of-patients-and-others.

2. Department for Constitutional Affairs. Mental Capacity Act 2005. Available from: https://assets.publishing.service.gov.uk/government/uploads/system/uploads/attachment_data/file/921428/Mental-capacity-act-code-of-practice.pdf.

Question2

Patient confidentiality: a partner's request not to tell the diagnosis

Balaji Varadhan

Question

You are a trainee working on a surgical ward. Mrs F recently complained of a change in bowel habits and was on your surgical ward as an inpatient the previous week and underwent various investigations including blood tests, colonoscopy and a computed tomography (CT) scan. In addition, a biopsy was taken during the colonoscopy.

The biopsy confirmed bowel cancer and the CT scan showed metastasis in the lungs and liver. Her case was discussed in the colorectal multidisciplinary team (MDT); the team decided that it was not surgically resectable, and to refer Mrs F to medical oncology for palliative chemotherapy. Her husband saw her GP when Mrs F was an inpatient in the hospital, and he was told these results and is aware of the bad prognosis.

Mrs F's partner has requested to see you in the hospital and asks you not to tell his wife the diagnosis.

Themes for discussion (▉ Table 1.2)

Table 1.2.	
Question themes	**What is expected from the candidate?**
1 The candidate greets the examiner.	Good body language and a presentable manner.
	If it is a role-play station, introduce yourself with your name and details, ask to whom you are speaking and confirm the identity and relationship of the person.
2 The examiner asks about the dilemmas in the scenario. (If it is a role-play station, the candidate will talk to the person who acts as the husband.)	The candidate gives details of the dilemmas in simple, straightforward language:
	• The partner has requested that his wife is not told of her diagnosis of cancer.
	• The candidate will enquire about the awareness of the husband and how he knew of the diagnosis.
	They listen empathetically and question the fears/worries of the husband.
	They explain to the partner that the patient has the capacity to make their own decisions. Therefore, you can discuss the diagnosis with the patient and the partner (with the patient's consent).
	The candidate explains the risks involved of not disclosing the information to the patient.
3 The candidate has good knowledge of the ethical issues involved.	Patient confidentiality: has a clear understanding and is aware of the importance.
	Doctor and patient relationship to maintain confidentiality.

Table 1.2.

	Question themes	What is expected from the candidate?
4	What happens if confidentiality is breached?	Trust fails between patient and doctor.
		The legality surrounding the confidentiality breach.
		Risks involved in breaching confidentiality.
5	GMC regulations.	All doctors should follow GMC guidelines and cannot breach confidentiality. The candidate shows an awareness of the GMC's 'Ethical guidance' and quotes it.
6	Four pillars of medical ethics.	Autonomy, beneficence, non-maleficence and justice.
		Able to clearly define the four pillars of medical ethics and relate these to the present scenario.
7	How do you apply medical ethics to this scenario?	Able to explain and justify the four pillars within this case scenario; correlates them appropriately.
8	Where can we find confidentiality and good practice in handling patient information guidelines?	The GMC's 'Good medical practice' guidance. The GMC's 'Ethical guidance'.
9	Conclusion.	The candidate concludes and summarises the station.
		The candidate thanks the examiner.
		If it is a role-play station, the candidate enquires if the actor (husband) has any other worries; the candidate explains that, if there are any other questions, they are happy to talk again and explain or clarify any doubts. The candidate thanks them for their time and opportunity to explain the facts.

Discussion

As in any ethical scenario question, there are pros and cons. However, patient confidentiality is key in this question. The patient has a legal and ethical right to know about their condition. At the same time, this must be explained empathetically to the family member and the need for the patient to be aware must be stressed. Patient safety and confidentiality are the priority in any scenario, and this must be mentioned clearly in the answer so that the examiner clearly hears this point from the candidate.

Key Points

- The candidate should be aware of the pros and cons.
- The candidate should stress the importance of patient confidentiality.
- The candidate can use the framework of the four pillars of ethics to explain the answer.
- The candidate can quote the GMC's 'Ethical guidance' and 'Good medical practice' guidance.

References

1. General Medical Council. Good medical practice. Available from: https://www.gmc-uk.org/-/media/documents/good-medical-practice---english-20200128_pdf-51527435.pdf.

2. General Medical Council. Disclosures for the protection of patients and others. Available from: https://www.gmc-uk.org/ethical-guidance/ethical-guidance-for-doctors/confidentiality/disclosures-for-the-protection-of-patients-and-others.

3. General Medical Council. Ethical guidance. Available from: https://www.gmc-uk.org/ethical-guidance.

Question 3

Patient confidentiality: a teenager asking for testing for STDs

Hema Kannappan

Question

You are a GP trainee working in your surgery. Andrea, who is 15 years old, presents with complaints of headaches. During the consultation, she discloses she has recently become sexually active and asks you to test her for sexually transmitted diseases (STDs). The following station will discuss the ethical dilemmas in this situation.

Themes for discussion (■ Table 1.3)

Table 1.3.

	Question themes	What is expected from the candidate?
1	The candidate greets the examiner.	Good body language and a presentable manner.

Table 1.3.

	Question themes	What is expected from the candidate?
2	The patient has disclosed a sexual relationship and is worried about STDs.	How long has the patient been sexually active? Explore the history in an empathetic manner. Why is she worried about STDs? Has she got reasons for her worries? Any significant history? What does she know about STDs? Assess her knowledge and need for education regarding safe sexual practice. Do the parents know? Assess the awareness and communication situation.
3	Awareness of risks.	Is she aware of the risks involved with unprotected sexual intercourse? Child protection and abuse: issues to be assessed.
4	Ethical issues involved.	Patient confidentiality: the candidate shows that they have a clear understanding regarding the duty of confidentiality. Doctor and patient relationship to maintain confidentiality.
5	What happens if confidentiality is breached?	Doctor and patient trust fails. The legality surrounding a confidentiality breach. Risks involved.
6	GMC regulations.	All doctors should follow the GMC guidelines and cannot breach confidentiality.

Table 1.3.

	Question themes	What is expected from the candidate?
7	Four pillars of medical ethics.	Autonomy, beneficence, non-maleficence and justice.
8	How do you apply medical ethics to this scenario?	The candidate can explain and justify the four pillars of medical ethics within this case scenario/context. Then, they apply these principles in a practical way.
9	Where can we find confidentiality and good practice in handling patient information guidelines?	The GMC's 'Good medical practice' guidance.
10	Conclusion.	The candidate concludes and summarises the station; they also thank the examiner.

Discussion

Please make sure that you can explain the pros and cons in clear, simple language. Explain ethical dilemmas to the examiner to ensure they have confidence that you understand; it is key in this station.

This station has the complexity of exploring the understanding of sexual practice in the teenager but, at the same time, advising appropriately on safe practice. The clinician has to find out whether the teenager's parents are aware of the practice, but at the same time assure patient confidentiality and give confidence to the patient.

Key Points

- Any ethical dilemma has pros and cons; the candidate must be aware of both.
- The candidate should be able to come to a clear conclusion and explain the reasoning behind this decision.
- Quote the UK General Medical Council's code of ethics/'Good medical practice' document to show you know the ethics behind the scenario.

References

1. General Medical Council. Disclosures for the protection of patients and others. Available from: https://www.gmc-uk.org/ethical-guidance/ethical-guidance-for-doctors/confidentiality/disclosures-for-the-protection-of-patients-and-others.

Question 4

Patient confidentiality: a partner refusing to disclose HIV status

Vijaianitha Nallendran

Question

You are a GP and a pregnant lady has come to see you after her screening blood tests. Unfortunately, she is positive for HIV. You gave the diagnosis and advised her to disclose the information to her partner. However, the patient refuses to disclose the information. The next station will discuss these issues and your opinion in this situation.

Themes for discussion (■ Table 1.4)

Table 1.4.	
Question themes	**What is expected from the candidate?**
1 The candidate greets the examiner and has good body language.	The candidate is presentable and uses good communication skills; always recommended in any station.

Table 1.4.

Question themes	What is expected from the candidate?
2 Is it right for doctors to disclose the information with the partner?	The candidate gives a good opening statement of the understanding of the situation.
3 The candidate volunteers the cons of disclosing the information without the patient's approval.	The candidate clearly understands the cons for disclosing information: • Trust is an essential part of the doctor-patient relationship and confidentiality is central to this. • Women may avoid attendance at the clinic and not receive appropriate care. • This will increase the risk of disease progression in her case. • There is an increased risk of vertical transmission, increasing the risk of infection to the fetus. • The partner will continue to be infected. • The patient and the overall community's trust in doctors will be reduced if confidentiality is breached. • It can deter other patients who are pregnant from undergoing an HIV test.

4 The candidate also explains the pros of disclosing the information.	The candidate clearly understands the pros for disclosing the information:
	
	 • The partner is at risk of infection with HIV, which has serious consequences for his health.
	 • The GMC recommends that doctors may disclose information to a person who has close contact with a serious communicable disease if the doctor has reason to think that:
	     - the person is at risk of infection that is likely to result in serious harm;
	     - the patient has not informed them and cannot be persuaded to do so.

Table 1.4.

	Question themes	What is expected from the candidate?
5	What actions does the doctor need to take in this situation?	• Explore the reasons why the patient does not want to disclose the information. • Give advice regarding practical measures that should be taken to reduce infection of the partner. • Continue to persuade the patient to disclose the information to her partner. • If the patient continues to refuse, inform the patient that you are going to disclose the information as it is your duty.
6	Do you know the situations when confidentiality can be overridden?	The candidate understands the GMC recommendations. Doctors may disclose personal information without breaching duties of confidentiality when the following circumstances apply: • The disclosure is of overall benefit to a patient who lacks the capacity to consent. • Disclosure is required by law. • Disclosure has been approved under a statutory process that sets aside the common law duty of confidentiality. • Disclosure can be justified in the public interest.
7	What factors must be considered if disclosing personal information without consent?	• Potential harm or distress to the patient from disclosure. • Potential harm to trust in doctors generally. • Potential harm to others if information is not disclosed. • Potential benefits to the individual/society from the release of information. • Nature of the information that is being disclosed and views expressed by the patient. • Whether harm can be avoided or benefit gained without breaching patient privacy or with minimal intrusion.

Table 1.4.

Question themes	What is expected from the candidate?
8 Do you know the people you can get advice from in the trust?	• Caldicott guardian. • Trust legal advisers. • Senior clinicians in the case of junior doctors. Hospitals have an ethical committee that can be approached for advice and practicalities in ethical dilemmas. For complex legal issues, medicolegal defence unions also provide clear advice on how to proceed. It is a requirement for all practising clinicians to have membership of a medical defence union.
9 Judgement and clarity.	The candidate has clarity in their answer and can explain the pros and cons, concluding clearly. A clear presentation, smiling throughout and avoiding repetition — these steps can increase the scores in this station.
10 Conclusion.	The candidate concludes the session and thanks the examiner at the end. This gains the candidate extra bonus points.

Discussion

Please ensure that you can explain the pros and cons and are confident in choosing one side and explaining the reasons for this stance. Explaining ethical dilemmas is key in this station.

The UK General Medical Council has clear guidance on what actions doctors should take when dealing with situations that carry ethical dilemmas. This guidance helps us to care for our patients in the best possible way without breaking trust and at the same time protecting other individuals and society.

British HIV Association (BHIVA) guidance is an excellent resource that discusses in detail how to manage this challenging situation and emphasises the need not to take disclosure lightly as it prevents the patient from engaging with healthcare. BHIVA guidance can be summarised as below in this complex scenario:

'Breaking confidentiality in order to inform a sexual partner of the index patient's positive HIV status is sanctioned as a 'last resort' by the World Health Organization (WHO) and GMC. However, it is not to be taken lightly as it could have the negative impact of deterring others from testing because of the fear of forced imparting of HIV status and loss of trust by patients in the confidential doctor-patient relationship. The MDT should manage cases with challenging issues around sharing of HIV status. It is important to record discussions and management strategies in these cases accurately. Timely partner testing during the pregnancy should be encouraged where possible and support given.'

Key Points

- Any ethical dilemma has pros and cons; the candidate must be aware of both.
- The candidate should be able to conclude and explain their reasoning clearly.
- Quote the UK General Medical Council's code of ethics/'Good medical practice' document to show you know the ethics behind the scenario.

References

1. General Medical Council. Disclosures for the protection of patients and others. Available from: https://www.gmc-uk.org/ethical-guidance/ethical-guidance-for-doctors/confidentiality/disclosures-for-the-protection-of-patients-and-others.

2. British HIV Association guidelines for the management of HIV in pregnancy and postpartum 2018 (2020 third interim update). Available from: https://www.bhiva.org/file/5f1aab1ab9aba/BHIVA-Pregnancy-guidelines-2020–3rd-interim-update.pdf.

Question5

Ethical issues: a Jehovah's Witness patient for preoperative preparation

Satya Francis

Question

A patient scheduled for elective surgery has come in for a pre-assessment. One team nurse tells you that this patient is a Jehovah's Witness. The following station will discuss the ethical dilemmas in this scenario.

Themes for discussion (■ Table 1.5)

Table 1.5.	
Question themes	**What is expected from the candidate?**
1 The candidate greets the examiner and has good body language.	The candidate is presentable and uses good communication skills; always recommended in any station.

Table 1.5.

	Question themes	What is expected from the candidate?
2	What do you know about Jehovah's Witnesses?	The candidate gives a good opening statement: Jehovah's Witnesses belong to the Christian faith in which the followers refuse blood transfusions and treatment with any blood-related products. They consider this as a violation of their faith.
3	Do they all refuse blood transfusions?	Not all of them refuse, but the majority do. Some individuals are happy to accept their own blood, also referred to as cell salvage; this is the process by which blood collected from the surgical field is filtered, washed and returned to the patient through a drip. Derivatives of primary blood components may be acceptable to some.
		The patient needs to understand the consequences of refusing blood and blood products when these are needed to save their lives and/or improve their clinical condition/status, and clinicians must inform patients accordingly.
		Options can be discussed for improving their blood content before surgery.
4	How would you get information about their wishes?	• From the patients themselves. • They may carry a card or an advanced directive that will explain their wishes. • From their clinical notes. • The clinician can speak to the patient's relatives and carers if the information is not available.
5	What would you do if no information is available?	Medical treatment can be given without consent in an emergency, but only when there are no other ways to determine the patient's wishes.
		Even in an emergency we should discuss this option with senior team members and the hospital administration/ethical team.

Table 1.5.

	Question themes	What is expected from the candidate?
6	What code(s) of ethics is/are involved in these ethical dilemmas? The candidate understands the code of ethics.	Autonomy and beneficence. Non-maleficence.
7	Could you explain patient autonomy?	An adult with capacity has the ability to make decisions after discussion with the doctors and healthcare workers about the benefits and risks of treatment. If the patient refuses treatment, healthcare professionals should respect their decision.
8	How is beneficence relevant in this situation?	As a doctor, we have a duty of beneficence. Therefore, if the patient has made a decision, the only important thing to ensure is that they fully understand all the facts and consequences of not accepting a blood transfusion when needed.
9	Judgement and clarity.	The candidate has clarity in their answer; smiling throughout and avoiding repetition — these steps can increase the scores in this station.
10	Conclusion.	The candidate must explain that this is a difficult situation. It is important for the candidate to understand the GMC's code of ethics. The candidate should be aware of a patient's autonomy and the relevance of beneficence in an emergency scenario when no information about the patient's wishes is available.

Discussion

Explaining ethical dilemmas such as patient autonomy and beneficence is important in this station.

Understanding the patient's wishes, and what they will accept is important; this will be tested if this is a role-play station, in which an actor will act as a Jehovah's Witness patient. Sometimes, they might carry an advance directive card and the candidate must ask for this.

Key Points

- Any ethical dilemma has pros and cons; the candidate must be aware of both.
- The candidate should be able to explain the importance of the patient's autonomy and the healthcare workers' duty to respect their wishes in decision making.
- Quote the UK General Medical Council's 'Ethical guidance'.

References

1. General Medical Council. Good medical practice. Available from: https://www.gmc-uk.org/ethical-guidance/ethical-guidance-for-doctors/good-medical-practice.

2. Woolley S. Jehovah's Witnesses in the emergency department: what are their rights? *Emerg Med J* 2005; 22(12): 869-71.

3. Lawson T, Ralph C. Perioperative Jehovah's Witnesses: a review. *Br J Anaesth* 2015; 115: 676-87.

Question 6

Ethical issues: parents not allowing treatment for a child

Hema Kannappan

(Question 11 in this section is similar but, rather than role play, it will explore the discussions following the refusal of treatment.)

Question

You are a trainee in a paediatric rotation currently working at night as the on-call resident doctor. You are called to A&E to review Joshua, a 4-year-old patient admitted with a fever and non-blanching rash. You suspect meningococcal sepsis and want to treat him with antibiotics as per the hospital protocol.

However, Joshua's parents are refusing treatment as one of the child's cousins was given antibiotics and died recently. So you must talk to them; this station is a role play and will be followed by questions by the examiner.

Themes for discussion (■ Table 1.6)

Table 1.6.

Question themes	What is expected from the candidate?
1 The candidate greets the examiner.	Good body language and a presentable manner. In role-play stations, it is important also to greet the actor who acts as the mother.
2 The candidate greets the parents and checks the identity of the patient.	Asks any nurse or other family member to be present whilst reviewing the patient. When applicable, checking the patient's identity after introducing themselves is important in all scenarios.
3 The candidate explains the differential diagnosis and treatment plan.	Explain to the parents why their child needs admission and antibiotics urgently. The candidate must talk in simple language, avoiding medical jargon, but making sure that the parents understand the seriousness of the situation and the need for treatment.
4 Mother's concern regarding the antibiotics.	Explore the mother's concerns. This must be done empathetically and the candidate should listen to the mother's worries. Reassure the parents and explain why antibiotics are a lifesaving option for this condition. Explain that each case is different and that the incidence of allergy is rare. The candidate should explain honestly the risks of not giving antibiotics to the patient.

Table 1.6.

	Question themes	What is expected from the candidate?
5	Communication with the parents.	The candidate should talk slowly and clearly.
		The candidate should allow sufficient time and ask if the parents understand the explanation; they could be anxious, and it is essential to be clear and empathetic, and appreciate the emotions and anxieties of the parents.
6	Mother still declines antibiotics.	The candidate should explore the ethical principles behind this complex problem. The candidate can explore who has parental responsibility and ask if both parents are refusing the treatment. If both parents refuse, social services might need to be involved, in the best interest of the child. Discussing the issues with the nurses, colleagues and the multidisciplinary team and engaging with parents to explain the team's decision might help this situation.
		Discuss child protection and the patient's best interest if the parents still refuse treatment.
7	Medical ethics.	Autonomy, beneficence, non-maleficence and justice.
		Ability to clearly define the four pillars of medical ethics.
8	Conclusion.	The candidate can summarise the station and explain that the child's safety is the priority.
		The candidate concludes by saying thank you to both the role player and the examiner.

Discussion

Ethical dilemmas are very complex, and the examiner does not expect the candidate to solve the complex problem immediately; however, being empathetic, understanding the concerns of the parents/child, explaining why treatment is needed in simple language that the parents can understand, understanding the ethical principles and knowing where to get the help in this situation are all vital parts of the assessment of this scenario.

Key Points

- In a role-play station, the candidate should listen to the patient and try to understand the concern of the patient/parent.
- Patient safety (in this case, a child's safety) is of prime importance.
- Empathetic discussions, understanding parents' concerns, and reflecting on them so that there is a good rapport will help in this station.
- Quote the UK General Medical Council's 'Ethical Guidance' if needed/if possible.

References

1. General Medical Council. Good medical practice. Available from: https://www.gmc-uk.org/ethical-guidance/ethical-guidance-for-doctors/good-medical-practice.

Question 7

Ethical issues: euthanasia

Siva Thanthullu

Question

This station will discuss the ethical principles of euthanasia. The examiner will ask questions on this theme to explore the candidate's understanding.

Themes for discussion (■ Table 1.7)

Table 1.7.	
Question themes	**What is expected from the candidate?**
1 The candidate greets the examiner.	A good introduction and good body language set the station in a positive way. We request this in all stations, although some might not have specific scores for this point. A good doctor should have good communication skills, and this will be marked positively in all the MMI stations.

Table 1.7.

	Question themes	What is expected from the candidate?
2	What is euthanasia? What is assisted suicide? What are the types of euthanasia?	Euthanasia or mercy-killing is the act of deliberately ending a person's life to relieve suffering.
		Euthanasia is ending the life of a person who is terminally ill; assisted suicide refers to a physician assisting a person in ending their life.
		Assisted dying is a sub-term in which the patient is terminally ill and dying.
		Euthanasia can be voluntary or non-voluntary.
		Euthanasia can be active (when acting deliberately to end life) or passive (withholding or withdrawing necessary treatment).
3	What does the UK law state with regard to euthanasia?	Euthanasia and assisted suicide are illegal under the law in the UK.
		Euthanasia can be considered as either manslaughter or murder; this could lead to a maximum penalty of life imprisonment in the UK.
		In addition, assisted suicide is illegal under Section 2 of the Suicide Act (1961) (amended by the Coroners and Justice Act 2009) and is punishable by up to 14 years imprisonment. However, suicide is not illegal in the UK.
		In the USA, euthanasia is allowed in a few jurisdictions including Oregon, Washington DC, Hawaii, Washington, Maine, Colorado, New Jersey, California and Vermont.

Table 1.7.

Question themes	What is expected from the candidate?
4 What are the ethical issues regarding euthanasia?	Supporters of euthanasia quote the Human Rights Act to support them in dying with high-quality care rather than succumbing to a terminal disease. However, opponents oppose ending a life and giving the doctor control over who will live.
	In this ethical debate, the cons include the slippery slope on how to decide the worthiness of living and who decides it; this can be arbitrary and there is no fixed definition of this process.
5 What are the legal challenges in euthanasia?	In 2015, the House of Commons rejected a bill to support assisted suicide in patients who were terminally ill.
	There have been high-profile cases in the news in recent times challenging the legal stance of euthanasia; it would be wise to quote one of these and explain the dilemma.
6 Is euthanasia legal in other parts of the world?	As mentioned in point no. 3, some jurisdictions in the USA allow euthanasia. It is legal in Switzerland, Germany, The Netherlands, Canada, and a few other countries.
7 What is the doctor's duty with regard to euthanasia?	The candidate realises that euthanasia is illegal in the UK. The doctor's duty is to safeguard and protect life, not to end it; however, it is justifiable to alleviate suffering in dying patients.

Table 1.7.

Question themes	What is expected from the candidate?
	Discuss this point on the basis of the four pillars of medical ethics: • Autonomy — giving the right to the patient to decide; the patient's dignity and whether the state should interfere in their personal choice. • Beneficence — duty of doing good, in the interest of the patient, to alleviate their suffering. • Non-maleficence — doing no harm; it can be argued that assisted suicide is deliberately harming the patient. • Justice — acting without discrimination. Keeping someone alive after brain-stem death could mean losing resources, which can be expensive. This money could be diverted to use where the results could be beneficial.
8 What is brain-stem death?	For patients in a coma who are on ventilatory and other support, it is essential to confirm brain-stem death by two medical practitioners before stopping treatment. For this: • There should be no reversible causes. • The patient must not breathe spontaneously. • The brain-stem respiratory centre should be destroyed.
9 For the palliative care of a dying patient, what are the rights to having high-quality end-of-life care?	For palliative end-of-life care: • The patient should have access to pain relief and relief of symptoms. • Strategies to cope with the terminal diagnosis should be offered. • The patient can make a legally binding advance decision to refuse treatment.

Table 1.7.	
Question themes	**What is expected from the candidate?**
	• The patient can create a lasting power of attorney for a friend or family they trust to make decisions for them if they lose this capacity.
10 Conclusion.	The NHS allows the withdrawal of life-sustaining care in palliative care dying patients, and this should not be confused with passive euthanasia.
	The candidate concludes and summarises the station; they also thank the examiner.

Discussion

Euthanasia is a common topic that is discussed in MMIs. The candidate should be well prepared to discuss the pros and cons, and then give their opinion and support why they took this option.

Euthanasia is a controversial topic, and the medical fraternity is divided amongst themselves regarding whether or not it should be allowed. The British Medical Association (BMA) recently conducted one of the largest polls to monitor the views of its members (February, 2020); the BMA has a neutral position on a change in the law on assisted dying. In this survey, 50% of the members supported a change in the law on prescribing drugs for eligible patients to self-administer to end their own life, whilst 39% opposed and 11% were undecided.

Key Points

- The candidate should demonstrate that they have an understanding of euthanasia.
- They should be aware of the law in the UK (or their respective country) and what it states concerning euthanasia.
- They should be able to explore the debate on the pros and cons of euthanasia.
- Being confident, but at the same time, explaining both sides of the dilemma will help in this station.
- In conclusion, they should be able to give an opinion on whether or not they support euthanasia, with supporting arguments.
- The commonest mistake in this debate includes staying on one side of the debate without appreciating the opposite view.

References

1. General Medical Council. Good medical practice. Available from: https://www.gmc-uk.org/ethical-guidance/ethical-guidance-for-doctors/good-medical-practice.

2. NHS UK. Euthanasia and assisted suicide. Available from: https://www.nhs.uk/conditions/euthanasia-and-assisted-suicide.

3. Legal Information Institute. Euthanasia. Available from: https://www.law.cornell.edu/wex/euthanasia.

4. British Medical Association. Physician-assisted dying survey. Available from: https://www.bma.org.uk/advice-and-support/ethics/end-of-life/physician-assisted-dying/physician-assisted-dying-survey.

Question 8

Ethical issues: rationing cancer treatment funding

Balaji Varadhan

Question

As you may be aware, some cancer treatments are managed under the Cancer Drugs Fund. Some drugs are not accessible to patients with cancer due to insufficient evidence. The general public is always confused about the process of how and why access to these drugs is obtained.

In this station, the examiner will question the reason behind rationing cancer treatment funding.

This station can also be given in the form of role play, with a patient frustrated that a drug is unavailable; if so, being empathetic, and listening to the patient before explaining is helpful.

Themes for discussion (■ Table 1.8)

Table 1.8.	
Question themes	**What is expected from the candidate?**
1 The candidate greets the examiner.	Good body language and a presentable manner.
2 What is the Cancer Drugs Fund (CDF)?	The Cancer Drugs Fund helps to access new treatments via access programmes whilst further evidence is collected to address clinical uncertainty. This aids patients with cancer to gain access to these treatments many months earlier from when the efficacy is proven.
3 Benefits of the CDF.	The candidate explains that it is a fast-tracked process to get access to drugs; this allows earlier access to drugs.
	The fund aims for clearer and faster decisions on which drug is available for cancer.
4 Why are drugs accessed through the CDF and there is no direct process of getting access to all drugs?	The NHS has limited resources, and these should be rationed based on clinical efficacy.
	The CDF helps to maximise the use of resources for benefit to the majority.
	The candidate can use the ethical pillars of beneficence and justice in this argument.
5 The examiner questions why a patient is not allowed to use this drug when a pharmaceutical company clearly says that it helps.	Evidence-based practice uses interventions based on the best evidence and research; this approach also ensures the treatment is cost-effective. Efficacy is usually measured in terms of improvement in quality-adjusted life years (QALY) and the cost needed to improve this.
	The CDF aims to act to maximise the benefit for most patients.

Table 1.8.

	Question themes	What is expected from the candidate?
6	Four pillars of medical ethics.	Autonomy, beneficence, non-maleficence and justice.
7	How do you apply medical ethics to this scenario?	The candidate should clearly define the four pillars of medical ethics; use all four pillars to explain the ethical dilemma in this case.
8	Where can we find ethical guidelines for doctors?	The GMC's 'Good medical practice' guidance. The GMC's code of ethics. In other countries apart from the UK, it is wise to know the local Medical Council guidelines to quote in exams.
9	Conclusion.	The candidate thanks the examiner and concludes the station.

Discussion

Rationing medical interventions can cause ethical dilemmas; in role-play stations, the patient can be angry or frustrated. Quoting recent newspaper articles or legal dilemmas can help the candidate answer this station.

The ethical dilemma of a postcode lottery (the availability of an intervention based on the geographical allocation of funding) can be approached using the four pillars of medical ethics; beneficence and justice play a more significant role in explaining and dealing with this problem.

Value to this answer could be added if the candidate has a basic knowledge of how the National Institute for Health and Care Excellence (NICE) approves medical interventions based on QALY and evidence.

Key Points

- The candidate should understand that there is a finite pot of resources and that this pot should be used efficiently for patient care.
- Beneficence and justice are ethical pillars that should be used in this station.
- Use the terms QALY, evidence-based approach, and cost-effectiveness in this question.

References

1. General Medical Council. Good medical practice. Domain 4: Maintaining trust. Available from: https://www.gmc-uk.org/ethical-guidance/ethical-guidance-for-doctors/good-medical-practice/domain-4---maintaining-trust.

2. General Medical Council. Good medical practice. Domain 1: Knowledge skills and performance. Available from: https://www.gmc-uk.org/ethical-guidance/ethical-guidance-for-doctors/good-medical-practice/domain-1---knowledge-skills-and-performance.

3. American Medical Association. Code of Medical Ethics overview. Available from: https://www.ama-assn.org/delivering-care/ethics/code-medical-ethics-overview.

4. National Institute for Health and Care Excellence. Available from: https://www.nice.org.uk.

Question 9

Ethical issues: abortion

Vijaianitha Nallendran

Question

A nurse in the termination of pregnancy clinic is seeing a 15-year-old girl who is now 16 weeks pregnant and requesting an abortion. The nurse has conscientious objections on moral grounds to providing abortion care.

The next station will discuss the ethical issues and your opinion in this situation.

Themes for discussion (■ Table 1.9)

Table 1.9.	
Question themes	**What is expected from the candidate?**
1 The candidate greets the examiner and has good body language.	The candidate is presentable and uses good communication skills; always recommended in any station.

Table 1.9.

Question themes	What is expected from the candidate?
2 Do women have the right to abortion?	The candidate gives a good opening statement showing that they understand the situation. The candidate understands the problems in this scenario, focusing on the rights of the mother and the rights of the fetus.
3 The candidate volunteers the reasons why they consider that women have rights to abortion.	The candidate has knowledge of and is able to discuss issues around: • Rights of the fetus versus the mother. • The Abortion Act 1967 renders providing abortion services lawful that would otherwise constitute a crime under the Offences Against The Person Act 1861. • In a legal setting where sterile facilities are available, abortion is a safe procedure for which major complications and mortality are rare at all gestational ages. • Aborting an unwanted pregnancy has less adverse psychological sequelae when compared with carrying that pregnancy to term.
4 The candidate understands the considerations needed for a 15-year-old patient.	• Need to check Gillick competence. • Aware of the duty to encourage young people to involve their parents. • Aware that the young person has the right to confidentiality.
5 Do medical professionals have the right to refuse to provide abortion services?	• The candidate gives a good opening statement showing that they understand the situation. • The candidate presents for and against arguments for this dilemma; see below.
6 The candidate volunteers the reasons why they consider that medical professionals have the right to refuse.	The candidate has knowledge that is demonstrated as follows: • The Abortion Act has a conscientious objection clause that permits doctors to refuse to provide treatment if it conflicts with their religious or moral beliefs.

Table 1.9.

Question themes	What is expected from the candidate?
	• The candidate understands that refusing does not extend to participating in paperwork/administration and routine care connected with abortion. • They are aware that it is the medical professional's duty to inform women of their right to see another doctor and provide them with information on how to access alternative services.
7 Do you know about the Abortion Act 1967?	The candidate has knowledge of the Abortion Act. Abortion is legal if it is performed by a registered medical practitioner and if it is authorised by two doctors, acting in good faith on one or more of the four grounds.
8 Do you know about the Human Fertilization and Embryology Act 1990?	It amended the Abortion Act 1967. It introduces a time limit on most abortions of 24 weeks' gestation, but permits termination at any gestation period on the grounds of serious fetal anomaly.
9 Judgement and clarity.	The candidate provides clarity in their answer and can explain the pros and cons, concluding clearly. A clear presentation, smiling throughout and avoiding repetition — these steps can increase the scores in this station.
10 Conclusion.	The candidate concludes the session and at the end thanks the examiner. This might gain the candidate extra bonus points.

Discussion

It is important to understand that women have the right to request an abortion and medical professionals have the right to refuse abortion treatment. However, medical professionals have a duty to refer women to alternative services/colleagues who can provide the service immediately.

Knowledge about the ethical issues surrounding abortion — the rights of the fetus, the rights of the woman and the legality surrounding the provision of abortion care — enables you to answer this question with clarity.

Key Points

- Awareness of the rights and the duty of the medical professional and the rights of the patient; the candidate must be aware of both.
- Awareness of Gillick competence for young people.
- Quoting the Abortion Act 1967 shows that the candidate understands the legality surrounding abortion.
- Awareness of the ethics surrounding the provision of abortion.

References

1. Abortion Act 1967. Available from: https://www.legislation.gov.uk/ukpga/1967/87/contents.

2. Royal College of Obstetricians and Gynaecologists. The care of women requesting induced abortion (Evidence-based clinical guideline no. 7). Available from: https://www.rcog.org.uk/guidance/browse-all-guidance/other-guidelines-and-reports/the-care-of-women-requesting-induced-abortion-evidence-based-clinical-guideline-no-7.

3. Bewley S, Lupton M. Ethical frameworks for obstetrics and gynaecology. *Obstet Gynaecol* 2003; 5(4): 208-13.

Question 10

Organ donation: opt in or opt out

Satya Francis

Question

One of your relatives is unsure about the organ donation law in England and would like to obtain more information before registering their interest. On 20 May 2020, the law around organ donation in England was changed to allow more people to save more lives.

The next station will discuss these issues and your opinion in this situation.

Themes for discussion (■ Table 1.10)

Table 1.10.	
Question themes	**What is expected from the candidate?**
1 The candidate greets the examiner and has good body language.	The candidate is presentable and uses good communication skills; always recommended in any station.

Table 1.10.

	Question themes	What is expected from the candidate?
2	What do you understand by the term 'organ donation'?	The candidate gives a good opening statement showing that they understand organ donation. It is the act of giving an organ to someone in need of a transplant. Certain organs such as the kidney can be donated whilst one is alive, but most other organs come from people who have died.
3	What are the challenges with organ donation?	The demand for an organ transplant is higher than the supply; there is a need for organs. The waiting list can be problematic as the organs must be matched for the donor and recipient. The candidate also understands the reasons preventing people from donating organs: lack of education, religious beliefs, ethical dilemmas, psychological factors, fear of not understanding the process, etc.
4	What do you understand by an opt-in or opt-out system?	Opt in is when the person voluntarily registers to be an organ donor. Opt out is the current law in England, which states that if a person has not registered their decision to opt out, they are considered to have no objection to being an organ donor after death if they are not excluded for other reasons. This law was introduced on 20 May 2020. In Wales, the legislation is 'deemed consent'; if a person has not registered an organ/tissue donation, they will be considered as having no objection to becoming a donor. In Scotland, the legislation is 'deemed authorisation'; if one has not confirmed whether they want to donate, they will be considered to be willing to donate organs and tissue when they die.

Table 1.10.

Question themes	What is expected from the candidate?
	In Northern Ireland, the law was opt in, but it recently changed to an opt-out system, which was approved in February 2022 and will become law in spring 2023.
5 Who belongs to the excluded group?	Everyone will be considered to be in favour of donating their organs and tissues unless: • They have opted out. • They are in one of the excluded groups (under the age of 18, resident in England for less than 12 months before their death, lack mental capacity). • Or they have appointed someone to decide for them after their death.
6 Why was the opt-out law introduced?	A survey implied that more people were willing to donate, but only a few had registered for the donation. The law aims to improve the number of people on the NHS Organ Donor Register; this can save a greater number of lives. In addition, more education is needed to create awareness of the need for organ donation, and the law can help in this process.
7 What are the ethical issues?	Some would argue that opt in is the best way as they have willingly registered to become an organ donor, but others might say the opt-out system will lead to a greater number of people on the register and would save more lives. The candidate needs to be aware of both sides of the argument; they should base their opinion with support of the four pillars of medical ethics: autonomy, beneficence, non-maleficence and justice.

Table 1.10.

	Question themes	What is expected from the candidate?
8	How would you overcome the hurdles in organ donation?	The candidate should give a few practical ideas that could include:
		• Education and awareness through campaigns; for example the 'Pass it on' campaign aims to improve the understanding of organ donation in the UK.
		• Working with faith leaders and community leaders, to overcome the obstacle of spiritual reasons and ethnic reasons.
		• For hesitation among the ethnic minority population, involving religious leaders to explain organ donation in line with religious beliefs.
		• Research into ways to use artificial organs, stem cells and genetically engineered solutions.
9	Judgement and clarity.	The candidate has clarity in their answer; they can explain opt in and opt out and can conclude clearly. A clear presentation, smiling throughout and avoiding repetition — these steps can increase the scores in this station.
10	Conclusion.	The candidate concludes the session and thanks the examiner at the end. This might gain the candidate extra bonus points.

Discussion

Organ donation — opt in or opt out — is an important debate that often comes up in MMI stations.. Therefore, the candidate should be well prepared to give a schematically organised answer and be able to give their personal opinion and support the answer.

As in any other ethical dilemma, there is no right or wrong answer, but awareness of organ donation legislation is necessary. In addition, the candidate should have knowledge of the reasons for the obstacles in obtaining organs and how to overcome them.

Key Points

- Any ethical dilemma has pros and cons; the candidate must be aware of both.
- The candidate should be able to explain the current situation with organ donation.
- Awareness of the legal aspects of opt in and opt out is essential.

References

1.   NHS UK. Blood and transplant. Organ donation. Available from: http://www.organdonation.nhs.uk.

2.   NHS UK. Blood and transplant. Organ donation laws. Available from: https://www.organdonation.nhs.uk/uk-laws.

3.   Byrne MHV, Ashcroft J. Organ donation: educating the public about the "opt-out" system is crucial. *BMJ* 2020; 368: m1207.

Question 11

Refusal of treatment: discussion

Balamurugan Nambi

(This question is similar to Question 6, but explores the discussion with an examiner rather than role play.)

Question

This is a clinical ethics discussion station; you must speak to the examiner who will discuss an ethical dilemma and ask questions.

In this scenario, you have advised treatment for a child; when they come back after 2 months, you find that the mother has not yet given the treatment. The examiner will discuss how you would approach this complex scenario.

Themes for discussion (■ Table 1.11)

Table 1.11.

Question themes	What is expected from the candidate?
1 The candidate introduces themselves.	The candidate greets the examiner and confirms their role in this scenario as a doctor.
2 Body language and empathy.	The candidate shows empathy and acknowledges the mother's concerns and says they will listen to her concerns. Body language and non-verbal skills should be appropriate. The candidate makes eye contact and actively listens.
3 Explains how they would discuss the situation with the mother; has a knowledge of ethical principles.	The candidate mentions that they would try to inform the mother of the benefits and drawbacks of taking the particular course of treatment and describes what will happen if treatment is not given.
	If the patient has capacity and Gillick competence, we must respect their autonomy. However, this scenario involves a young child, and so treatment should be in the child's interest. The candidate must ensure that the mother is fully informed of the need for treatment.
	The candidate could also probe into why the mother does not want the treatment to take place; if there are any misconceptions, it gives an opportunity to clear them. It is wise to check if she has an insight into what she is doing to the child by this action.
4 Gillick competence/parental consent.	As we are dealing with a child, the candidate would first assess the child's competence.
5 Assessing the social situation.	There is a need to explain to the mother the seriousness of the situation and the implications for the child.

Table 1.11.	
Question themes	**What is expected from the candidate?**
	In some situations, it is worth finding out any financial stress within the family in which the mother could not afford treatment; or whether any other factor or belief prevents the child from having this treatment.
	The candidate could also explain that they will liaise with her GP to find out the background social situation of the family and the child; particular concerns could be with regard to a previous history of neglect or safeguarding concerns within the family.
	The candidate could explain that they will also find out whether the mother has any underlying mental or physical health problem that impedes her decision-making process.
6 The candidate explores the mother's wishes.	It is very important to know what the mother wants in this situation and if she has expressed any wishes previously. Being empathetic and explaining the importance of adhering to a treatment plan based on the child's best interest is essential.
7 Acting in the best interests of the child.	This involves including the MDT discussions in the team and acting in the child's best interest. There might be a potential chance for the medic to escalate the concerns to social care. If the situation is life-threatening, this might necessitate seeking legal advice.
	It is important that the candidate discusses this answer based on the four pillars of medical ethics: autonomy, beneficence, non-maleficence and justice.

Table 1.11.

Question themes	What is expected from the candidate?
8 Advises further discussion with the treating team and with other family members.	The candidate stresses that they will have further discussions with the hospital team and the social care team; liaising with the GP or family doctor is also important. The family should be actively involved at all stages. This could include exploring the availability of psychological/pastoral support.
9 Closure of the station.	The candidate concludes the station and explains that they will be empathetic and allow the mother to ask questions and contact them again if needed. They thank the examiner for the opportunity.

Discussion

This station can easily be presented as a role-play station in which an actor acts as the mother and the examiner stands nearby to score the station. Being empathetic and listening are the key communication skills in this scenario. If the candidate has listened and explored why the mother is refusing the treatment, they should score good points in this role-play station.

In rare situations, doctors and parents can have disagreements about a child's medical treatment. The 'zone of parental discretion' is a tool to assist doctors in deciding whether a parental choice should be overridden; this tool looks at ethical aspects of treatment plans and looks at achieving the best possible treatment. This approach focuses on the potential harm caused by the parents' decision rather than trying to identify and insist on the option in the child's best interests.

Usually, parents know their children best. Parents also bear the primary burden of the medical decisions made for their children, caring for them in the long term. But the parental right to make medical decisions is not unlimited. Their choice could be due to a lack of knowledge, an irrational fear of side effects, a rational fear of known effects, or various beliefs. Their decision-making role is sometimes questioned when they disagree with the recommended treatment for their child. There are many ways in which parents may do this. Doctors should balance the child's well-being and the parents' autonomy by accepting choices that may be suboptimal for the child, if they are not harmful.

In these situations, it might be worth seeking advice from the clinical ethics committee in the hospital; these are available in the UK and USA and are also developing in other countries.

Some parental choices do not optimise the child's well-being but will not harm the child. For example, the parents' preferred form of surgery may not be the best available, but may still be very likely to treat the child's condition effectively. Such decisions fall within the boundary of the parents' discretion and should not be overridden. The outer boundary of the zone of parental discretion is harm to the child. For example, if parents refuse the physiotherapy necessary to ensure their child will walk again, this choice is outside the zone of parental discretion and should be overridden.

The clinician should respect and balance the two important values of parental autonomy and children's well-being.

Key Points

- Please remember that ethical dilemmas have no right or wrong answer, but the candidate should be aware of the problems and available options.
- Always discuss ethical scenarios based on the four pillars of medical ethics: autonomy, non-maleficence, beneficence and justice.
- In scenarios in which treatments are refused, be empathetic and talk to the patient or parent and find out the reasons behind this decision.
- Appropriate education and explanation might be the solution in role-play stations.

References

1. Gillam L. The zone of parental discretion: an ethical tool for dealing with disagreement between parents and doctors about medical treatment for a child. *Clin Ethics* 2016; 11(1): 1-8.

2. McDougall RJ, Notini L. What kinds of cases do paediatricians refer to clinical ethics? Insights from 184 case referrals at an Australian paediatric hospital. *J Med Ethics* 2016; 42(9): 586-91.

Question 12

A patient with depression refusing treatment for suicidal ideas

Balamurugan Nambi

Question

This is a role-play station. You are the resident doctor in the admissions ward of the hospital and are asked to see a 28-year-old patient with depression refusing treatment for suicidal ideas.

You must talk to the patient in the next station. The examiner will observe and score the station.

Themes for discussion (■ Table 1.12)

Table 1.12.	
Question themes	**What is expected from the candidate?**
1 The candidate introduces themselves.	The candidate greets the patient and the examiner; the candidate introduces themselves. They check the identity of the patient before starting the consultation.

Table 1.12.

Question themes	What is expected from the candidate?
2 Body language and empathy.	The candidate shows empathy and acknowledges the patient's concerns by listening actively. They ensure that body language and non-verbal skills are appropriate. The candidate should make eye contact with the patient. The candidate acknowledges what was said to him by the patient by appropriate repeat feedback to check whether their understanding is correct.
3 Explores more about the condition.	The candidate gently probes into the patient's condition and asks relevant questions sensitively to ensure that they get a clear understanding of the patient's condition.
Assessment of the degree of depression.	If the actor has stopped talking, the candidate can ask about sleep, appetite, energy level, hobbies, anhedonia, concentration, suicidal ideas, and self-confidence.
4 Suicidal ideations.	The candidate approaches the topic of suicidal ideation and asks about this in various ways: • How long have they had suicidal ideas? • What are these thoughts/ideas? • Have they any plans to end their life? • Have they made any previous attempts? The candidate then explores the support structure including: • Social history: to explore their family circumstances. • Family history: married or single; have they any children? • Financial history: any financial stress? Any stress with their job? • Physical history: any physical health problems?

Table 1.12.

	Question themes	What is expected from the candidate?
5	To assess insight into their condition.	• Do they acknowledge that they have a mental illness? • Do they realise that they need treatment for their mental illness? • Is he willing to accept help?
6	Mild-to-moderate depression with suicidal ideations. (The patient has capacity.)	If the patient has moderate depression and has insight into their condition, the doctor cannot force treatment provided they do not have any plan to end their life. The candidate can make sure that this patient with depression is aware of self-help groups, support groups, and other local and national resources.
7	Severe depression with a suicidal plan and intent and lacks capacity.	If the patient has severe depression with suicidal intent and lack of capacity, the candidate will call a senior colleague for help. He should be assessed under a legal framework such as the Mental Capacity Act or Mental Health Act. Awareness of the crisis helpline in the mental health team is needed. The candidate should be aware of the implications of the severity of depression.
8	Advises further discussion with the treating team and with other family members.	This involves including the multidisciplinary team and acting in the patient's best interest. The candidate explains that they will give verbal and written information about the help available for depression. The candidate can also mention that they will signpost the appropriate psychological services that can help with addressing stigma and treatment for depression.
9	Closure.	The candidate explains to the patient that they can contact them if they prefer to do this and explains that the team is there to support him. They give the opportunity for further questions, explain that they will discuss with the team and come back, and concludes the session by thanking the patient.

Discussion

Depression is one of the predominant mental health problems in the world. In 2014, the incidence of anxiety and depression was 19.7% of people in the UK aged 16 and above. Depression is not a sign of weakness. It can happen to anyone; even famous people, athletes and celebrities can experience depression. The good news is that most people with depression will get better on their own by doing things to help themselves.

Signs of depression include a hopeless outlook, loss of interest, concentration difficulties, change of appetite, increased fatigue and sleep problems, irritability, low energy levels, feeling suicidal, uncontrollable emotions, and feeling guilty and unworthy.

Depression can be triggered by life events, personal circumstances, childhood trauma, alcohol and drug use, genetic factors, etc. It can also be triggered by a stressful or distressing event, such as a bereavement, relationship breakdown, or job loss. Regular heavy drinking or using drugs such as cannabis can make you more likely to become depressed in the long term.

Patients should immediately get help if they think of hurting themselves or someone else. They should also get help if symptoms are persistent and affect their day-to-day activities.

A patient can help themselves by eating healthily, keeping active, avoiding alcohol/drugs, socialising with friends and families, being kind to themselves, doing things they enjoy, and being involved in a support group for depression.

Depression is treatable; 80%-90% of affected patients respond to treatment. Cognitive behaviour therapy (CBT) and talking therapies can help with depression either as individual sessions or as group programmes, depending on the patient. Anti-depression medications have a role in some patients.

Key Points

- Engage in creating a rapport with the patient.
- Be empathetic; listen to the patient and feed back that you have listened.
- Non-verbal cues are important communication skills that should be practised.
- The candidate should gently explore the extent of suicidal ideas.
- Check if the patient has insight into the medical condition.

References

1. NICE (National Institute for Health and Care Excellence). Depression in adults: recognition and management. Clinical guideline [CG90]. Available from: https://www.nice.org.uk/guidance/cg90.

2. Ferguson JM. SSRI antidepressant medications: adverse effects and tolerability. *Prim Care Companion J Clin Psychiatry* 2001; 3(1): 22-7.

Question 13

A colleague prescribes the wrong dose of medicine

Satya Francis

Question

You find out that a colleague has prescribed a patient the wrong dose of medication. The next station will assess how you would approach this complex scenario. The examiner will ask questions on this theme.

Themes for discussion (■ Table 1.13)

Table 1.13.

Question themes	What is expected from the candidate?
1 The candidate greets the examiner and has good body language.	The candidate is presentable and uses good communication skills; always recommended in any station.

Table 1.13.

	Question themes	What is expected from the candidate?
2	How would you approach this?	Obtain the facts about what happened; these can be obtained from medical notes, prescription charts and by speaking to the colleague.
		Colleagues deserve the chance to correct mistaken assumptions.
		A patient-centred approach: patient safety is key in this scenario.
		Communication with the patient — explain honestly and say sorry for any mistake.
3	What guidance is the candidate aware of regarding this?	The candidate clearly understands the GMC's guidance, 'Good medical practice'; this scenario involves:
		• Domain 2 — Safety and quality.
		• Domain 3 — Communication.
		• Domain 4 — Maintaining trust.
4	What would you do next?	The candidate clearly understands the importance of patient safety:
		• Patient-centred care is the aim of healthcare. Being honest and accepting mistakes and correcting them are vital.
		• Establish the patient's well-being and ensure no harm has been done.
		• Establish if there were any side effects from the wrong dose of medication.
		• Ensure that the right treatment is prescribed to the patient.

Table 1.13.

	Question themes	What is expected from the candidate?
5	What is the goal of the discussion with the involved colleague?	To establish what happened, under what circumstances and any mistaken assumptions.
		If they agree there was a harmful error, knowledge of how to report this through hospital incident forms to reduce morbidity and mortality in the future.
		Ensure honest and open communication with the patient; involving senior colleagues is essential.
		If the colleague disagrees, the candidate should inform a mentor or a senior colleague to avoid critical incidents.
6	How would you disclose this to the patient?	It is the patient's right to have honest information. This should be shared with professionalism and compassion.
		This is one of the domains in 'Good medical practice' from the GMC.
7	What is the duty of candour?	Doctors have an ethical duty to tell patients when things have gone wrong. It is their duty to apologise and work towards putting things right in these situations.
8	How can this be prevented?	• Open discussion and finding the reasons for errors.
		• Clear documentation in the clinical notes.
		• Hospital incident forms (such as 'DATIX' forms) that help to record and analyse critical incidents.
		• Discussion in morbidity and mortality meetings/team meetings/audit meetings to analyse and prevent such events in the future.
		• Education of the team to create awareness.

Table 1.13.

	Question themes	What is expected from the candidate?
9	Judgement and clarity.	The candidate has clarity in their answer; they can explain the principles of the GMC's 'Good medical practice' guidance.
		A clear presentation, smiling throughout and avoiding repetition — these steps can increase the scores in this station.
		The candidate is empathetic and describes patient-centred care and the duty of candour.
10	Conclusion.	The candidate concludes the session and thanks the examiner at the end. This gains the candidate extra bonus points.

Discussion

It is important to practise similar stations as they recur in MMIs. Making mistakes is unavoidable and health services try to learn from these mistakes. In role play it is essential to explain the mistake honestly, apologise, and detail the steps to the patient that will be taken to correct the mistake and to prevent mistakes in the future.

Awareness of a duty of candour is important for a medical student and clinician. In all situations, probity and honesty are considered vital.

Key Points

- Patient-centred care and patient safety are the key.
- Be honest and maintain trust and integrity in patient care.
- Duty of candour: this is adopted in many countries including in the UK General Medical Council's 'Good medical practice' guidance and the American Medical Association's Code of Medical Ethics.

References

1.   General Medical Council. Good medical practice. Available from: https://www.gmc-uk.org/ethical-guidance/ethical-guidance-for-doctors/good-medical-practice.

2.   Gallagher TH, Mello MM, Levinson W, *et al.* Talking with patients about other clinicians' errors. *N Engl J Med* 2013; 369(18): 1752-7.

Question 14

Should psychoactive drugs be banned?

Balamurugan Nambi

Question

There is a debate on whether psychoactive drugs should be banned. Many of these drugs can cause harm. The examiner will assess how the candidate balances their views on this theme in the next station.

Themes for discussion (■ Table 1.14)

Table 1.14.	
Question themes	**What is expected from the candidate?**
1　The candidate greets the examiner and has good body language.	The candidate is presentable and uses good communication skills; always recommended in any station.

Table 1.14.

	Question themes	What is expected from the candidate?
2	Do you understand what is meant by the term psychoactive drugs?	Psychoactive substances are substances that, when administered, can affect mental processes such as cognition (World Health Organization). They comprise both legal and illegal substances. Many of these drugs can be abused for recreational use. Many of these drugs can be addictive.
3	What is the legal position on the use of psychoactive substances?	Psychoactive drugs can be legal or illegal. The position varies between different countries and even within regions in a country. The law that deals with this is based on the Misuse of Drugs Act 1971.
		The Psychoactive Substances Act 2016 states that it is an offence to produce, supply, offer to supply, possess with intent to supply, import or export psychoactive substances; the maximum penalty is 7 years' imprisonment.
4	Should psychoactive substances be banned?	The candidate clearly understands the problem and the ethical dilemma; he starts by giving an introductory statement and explaining the complexity.
5	The candidate gives reasons why the drugs should be banned.	The candidate gives reasons in clear, simple language supporting why these drugs should be banned: <ul><li>If not banned, it can lead to thousands of new users yearly and cause physical and mental damage to vulnerable people.</li><li>More individuals with a biological predisposition towards addiction will try to experiment with drugs if they are not banned.</li><li>More problematic and antisocial behaviour can arise in society.</li><li>Drug tourism can lead to more problems.</li></ul>

Table 1.14.

	Question themes	What is expected from the candidate?
		• The wrong message can be sent to young people that it is acceptable to take drugs. This can also create the wrong message that they are safe. • The cannabis industry is one of the fastest growing industries and can lead to more problems for users. The dose of cannabis varies in these preparations and is difficult to monitor.
6	The candidate gives reasons why some do not want the drugs to be banned.	The candidate explains reasons why they should not be banned: • Avoids criminalising people who abuse drugs, which could lead to more problematic behaviours. • Drug abusers have more chance of avoiding addiction if they are not caught up in the criminal justice system. • Addiction treatment and rehabilitation are less expensive than criminalising and jail sentencing; the courts can be freed up to do other vital work. • For example, Portugal has found that, since decriminalisation, both addiction and substance misuse rates have gone down. • The composition of these substances could be closely controlled; if illegal, the purity of substances and differences in strengths can lead to overdose and dangerous effects. • Legalising cannabis has increased tax revenue in many states in the USA; for example, Colorado raised more than US$1 billion in 2019. It has been suggested that legalising cannabis can raise more than £1.5 billion in the UK per year.
7	The candidate explains their position in this ethical dilemma.	The candidate has clearly explained the pros and cons of banning psychoactive substances; they have given examples from different countries. At the end, they conclude what they feel is right. They have a clear opinion and can substantiate these reasons with clarity.

Table 1.14.

Question themes	What is expected from the candidate?
8 The candidate explains their answer based on the four pillars of medical ethics.	The candidate uses the four pillars of ethics: autonomy, non-maleficence, beneficence and justice.
9 Judgement and clarity.	The candidate has clarity in their answer and can explain the pros and cons, concluding clearly. A clear presentation, smiling throughout and avoiding repetition — these steps can increase the scores in this station.
10 Conclusion.	The candidate concludes the session and thanks the examiner at the end. This gains the candidate extra bonus points.

Discussion

Legalising cannabis and banning psychoactive or psychotropic drugs, etc. are common ethical dilemma situations that can come up in MMI stations. The candidate should not feel that they are there to solve the problem but should show that they understand the problem and its complexity. They can reason why some support, and some oppose the situation. They should come to a clear opinion by themselves with reasoning.

Key Points

- Please remember that ethical dilemmas have no right or wrong answer, but the candidate should be aware of the problems and available options.
- The candidate must reason why they should be banned or not and give adequate evidence for both sides.
- They should explain from the healthcare side and also look at society, economy and community. They can detail the legal aspects and financial aspects to support their views.

References

1. Crown Prosecution Service. Psychoactive substances. Available from: http://www.cps.gov.uk/legal-guidance/psychoactive-substances.

2. Holland A. An ethical analysis of UK drug policy as an example of a criminal justice approach to drugs: a commentary on the short film Putting UK Drug Policy into Focus. *Harm Reduc J* 2020; 17(1): 97.

3. Gabbert G. Pros and cons of drug decriminalization. Mental Health Match 2021. Available from: https://mentalhealthmatch.com/articles/recovery/pros-and-cons-of-drug-decriminalization.

Question 15

A patient coming in for elective surgery: is it OK to tell them all the risks?

Satya Francis

Question

A patient is coming in for an elective planned surgery. Is it OK to tell them all the risks that can happen?

The examiner will question you on this scenario in the next station.

Themes for discussion (■ Table 1.15)

Table 1.15.	
Question themes	**What is expected from the candidate?**
1 The candidate greets the examiner and has good body language.	The candidate is presentable and uses good communication skills; always recommended in any station.

Table 1.15.

	Question themes	What is expected from the candidate?
2	What do you understand by consent in medicine?	The candidate has a good understanding of consent in healthcare management.
		A patient must give permission before they receive any medical treatment, investigation or examination. It must be voluntary and informed, and the patient must have capacity. It can be verbal, written or implied.
3	When is the consent valid?	It is valid when consent is given voluntarily based on the information received and understood. The patient should have the capacity to make the decision.
	Who could take the consent?	Consent should be taken by one with sufficient knowledge and qualification to provide the treatment, able to discuss the risks and benefits, and provides information on alternative management.
4	What is the Mental Capacity Act?	The Mental Capacity Act 2005 is a legal framework for acting and making decisions on behalf of adults who lack the capacity to make particular decisions for themselves.
6	Is informed consent needed?	It is ethical and required by law.
		The patient must have received and understood sufficient information about the diagnosis, proposed treatment, and the implications of the treatment. The patient must be informed of different options for treatment including the option of no treatment. The risks and benefits of each option must be given to the patient.

Table 1.15.

Question themes	What is expected from the candidate?
7 How could harm be avoided in healthcare management by appropriate consenting?	A healthcare professional should follow the key principles in consenting.
	All patients have the right to be involved in their treatment and care decisions and to make informed decisions if they can. The exchange of information between doctor and patient is essential for good decision making. Serious harm can result if the patient is not listened to or if they are not given the information they need.
8 Can we withhold information from the patient?	No, withholding information can be legally challenged. We should not withhold any information from the patient who needs to decide about their treatment.
	If a relative or caregiver asks a doctor to withhold information, a doctor should not do this as the patient needs to know everything needed about their care.
9 Judgement and clarity.	The candidate has clarity in their answer and has a good understanding of good medical practice, decision making and informed consent. A clear presentation, smiling throughout and avoiding repetition — these steps can increase the scores in this station.
10 Conclusion.	The candidate concludes the session and thanks the examiner at the end. This gains the candidate extra bonus points.

Discussion

Informed consent is an important topic that recurs in medical interviews. The candidate should be aware of the need for detailed consent. Awareness of mental capacity to take decisions is also vital.

The General Medical Council has issued guidance on decision making and consent; the candidate should be aware of this guidance. Shared decision making and consent are fundamental to good medical practice. As per this document, the seven principles of consent include:

1. All patients have a right to be involved in making decisions about their care and treatment; they should be supported to make these informed decisions.
2. Decision making is an ongoing process focused on meaningful dialogue; specific to the individual patient.
3. All patients have a right to be listened to, and given the information they need.
4. Doctors must try to find out what matters to the patients; they should offer reasonable alternatives, including the option of taking no action.
5. Start with the presumption that all adults have the capacity to make decisions. If a patient lacks capacity, that should be assessed as per legal requirements.
6. Choice of treatment must be of overall benefit to patients, and those close to them or advocating for them should be consulted.
7. The patient whose right to consent is affected by law should be supported to be involved in the decision-making process.

Key Points

- The candidate should be able to outline 'Good medical practice' set out by the General Medical Council with regard to decision making and consent.
- The candidate should show awareness of the Mental Capacity Act 2005.

References

1. General Medical Council. Good medical practice. Available from: https://www.gmc-uk.org/ethical-guidance/ethical-guidance-for-doctors/good-medical-practice.

2. General Medical Council. Decision making and consent. Available from: https://www.gmc-uk.org/ethical-guidance/ethical-guidance-for-doctors/decision-making-and-consent.

3. Royal College of Surgeons of England. Consent: supported decision-making. Available from: https://www.rcseng.ac.uk/standards-and-research/standards-and-guidance/good-practice-guides/consent.

4. Brannan S, Campbell R, Davies M, English V, Mussell R, Sheather JC. Ethics briefings. *J Med Ethics* 2015; 41(5): 429-30.

Question 16

A teenager asking for oral contraceptive pills

Hema Kannappan

Question

You are a foundation doctor in a GP practice.

A 14-year-old teenager, Sophie, asks for oral contraceptives and specifically requests that her parents are not told. In the next role-play station, you will be talking to Sophie about this request.

The examiner will question the candidate about the ethics in this station after this discussion.

Themes for discussion (■ Table 1.16)

Table 1.16.	
Question themes	**What is expected from the candidate?**
1 The candidate greets the patient and the examiner.	Good body language and a presentable manner.
	The candidate introduces themselves and confirms that they are talking to the right person.
2 The candidate asks the patient why she does not want her parents to be told.	The candidate starts by asking the patient about the problem and then empathetically questions their worries. The candidate lets Sophie talk and listens actively.
	The candidate should be able to elicit Sophie's emotions of fear and let her talk in this station.
3 The candidate confirms that the patient understands the risks and side effects of oral contraceptives.	The candidate asks the patient whether she understands the side effects and risks. They confirm that the patient has an understanding of the issues.
4 The candidate reassures the patient that confidentiality will be maintained.	The candidate has an understanding of patient confidentiality. They have a good rapport with Sophie so she understands that the doctor is acting in her best interest. Sophie is reassured that the doctor and patient relationship confidentiality will be maintained.
5 The candidate explores the relationship in the family and why the patient wants to keep it confidential.	The candidate has good communication skills and lets the patient talk about why they want to keep treatment confidential. Non-verbal cues of being empathetic and listening skills are important in this task.

Table 1.16.

	Question themes	What is expected from the candidate?
6	The examiner asks about the stance of UK legislation with regard to sexual relationships.	UK law clarifies that those aged under 16 are not able to give consent for sexual relationships. Given that Sophie is only 14, this raises concerns and the doctor should act in the patient's best interest.
7	The examiner questions the duty of doctors in this scenario.	The doctor should act in the best interest of the patient. They should: • Explain the risks and benefits of oral contraceptives. • Understand child protection and safety. • Confirm that Sophie understands the advice given. Doctors should explain clearly that they can breach confidentiality in the patient's best interest if there is a risk of abuse.
8	Four pillars of medical ethics.	Autonomy, beneficence, non-maleficence and justice. The candidate should be able to clearly define the four pillars of medical ethics and justify how to apply them in this scenario.
9	Where can we find confidentiality and good practice in handling patient information guidelines?	The candidate is aware of the 'Good medical practice' guidelines from the General Medical Council.
10	Conclusion.	The candidate concludes in an acceptable manner. They thank the patient and the examiner.

Discussion

Role-play stations should be practised well before the actual MMI. Appropriate introduction, confirming that you are talking to the right patient, and concluding is essential for all role-play stations. In addition, at the end, please do not forget to thank the examiner as they are observing your conversation with the patient.

It is a complex scenario, and the examiner is aware of the complexity and does not expect a solution for the problem. The examiner assesses how you communicate in the scenario, being empathetic, and understanding the safety issues with regard to confidentiality. The role of the doctor in putting patient safety first is important. If you feel confused in a particular ethics station, please start by applying the four pillars of medical ethics, which will help you structure the answer.

Key Points

- The candidate must understand the importance of patient confidentiality.
- The candidate should be aware of the law with regard to patients younger than 16 years old.
- The candidate should be clear that it is important to override patient confidentiality in the best interests of the patient, and honestly explain this to the patient.
- The GMC's guideline, 'Good medical practice', should be quoted.

References

1. General Medical Council. Good medical practice. Available from: https://www.gmc-uk.org/-/media/documents/good-medical-practice---english-20200128_pdf-51527435.pdf.

2. General Medical Council. Disclosures for the protection of patients and others. Available from: https://www.gmc-uk.org/ethical-guidance/ethical-guidance-for-doctors/confidentiality/disclosures-for-the-protection-of-patients-and-others.

Question 17

Intervention without patient consent in a near-death scenario

Priya Gauthama

Question

James is in a near-death emergency; the hospital performs surgery as James was not in the right frame of mind to decide, despite him not wanting surgery. He recovers and sues the hospital for performing surgery against his wishes.

The examiner will ask questions regarding how you will approach this complex ethical scenario. The next station will discuss these issues and your opinion on this situation.

Themes for discussion (■ Table 1.17)

Table 1.17.	
Question themes	**What is expected from the candidate?**
1 The candidate greets the examiner and has good body language.	The candidate is presentable and uses good communication skills; always recommended in any station.
2 Good opening statement.	The candidate gives a good opening statement showing that they understand the situation.

This should be a succinct summary of the ethical problems that could lead to further discussion. |
| 3 The candidate explains the scenario and its implication. | The candidate explains the following based on the priority of needs:

• Information gathering and confidential enquiry with this incident.
• To discuss with a senior member of the staff for further guidance. |
| 4 The candidate has a clear understanding of the issues. | • The candidate mentions the issues around consent, mental capacity and the ethical issues surrounding it.
• A clear understanding that this was an emergency, and that James was in a near-death situation.
• James was not in a clear frame of mind to make an informed decision in the emergency.
• The doctors performed surgery in James' best interests to save his life. |
| 5 The candidate has a clear opinion/conclusion. | The candidate summarises the issues involved and the importance of treating the patient in his best interests in an emergency scenario. |

Table 1.17.

	Question themes	What is expected from the candidate?
6	Four pillars of medical ethics.	The candidate can apply the four pillars of medical ethics in this scenario: autonomy, beneficence, non-maleficence and justice.
7	Do you know what the Hippocratic Oath is? — a doctor has an obligation to save lives.	The candidate has an understanding of the Hippocratic Oath. *'Primum non nocere* — first, do no harm.' This oath is incorporated and updated in the UK General Medical Council's 'Good medical practice' guideline and the American Medical Association's Code of Medical Ethics.
8	Do you know any guidelines for the duty of the doctor?	The candidate understands the guidelines such as from the General Medical Council in the UK and the American Medical Association's Code of Medical Ethics.
9	Conclusion.	The candidate concludes the session and thanks the examiner at the end. This gains the candidate extra bonus points.

Discussion

This is a question on ethical issues, mental capacity and informed consent.

In similar situations, please take some notes or prepare mentally in the 1-2 minutes given to prepare for this question before the actual station starts. Structure your answer and prepare a starting sentence that can impress the examiner.

Remember and correlate the four pillars of medical ethics that is a framework used for medical ethics issues:

1. Autonomy (giving the patient the freedom to choose when they can): the patient's autonomy is to respect their wishes or decisions. It is the patient's right to come to their own decisions about what is best for them. However, autonomy requires that the patient is competent and has the capacity to make a decision. If a patient lacks capacity, meaning that they cannot understand, retain, weigh up or communicate their decision due to a disorder of the brain or mind, their autonomy can be overruled by a doctor, as long as the doctor is acting in the patient's best interests. In this case, the hospital acted in the best interest of James to save his life in an emergency situation. In a non-emergency situation, doctors need to follow their patient's wishes after a detailed discussion of the situation, providing all the information available to help them to make an informed decision based on their choice. It is the patient's right to come to their own decisions about what is best for them even if these decisions are viewed as unwise by healthcare providers or wider society.

2. Beneficence (doing good): doctors should always act for the benefit and best interest of the patients.

3. Non-maleficence (to do no harm): health professionals should not harm the patients or do anything that can harm them.

4. Justice (ensuring fairness): assessing that it is important to save James' life in the emergency scenario was fair.

The classical Hippocratic Oath has been summarised as a solemn promise:

*   Of solidarity with teachers and other physicians.
*   Of beneficence (to do good or avoid evil) and non-maleficence ('do no harm') towards patients.
*   Not to assist suicide or abortion.
*   To leave surgery to surgeons.
*   Not to harm, especially not to seduce patients.
*   To maintain confidentiality and never gossip.

The classic Hippocratic Oath has been modified in modern medicine to suit the present day. Following the GMC's 'Good medical practice' guidance will fulfil the qualities needed for a doctor.

Key Points

- There are pros and cons to any ethical dilemma; the candidate has to be aware of both.
- The candidate should be able to clearly come to a conclusion and explain their reasoning.
- The candidate should quote the General Medical Council's 'Good medical practice' document or the American Medical Council's or a similar body's code of ethics to show that they are aware of the ethics behind the scenario.
- Quoting the Hippocratic Oath shows that the candidate understands the ethical duties of a doctor.

References

1. General Medical Council. Good medical practice. Available from: https://www.gmc-uk.org/ethical-guidance/ethical-guidance-for-doctors/good-medical-practice.

2. American Medical Association. Code of Medical Ethics overview. Available from: https://www.ama-assn.org/delivering-care/ethics/code-medical-ethics-overview.

3. Olejarczyk JP, Young M. Patient rights and ethics. Stat. Pearls Publishing 2022. Available from: https://www.ncbi.nlm.nih.gov/books/NBK538279.

4. Knott L. The hippocratic oath and good medical practice. Available from: https://patient.info/doctor/ideals-and-the-hippocratic-oath.

Question 18

Non-accidental bruising in a young child

Hema Kannappan

Question

You are a junior doctor working on a paediatric ward. You are examining a 3-year-old boy, Jamie, in the assessment unit for a lower respiratory tract infection. Whilst examining his chest, you notice that he is covered in bruises all over his body. In the next station, the examiner will ask questions about non-accidental injuries in a child and what you will do in these situations.

Themes for discussion (■ Table 1.18)

Table 1.18.

	Question themes	What is expected from the candidate?
1	The candidate greets the examiner.	Good body language and a presentable manner.

Table 1.18.

	Question themes	What is expected from the candidate?
2	The candidate succinctly summarises the situation.	The candidate explains the finding of non-accidental bruises discovered during a routine examination.
3	The examiner says the mother explained that the bruising is due to their common cultural practice.	What does she mean by 'common cultural practice'? The candidate understands the customs in some foreign cultures, but realises the seriousness of the situation and the need for child safety. Child safety is protecting all children from child abuse, managing the risks, providing support, and responding to incidents or allegations of child abuse.
4	What is child protection?	Child protection is part of the safeguarding process that focuses on protecting children identified as suffering or likely to suffer significant harm. The candidate is able to differentiate between accidental or non-accidental causes. Non-accidental injuries could be suggested by bruising over soft tissues, multiple bruises, bruises in the shape of an instrument or hand, burns suggestive of cigarette burns, etc.
5	Once identified, where will you get help?	Being a junior doctor, the candidate will immediately obtain help from a senior colleague. They will raise their concerns with the multidisciplinary team. They understand the seriousness of the situation. The candidate can then escalate the finding to social services if they are concerned with child safety. If asked, the candidate states that they will explain the concerns to the parents in the interest of child safety.

Table 1.18.

	Question themes	What is expected from the candidate?
6	GMC regulations.	All doctors should follow GMC guidelines and the candidate is aware of 'Good medical practice'.
7	Four pillars of medical ethics.	Autonomy, beneficence, non-maleficence and justice.
8	How do you apply medical ethics to this scenario?	The candidate should be able to explain and justify the four pillars within this case scenario.
9	Conclusion.	The candidate concludes and summarises the station; they thank the examiner.

Discussion

Child safety is a complex scenario to deal with, even for senior doctors; the examiner understands the limitations and will only be testing the candidate's awareness of the problems and the pathway to get help in needed circumstances.

In some MMIs, this can present as a role-play station with an examiner observing how the candidate communicates. Being calm, but realising the seriousness, and acting in the child's best interest are the criteria assessed in this role-play station.

Key Points

- The candidate must understand the concept of child safety.
- The candidate should be aware that they need to get help.
- They can quote the GMC's 'Good medical practice' guidance and use the four pillars of medical ethics to base their answer.

References

1. NSPCC Learning. Safeguarding children and child protection. Available from: https://learning.nspcc.org.uk/safeguarding-child-protection.

2. General Medical Council. Good medical practice. Available from: https://www.gmc-uk.org/ethical-guidance/ethical-guidance-for-doctors/good-medical-practice.

Question 19

A patient with alcoholism consuming hand sanitiser

Priya Gauthama

Question

You are a junior doctor on the medical ward; a patient named Wilson is admitted for the management of alcohol dependency. The nurse in the ward informs you that Wilson has stolen a bottle of hand sanitiser and consumed it.

How would you approach this? The next station will discuss these issues and your opinion on this situation.

Themes for discussion (■ Table 1.19)

Table 1.19.	
Question themes	**What is expected from the candidate?**
1 The candidate greets the examiner and has good body language.	The candidate is presentable and uses good communication skills; always recommended in any station.

Table 1.19.

	Question themes	What is expected from the candidate?
2	The examiner gives a good succinct opening statement.	The candidate gives a good opening statement showing that they understand the situation. This gives a good introduction to the clinical and ethical problems in this scenario.
3	The candidate explains the scenario and its implication.	The candidate explains the following points based on the priority of needs:

- Ensuring the safety of the patient and appropriate treatment as they have consumed hand sanitiser.
- Information gathering and confidential enquiry with the patient once they have recovered from the incident.
- Checking if this is a one-off incident or a repeated occurrence.
- Assessing the background medical condition of the patient such as mental health condition, other medical illnesses.
- Ascertaining the current treatment of his alcohol dependency and involving the appropriate professionals and agencies to support the patient.
- Loss of a sanitiser repeatedly can take a toll on infection control measures on the ward if not recognised.

4	The candidate clearly understands how to avoid this in the future.	

- If this is a repeated occurrence, prompt action to be taken to relocate the hand sanitiser to a safer place as it may compromise the well-being of others on the ward if they cannot use it. Extra monitoring should be put in place for Wilson during his next admission.
- Implement incident reporting and action to avoid similar incidents in the future.
- Discuss with a senior member of staff for further guidance.
- Discuss with the multidisciplinary team to create awareness and prevent recurrences.

Table 1.19.

Question themes	What is expected from the candidate?
5 The candidate has a clear opinion/conclusion.	• The candidate should explain that he will speak to Wilson to find out the reason behind this particular incident and talk to him in person confidentially. • Ensure that the patient has an appropriate support structure to help and to avoid such incidents in the future. • Check the patient's understanding of the risks posed to themselves and others on the ward. • Provide a follow-up appointment on discharge and refer the case to the appropriate professionals such as mental health professionals for further guidance and management.
6 Do you know what are the four pillars of medical ethics?	The candidate understands the medical ethics framework and can quote the four pillars of medical ethics.
7 Do you know of any guidelines outlining the duty of the doctor?	The candidate understands guidelines such as those from the General Medical Council (GMC) in the UK, the American Medical Association's Code of Medical Ethics, or specific national guidelines.
8 Conclusion.	The candidate concludes the session and thanks the examiner at the end.

Discussion

Ethical dilemmas are complex scenarios in MMIs; in this station, we advise candidates to take their time and use the preceding 1-2 minutes to frame their answers, if allowed. They should start with a good opening summary.

Remember and correlate the four pillars of medical ethics that is a framework used for medical ethics issues:

1. Autonomy (giving the patient the freedom to choose when they can): it is the patient's right to come to their own decisions about what is best for them, even if these decisions are viewed as unwise by healthcare providers or wider society. Autonomy enables the individual to make informed choices after being provided with all the information about their condition. Autonomy requires that the patient is competent and has the capacity to make a decision. It has to be noted that although patients are free to refuse any treatment or pick a treatment from a range of treatment options, they cannot demand a specific treatment or action that the doctor finds not suitable or is not competent to offer. Doctors cannot force patients to undergo particular management options, and patients have the right to decline treatment themselves. If a patient lacks capacity, meaning that they cannot understand, retain, weigh up or communicate their decision due to mental health issues or organic causes, a doctor can overrule their autonomy. For example, for a patient with dementia, a doctor can overrule their decision to refuse treatment as long as the doctor is acting in the patient's best interests.

2. Beneficence (doing good): this is doing what is best for a patient. Autonomy and beneficence may conflict, when a competent patient chooses an action that is not in their best interests. It considers the balance of benefits of any treatment against the risks involved. Doctors should always act to the benefit and best interest of the patients.

3. Non-maleficence (to do no harm): health professionals should not harm patients. Most treatments may have some side effects or cause harm, but professionals should ensure that the harm is not disproportionate to the benefits of the treatment.

4. Justice (ensuring fairness): this is the idea that any ethical decision should be considered as part of the wider context in society, distributing the benefits, risks and costs fairly.

Key Points

- There are pros and cons to any ethical dilemma; the candidate has to be aware of both.
- The candidate should be able to clearly come to a conclusion and explain their reasoning.
- The candidate should quote the General Medical Council's 'Good medical practice' document or the American Medical Council's or a similar body's code of ethics to show that they are aware of the ethics behind the scenario.
- Quoting the medical ethics framework shows that the candidate understands the ethical duties of a doctor.

References

1. General Medical Council. Good medical practice. Available from: https://www.gmc-uk.org/ethical-guidance/ethical-guidance-for-doctors/good-medical-practice.
2. American Medical Association. Code of Medical Ethics overview. Available from: https://www.ama-assn.org/delivering-care/ethics/code-medical-ethics-overview.

Question 20

A patient requesting syringes and needles

Thiagarajan Sridhar

Question

You are a junior doctor in a GP surgery; one of your patients is requesting needles and syringes, without any medical indication.

The examiner in the next station will discuss the problems that could arise in this scenario. You will be asked to opine whether you would give the needles and syringes or not. The examiner will assess your thinking process behind this decision.

Themes for discussion (■ Table 1.20)

Table 1.20.

	Question themes	What is expected from the candidate?
1	The candidate greets the examiner and has good body language.	The candidate is presentable and uses good communication skills; always recommended in any station.

Table 1.20.

	Question themes	What is expected from the candidate?
2	What do you think of this scenario?	The candidate gives a good opening statement showing that they understand the situation.
3	The candidate explores the request of the patient and the problems or issues.	The candidate considers various situations why the patient could have asked for needles and syringes: • The reason for such a request to be asked directly. • Any drug issues or intravenous drug abuse. • Any medical issues — recommended by the hospital in another country, for example, a diabetic on insulin. • For family member use.
4	The candidate understands the risks of refusing the request.	• Drug addiction will lead to access to needles by all means. • The patient can access unhygienic needles, increasing the risk of transmission of diseases. • Explore family/social support. • Other health issues. • Mental health issues.
5	The candidate is sensitive to the issue and offers support.	The candidate should be able to discuss this sensitive matter without bias. The candidate should not be patronising to the patient. They should be aware of the 'needle and syringe programme' that is available to avoid disease transmission by sharing needles.
6	What is your opinion about the needle and syringe programme?	The candidate explores the whole issue and gives their own opinion without prejudice; they look at the pros and cons of the request and look at other solutions also.

	Question themes	What is expected from the candidate?
7	Judgement and clarity.	The candidate has clarity in their answer and can explain the pros and cons, concluding clearly. A clear presentation, smiling throughout and avoiding repetition — these steps can increase the scores in this station. The candidate should show empathy and be willing to discuss difficult issues and support patients.
8	Conclusion.	The candidate concludes the session and thanks the examiner at the end. This gains the candidate extra bonus points.

Table 1.20.

Discussion

This question throws up many moral and social challenges. As a health professional, one should be sensitive to all the patient's needs. In addition to medical needs, doctors are often the first point of contact about social and emotional issues.

Doctors are expected to work with other professionals in a multidisciplinary way to support patients. Whatever one's personal opinion about social issues, doctors will be expected to act without prejudice in the best interests of the patient.

Needle and syringe programmes aim to reduce the transmission of viruses and other infections, such as HIV, hepatitis B and C, and bacterial infections, that can happen by sharing needles.

Key Points

- There are pros and cons to any ethical dilemma; the candidate must be aware of both.
- The candidate should be able to clearly explain their reasoning and always be empathetic to a particular situation.
- They should be able to quote/outline any professional body's documents/guidances.
- They should be sensitive to patients' requests and always explore options to help the patients.

References

1. NICE (National Institute for Health and Care Excellence). Needle and syringe programmes. Public health guideline [PH52]. Available from: https://www.nice.org.uk/guidance/ph52.

Question 21

A colleague offering a placebo to a patient

Prabhu Gandhimani

Question

You are a junior doctor in a GP surgery. Your colleague offers a placebo to a patient without telling her.

Is it right to offer a placebo without telling the patient? The next station will discuss the ethics behind this scenario.

Themes for discussion (■ Table 1.21)

Table 1.21.	
Question themes	**What is expected from the candidate?**
1 The candidate greets the examiner and has good body language.	The candidate is presentable and uses good communication skills; always recommended in any station.

Table 1.21.

Question themes	What is expected from the candidate?
2 What is a placebo and how does it work?	The candidate presents: • A definition of placebo and an understanding of the scientific basis, the mind-body interaction, and the context of receiving treatment (see the discussion below). • Knowledge of placebos in clinical trials. • Understanding that placebo responders are not malingerers.
3 What is a nocebo?	The candidate presents: • Understanding that placebo treatment can evoke a side effect although no active ingredient exists.
4 Why might a doctor have given a placebo?	The candidate clearly understands the pros of the placebo: • Acting in the best interest of the patient. • Wanting to please the patient by showing that the doctor has done something for him, without doing harm. • Also considering that the doctor might have given the placebo to avoid the patient making repeated consultations asking for treatment, therefore improving the efficiency of the healthcare system.
5 The candidate also explains the cons for the placebo.	The candidate clearly understands the cons of the placebo: • The doctor might ignore non-specific patient symptoms, but these symptoms could be from a serious underlying disease that might need investigation or might get worse in the future. • The patient might ignore further symptoms thinking that they have had treatment.

Table 1.21.

Question themes	What is expected from the candidate?
	• The patient might lose trust in the profession. • This action affects the doctor-patient relationship. • The GMC clearly states the need for honesty among doctors; this is a breach and has probity issues.
6 What are the ethical issues in this scenario?	The candidate talks about the four pillars of ethics: • The candidate knows the importance of informed consent to facilitate patient autonomy. • Beneficence — although a placebo can provide a clinical response this is not ideal as it does not treat the underlying cause. • Non-maleficence — by ignoring the patient's vague symptoms, the actual disease process could get worse. • Justice — it is arguable whether it will ensure fairness by reducing multiple appointments or unnecessary investigations.
7 Is it right for doctors to give placebos?	The candidate has a clear opinion/conclusion and explains their reasons. The candidate is clear that this is WRONG to give a placebo without informed consent.
8 Is it ethical to use a placebo in clinical trials?	The candidate is clear that there are no ethical issues as patients are consented before the trial. In research trials, patients will be told that they will be randomly separated into two groups, one given the research drug and another given a placebo; in this scenario, the patient is aware that there is a 50:50 chance they might be given a placebo. However, the patient has the right to withdraw from the research at any time, and they have the right to know which group they were in once the research is completed.

Table 1.21.

	Question themes	What is expected from the candidate?
9	Judgement and clarity.	The candidate has clarity in their answer and can explain the pros and cons, concluding clearly. A clear presentation, smiling throughout and avoiding repetition — these steps can increase the scores in this station.
10	Conclusion.	The candidate concludes the session and thanks the examiner at the end. This gains the candidate extra bonus points.

Discussion

Placebo is a Latin word meaning 'I will please'; it refers to a treatment or a drug without any active ingredients and therefore should be of no therapeutic benefit. Although, there is no active treatment, placebos have been scientifically proven to have a positive impact on the health and psychological well-being of a patient.

The nocebo effect refers to the negative effect or side effect that a patient can experience when treated with a placebo. Even without the active ingredient, side effects can happen.

Both placebo and nocebo are thought to be mediated by brain-body responses to the context in which the treatment is delivered and the expectation of the patient that the treatment given is going to make them better. The idea of using placebos for treatment is as old as the history of medicine itself, and initially they were used to treat psychosomatic illness and placebo responders were thought to be malingerers. But available evidence shows that these responses are real and have a sound scientific basis.

Placebos are often used in clinical trials as 'control treatments' to 'blind' the subject or the researcher to whether someone is receiving an active treatment. The placebo medicine looks exactly the same as the treatment medicine in size, colour, smell and texture but lacks the active ingredient. This helps to eliminate bias and makes the study more rigorous. In fact, a randomised controlled double-blinded clinical trial is the gold standard in medical research.

However, prescribing a placebo without patient knowledge might mean that you are withholding information and not allowing the patient to make an informed decision about their treatment. It could be regarded as unethical, as it takes away patient autonomy and is a violation of the trust a patient has in a doctor and can make a patient lose faith in the doctor and even the medical profession overall. There is a widespread belief that placebos will only work if the patient does not know that they are being given a placebo, but recent evidence shows that they work even if the patient knows they are taking a placebo.

Although the doctor might have acted in the best interests of the patient when giving the placebo, doing so without the knowledge of the patient is unethical and voids the consenting process. Before any trials of medicines involving placebos, ethics committee approval has to be sought to ensure that the patients are not put in any harm by the trial and are given adequate information regarding the trial. They are made explicitly aware that the treatment they receive might be a placebo and so there are no ethical issues about using a placebo in clinical trials.

Key Points

- Knowledge about placebos is a must to answer this question.
- There are pros and cons to any ethical dilemma; the candidate has to be aware of both.
- The candidate should be able to clearly come to a conclusion and explain their reasoning.
- A doctor's prime duty is to be open, honest, act with integrity to maintain trust in the profession and involve patients in the decision-making process.

References

1. Wager TD, Atlas LY. The neuroscience of placebo effects: connecting context, learning and health. *Nat Rev Neurosci* 2015; 16(7): 403-18.

2. Miller FG, Colloca L, Kaptchuk TJ. The placebo effect: illness and interpersonal healing. *Perspect Biol Med* 2009; 52(4): 518-39.

3. American Medical Association. Placebo use in clinical practice. CEJA; 2006.

4. Kaptchuk TJ, Friedlander E, Kelley JM, *et al.* Placebos without deception: a randomized controlled trial in irritable bowel syndrome. *PLOS ONE* 2010; 5(12): e15591.

Question22

A patient travelling abroad for assisted suicide

Thiagarajan Sridhar

Question

You are a junior doctor; one of your patients has advanced cancer and tells you that she is travelling abroad for assisted suicide. She says that her partner is arranging this and is fully supportive of her decision.

In the next station, the examiner will discuss the ethics of assisted suicide with regard to this scenario.

Themes for discussion (■ Table 1.22)

Table 1.22.	
Question themes	**What is expected from the candidate?**
1 The candidate greets the examiner and has good body language.	The candidate is presentable and uses good communication skills, demonstrating confidence in dealing with a very difficult situation such as this.

Table 1.22.

Question themes	What is expected from the candidate?
2 The examiner asks the candidate to describe the scenario.	The candidate shows a good understanding of the situation. The candidate sets the scene with a good opening statement about the complexities of this scenario.
3 The candidate offers to listen to the patient's concerns and explores why the patient and her partner are taking this path.	The candidate explores the current situation: • The patient has a terminal illness with limited life expectancy. • The candidate should be empathetic to the patient's needs. • The candidate explores the underlying clinical issues that could be better supported by other treatments. • The candidate explores the main reasons for such a request, for example, it could be recent discussions with a healthcare professional about prognosis, burden on the family, untreated pain or nausea, etc. • The candidate also explores if the patient clearly understands this and has sufficient capacity to make the decision (e.g. there are no underlying issues such as a learning difficulty).
4 The candidate explains the ethical rules and the legal aspects of such a request in the UK or a different country.	• Euthanasia is illegal in the UK. • Assisted suicide is illegal in the UK and carries a maximum of 14 years. • Depending upon the circumstances, euthanasia is considered as manslaughter or murder. • The candidate should discuss symptom control and palliative care support, or other supportive treatment that might be needed. • They clearly explain that the patient's partner or family could potentially face legal problems if options outside the UK are pursued. • Whilst they are sympathetic to the patient's need, they should not propose anything outside the current legal framework.

Table 1.22.

	Question themes	What is expected from the candidate?
5	What is your opinion about euthanasia? Do you support it or not?	The candidates are allowed to have a personal opinion, but they also understand their responsibilities under the legal framework.
		If they support euthanasia, they should have persuasive arguments, about quality of life, distress to the family, human rights and freedom to decide. They should not mention the burden to the taxpayer or the NHS as the main criteria.
		If they do not support euthanasia, then they should explain using reasons such as pro-life, the doctor's role to save lives, the risks of vulnerable patients being pushed into taking decisions without medical/legal support, etc.
		It might be worth remembering the British Medical Association's (BMA) stance in this dilemma: it is currently neutral and neither opposes nor supports it; in the past, the BMA had strongly opposed it.
6	If the government decides to change the law to make euthanasia legal, what are the safeguards that could be built in?	Support and training for the medical team.
		Support for the patient and family.
		An independent medical and legal team to validate the request.
		Rigorous governance and audit of such decisions.
		Involvement of religious institutions and other human rights charities.

Table 1.22.	
Question themes	**What is expected from the candidate?**
7 Judgement and clarity.	The candidate has clarity in their answer; they clearly understand the gravity of the situation but handle it well with confidence. The candidate should be empathetic to the patient's needs.
8 Conclusion.	The candidate concludes the session and thanks the examiner at the end.

Discussion

There is a clinical, ethical and moral dilemma in this question. Candidates are free to air their opinion but should understand the legal framework currently in the UK.

They should be able to independently discuss the pros and cons and should be able to give a balanced view.

Candidates would be expected to deal with a very tricky and difficult situation without any bias. They should be fully aware of the legal pitfalls and should follow the current legislation. They should also exhibit an insight that rules could change in the future, but there is no guarantee that this will happen and they should not be giving patients unrealistic expectations.

Key Points

- There are pros and cons to any ethical dilemma; the candidate must be aware of both.
- The candidate should be able to clearly conclude and explain their reasons.
- The candidate should quote the General Medical Council or any national guidelines that regulate this scenario; the candidate should be aware that rules are different in different countries.
- They should understand the guiding principle of 'do no harm'.
- Candidates should always be aware of the need to seek further legal opinion.

References

1.   British Medical Association. Physician-assisted dying. Available from: https://www.bma.org.uk/advice-and-support/ethics/end-of-life/physician-assisted-dying.

2.   NHS UK. Euthanasia and assisted suicide. Available from: https://www.nhs.uk/conditions/euthanasia-and-assisted-suicide.

3.   UK Parliament. Parliamentary bills. Assisted dying bill [HL]. Available from: https://bills.parliament.uk/bills/2875.

Question 23

A patient demanding painkillers

Kodaganallur Parthasarathi Krishnan

Question

You are a junior doctor in a GP surgery. A patient of yours, Mr Jones, is demanding strong painkillers and you decline his request as there is no indication. He now threatens you that he is going to obtain illegal drugs and inject himself. How will you manage this?

This is a role-play station with an actor; the actor will take the role of the patient. There will be an examiner observing and assessing this station.

Themes for discussion (■ Table 1.23)

Table 1.23.	
Question themes	**What is expected from the candidate?**
1 The candidate introduces themselves.	This is a complex scenario; the candidate understands this complexity but stays calm and has a good approach. They should introduce themselves clearly. They should show empathy with their body language, and speak clearly but calmly.
2 The candidate confirms that they are speaking to the right patient — named Mr Jones.	It is important to check that the correct patient is being spoken to. In real life, the date of birth and address should also be checked.
3 The candidate shows an understanding of the theme.	The candidate seeks a detailed background history from the patient with special emphasis on focusing on the theme.
4 The candidate reviews the drug history of the patient.	The candidate questions the patient's presenting complaints; the candidate assesses the patient for signs and symptoms including pain scores, reviews their existing drug history, and reassures the patient that all necessary medications have already been prescribed.
5 The candidate probes the need for strong painkillers.	They explore the need and the understanding for strong painkillers (opioids), explore any previous drug history, explain the side effects and dissuade the patient. Firmness is shown in not offering what the patient demands.
6 The patient becomes angry and agitated now. They threaten the candidate that they will now resort to seeking these drugs illegally.	This is a tricky and challenging situation for any doctor. The candidate can show varying emotional responses to this based on their personality. As part of the interview process, they are expected to stay calm and show empathy, with the patient taking them into their confidence without succumbing to the threat posed.

Table 1.23.

	Question themes	What is expected from the candidate?
7	Discussion with the patient regarding the side effects of illegal drugs.	The candidate then goes on to explain the need to stay away from illegal drugs and the harm that these do, including physical, social and psychological derangements. Furthermore, they could mention that obtaining drugs in this way is against the law.
		The candidate can explain that they will discuss this with their senior mentor/colleague if they are still not happy; they can offer a second opinion with a senior colleague if the patient accepts. They should be empathetic, and offer apologies that they could not meet the expectations of the patient.
8	Explains to the examiner what further steps need to be done.	The candidate admits that this is a complex scenario not faced before. They will seek help from senior colleagues, as well as the multidisciplinary team, including the nurse and allied staff.
9	Examiner to probe what groups are available in these scenarios in this clinical setting.	Multidisciplinary teams, psychiatry liaison groups, psychologists, adult safeguarding groups, and addiction prevention leaflets including websites and local addresses can be used.
10	Conclusion.	The candidate can demonstrate control of the situation both in terms of assuring the patient, also showing knowledge of actions necessary to guide the patient to stay away and seek appropriate help.

Role play for the actor

The actor was told to act as Mr Jones. He had to act with discomfort and pain, being unhappy with existing medications. When probed further, the actor will forcefully demand stronger pain medicines.

The candidates are expected to say no to this. Following on, actors are advised to threaten the candidate that they would go and procure these drugs illegally and inject themselves. Actors should continue to maintain this stance and show their displeasure all the time.

Discussion

Some of the MMI stations can have an angry or unsatisfied patient; these are complex, but a good candidate can calm the patient and listen to their history. This station checks whether the candidate can listen, communicate and show empathy. The unique situation in this station is that the candidate is not in a position to comply with the patient's demand; they should advise him of the unwanted effects of such illegal drugs and also stop them from taking them by seeking help from relevant bodies in the trust.

The UK General Medical Council's (GMC) 'Good medical practice' guidance (Domain 2: Safety and quality) clarifies the need to respond to concerns openly and safely. Domain 3 (Communication partnership and teamwork) stresses that doctors must listen to patients, take account of their views, and respond honestly to their questions. GMC guidance for medical students also promotes the same messages but advises them to inform supervisors involved in the care.

One of the key aspects of this station is to stay calm but show empathy at the same time. Listening is an active skill and needs to be developed; at the same time, most stations last for 5-7 minutes, and the candidate must apologise and convince the patient of the task. Practising repeatedly with mock actors can build confidence in the candidate to face real MMI scenarios.

Key Points

- In a patient role-play scenario, it is important to introduce yourself and confirm that you are speaking to the right patient.
- An empathetic approach and keen listening are vital in these situations.
- If the patient calms down, this will lead to successful communication.
- Always conclude the session; if it is a patient role play, do not forget to ask if there is anything else that the patient wants.

References

1. General Medical Council. Good medical practice. Domain 2: Safety and quality. Available from: https://www.gmc-uk.org/ethical-guidance/ethical-guidance-for-doctors/good-medical-practice/domain-2----safety-and-quality#paragraph-22.

2. General Medical Council. Good medical practice. Domain 3: Communication partnership and teamwork. Available from: https://www.gmc-uk.org/ethical-guidance/ethical-guidance-for-doctors/good-medical-practice/domain-3---communication-partnership-and-teamwork#paragraph-31.

3. General Medical Council. Achieving good medical practice: guidance for medical students. Domain 4 Maintaining Trust. Available from: https://www.gmc-uk.org/education/standards-guidance-and-curricula/guidance/student-professionalism-and-ftp/achieving-good-medical-practice/domain-4-maintaining-trust#act-with-honesty-and-integrity.

4. National Institute on Drug Abuse. Preventing drug misuse and addiction: the best strategy. Available from: https://nida.nih.gov/publications/drugs-brains-behavior-science-addiction/preventing-drug-misuse-addiction-best-strategy.

5. NHS UK. Drug addiction: getting help. Available from: https://www.nhs.uk/live-well/addiction-support/drug-addiction-getting-help.

Question 24

A mother refusing blood transfusion for a child

Balamurugan Nambi

Question

You are the on-call junior doctor (FY2) in the A&E department of the hospital; a 14-year-old boy was brought in by ambulance following a horseback riding injury and he has profuse bleeding. He is fully conscious and needs an urgent blood transfusion, but his mother demands that you should not go ahead with the blood transfusion.

In the next station, the examiner will ask questions on how you will deal with this scenario.

Themes for discussion (■ Table 1.24)

	Question themes	What is expected from the candidate?
1	The candidate introduces themselves.	The candidate greets the examiner and introduces themselves.
2	Body language and empathy.	The candidate shows empathy for the situation and acknowledges the concerns of the mother and explains that they will listen to her concerns. Body language and non-verbal skills should be appropriate. The candidate should make eye contact and actively listen.
3	Explores more about the child's condition.	The candidate explains that they will assess the child's condition; confirming that there is an urgent need for a blood transfusion.
4	Gillick competence/parental consent.	The candidate should assess whether the child is mature enough to understand the blood transfusion process and the risks associated with it, based on Gillick competence. If the child is deemed Gillick competent, the doctor should accept the consent and proceed with the transfusion. However, the candidate will try to involve the family and obtain consent when possible. They should discuss the situation with the team and senior colleagues in this complex scenario.
5	If the child is not competent.	It is very important to obtain parental consent before proceeding with the transfusion. The seriousness of the situation and the implications to her son's life need to be explained to the mother.

Table 1.24.

Table 1.24.

	Question themes	What is expected from the candidate?
6	Explain blood transfusions, their benefits and risks, in simple understandable language.	The candidate starts by explaining the blood transfusion process: a blood transfusion is a common procedure in which donated blood or blood components are given through an intravenous line and this can be lifesaving. A blood transfusion is given to replace blood and blood components that may be too low, which is secondary to the horseback riding injury. Typically, the blood comes from an anonymous person who has donated blood for use as hospitals see fit. A blood bank holds the blood until it is needed for transfusion. Donated blood is tested according to national guidelines. If there are any concerns that the blood is not safe, it is discarded.
7	Explores the wishes and concerns of the mother; check if there are religious reasons such as being Jehovah's Witnesses.	The candidate expresses that they will be empathetic and explain the blood transfusion process and reassures the parent. It is very important to know the wishes of the patient's mother in this situation and if she has expressed any wishes previously. Is she worried about infection or has she had any past experience of bad reactions to blood transfusions in the family or religious objections as Jehovah's Witnesses?
8	Acting in the best interests of the child.	This involves including the MDT in the team and acting in the child's best interests. There might be potential for the parent to proceed with legal challenges in court. For emergencies, it is vital to discuss the situation with the MDT and ethical and legal team before proceeding if the situation is life-threatening.

Table 1.24.	
Question themes	**What is expected from the candidate?**
9 Advises further discussion with the treating team and with other family members.	The candidate advises further discussion with the hospital team. They should explore the availability of psychological/pastoral support.
10 Closure and conclusion.	The candidate concludes the session and thanks the examiner.

Discussion

This question can easily be made a role-play station in the MMI, in which the communication skills of the candidate could be tested. Being empathetic and listening to the patient or parent are key skills in any communication station.

Exploring the concerns of the mother and finding out why she does not want blood transfusions for her son is essential; obtaining a history in an empathetic manner will help to find a solution to this ethical dilemma.

Gillick competence applies if a child or young person under the age of 16 years wants treatment, but their parents or carers refuse it. Professionals need to consider several aspects whilst assessing needs; these include:

- Child's age, maturity and mental capacity.
- Their understanding of issues and their effects.
- Risks, implications and consequences.
- How well they understand the information.
- Their understanding of alternative options.
- Their ability to explain the rationale around decision making.

Young people also have the right to seek a second opinion from another medical professional. Gillick competency can also be used when young people refuse medical treatment. In all cases, the child's safety and well-being are paramount.

Key Points

- Communication skills are tested in this scenario.
- The candidate should be keen to find out the concerns of the mother.
- The patient's well-being is the primary concern of the doctor.
- Awareness of Gillick competence is assessed.

References

1. General Medical Council. Good medical practice. Available from: https://www.gmc-uk.org/-/media/documents/good-medical-practice---english-20200128_pdf-51527435.pdf.

2. NSPCC Learning. Gillick competency and Fraser guidelines. Available from: https://learning.nspcc.org.uk/child-protection-system/gillick-competence-fraser-guidelines#heading-top.

Question 25

Relatives refusing to stop intensive care treatment

Selvakumar Panchatsharam

Question

Your friend's mother is on a ventilator with a 'Do Not Resuscitate (DNR)' status. Your friend asks you for advice and states that she wants to continue all treatments for her mother despite the poor prognosis and against the intensive care doctors' advice. In the next role-play station, you must talk to her and make her understand the seriousness of the situation.

Themes for discussion (■ Table 1.25)

Table 1.25.	
Question themes	**What is expected from the candidate?**
1 The candidate introduces themselves.	The candidate greets the examiner and confirms their role in this scenario as a doctor and as a friend of a distressed relative whose mother is currently in intensive care, on a ventilator, receiving life support.

Table 1.25.

	Question themes	What is expected from the candidate?
2	Body language and empathy.	The candidate shows empathy and acknowledges the concerns of the friend by listening to her concerns. The body language and non-verbal skills should be appropriate, similar to a breaking bad news scenario. The candidate makes eye contact and actively listens.
3	Explores more about the relative's condition.	The candidate gently probes into the patient's condition. They ask relevant questions sensitively to ensure that they have a clear understanding of the patient's condition.
4	Explains cardiopulmonary resuscitation (CPR), the benefits and risks.	They start by explaining CPR, how and when it is performed. They explain that it is performed in a cardiac arrest by compressing the chest by a third to allow blood circulation along with ventilation, delivering electrical shock (if necessary) and by injection of drugs, until the patient shows signs of life. It is an invasive procedure that can be beneficial to restore circulation in some circumstances when the underlying cause of the arrest is reversible. However, it also carries a significant burden of damage to internal organs, rib fractures, potentially brain damage due to lack of oxygen, and disability. If CPR is unsuccessful, it carries the risk of potentially causing a traumatic and undignified death. A 'Do Not Resuscitate (DNR)' decision is made by the treating hospital team, if cardiac arrest is expected to be part of the dying process, or if the doctors feel that after resuscitation, even if circulation is restored, it would lead to a poor outcome and there is no overall benefit in performing CPR.

Table 1.25.

	Question themes	What is expected from the candidate?
5	Difference between a DNR notice and withdrawal of life support.	The candidate should have a clear understanding of the differences between a DNR notice and withdrawal of life support. Simply having a DNR notice does not equate to stopping treatment. A DNR decision only applies to not performing CPR if her mother develops a cardiac arrest, as they deem that there is no overall benefit and may do more harm than good if it is performed. Although this is a medical decision, they would discuss it with people close to them (as in this situation if the patient is unconscious) to ensure that they understand the reasons for this decision. Also, the medical team may consider revisiting the decision if there is a substantial change in her condition. Reassure the friend that they would be continuing other supportive treatment to help her mother get better.
6	Benefits and harm of CPR and DNR may be appropriate in certain circumstances.	The candidate should explain that CPR is a very effective treatment if performed immediately after cardiac arrest and that the underlying cause of the cardiac arrest is immediately reversible. They should differentiate between the two broad types of cardiac arrests either due to abnormal heart rhythm, a primary heart problem, usually reversed by an electric shock along with CPR, or cardiac arrest due to other organ systems failure. They explain that the former has a better outcome compared with the latter. In intensive care, whilst on life support the latter is more common, and usually has a low chance of success and often leads to a worse outcome. This is because patients are already very unwell and cardiac arrest is a consequence of other organ systems failure. Even in the small proportion of patients whose hearts recover after cardiac arrest, this could still result in brain damage or prolong their hospital stay, which could result in a worse quality of life after discharge from the hospital.

Table 1.25.

	Question themes	What is expected from the candidate?
7	Explores the mother's wishes.	It is very important to know what her mother would want in this situation and if she has expressed any wishes previously. Also, it is important to ask if she has an advance directive in place for decisions relating to healthcare. It is worth asking if she has appointed a lasting power of attorney and if they have been consulted.
8	Acting in the best interests of the patient.	The candidate should explain that because her mother is being ventilated in intensive care, she is likely to be on sedative medications that could impair her consciousness and may lack the mental capacity to make decisions. Therefore, the hospital team in this situation will usually consult the people close to her to establish her beliefs and wishes to ascertain her best wishes or in other words 'what she would want'. The decision to DNR would have been taken in her 'best interests' as they perceive there is no overall benefit in performing CPR or CPR may be futile or could cause more harm than benefit.
9	Advises further discussion with the treating team and with other family members.	The candidate should ask if she has any further queries and advise discussion with other family members to ascertain her mother's likely wishes and best interests and advises further discussion with the hospital team.
		The candidate should explore the availability of psychological/pastoral support. They can request more time for the family to come to terms with the decision or to seek a second opinion if they disagree.
10	Conclusion.	They explain to the friend that they can contact them if they prefer to do so, and that they are there to support them. At the end, the candidate thanks the actor and the examiner.

Role play for the actor

The actor was told to act as a friend of the candidate who is in distress about her mother's condition. She found out about the DNR order from her father and is clearly very upset. She thinks that the doctors treating her mother are 'giving up' on her. She feels that she has not been consulted to seek her consent about CPR.

When asked about her mum's condition, she explains that her mum was admitted to the intensive care unit (ICU) 1 week ago due to pneumonia and sepsis. She is currently on a ventilator on life support. They have informed her that she is critically ill. Also, her mother's overall condition has been deteriorating in the past year and she is struggling to carry out her day-to-day activities.

When asked about an advance directive form, she is not aware of her mother having this in place. There is no lasting power of attorney. However, her mother's general health has been declining and she has been refusing to see her GP. She has also expressed her wishes in the past that she would not accept a poor quality of life.

Discussion

CPR is a medical intervention performed in the event of cardiac arrest. It is an invasive intervention involving chest compression, ventilation of the lungs, electric shocks and injection of drugs. There are two broad types of cardiac arrest. The first one is when patients develop an abnormal heart rhythm when a direct electric current is applied to stun the heart and reverse the abnormal rhythm. The second type of arrest is due to non-cardiac causes due to several conditions. Although chest compressions are performed in both types of arrest, the outcome of a cardiac arrest depends on the duration of the arrest, prompt initiation and most importantly the underlying cause of the arrest.

Critically ill patients in ICU receiving life support have already experienced multi-organ failure. Performing CPR in this context can be unsuccessful or futile and carries the risk of causing distress and trauma to the dying person.

Clinicians make decisions for the patients based on balancing the benefits versus harm of the proposed treatment. When this decision is made, the patient's legal proxy or someone close to the patient must be consulted to ascertain the patient's wishes or beliefs, and if there are any advance refusals for treatment in place, unless it is not practical or appropriate to do so.

DNR decisions are commonly perceived by the public as 'stopping treatment'. It is important to understand and emphasise the difference between the two. DNR simply means not performing CPR in the event of a cardiorespiratory arrest. It does not constitute decisions relating to other aspects of care.

The key laws relevant to DNR are:

1. The Mental Capacity Act (MCA) 2005 is an act that underpins the decisions made, including hospital settings, for adults who lack mental capacity. There are five pillars of the MCA: presumed capacity, support decision making, respect unwise decisions, work in best interests, and choose the least restrictive option. The key pillar for intensive care patients is 'best interest'.
    Often, but not always, patients who are on ventilators are on sedative medications that can impair their consciousness and therefore their capacity. In such circumstances, the treating physician and the team make decisions based on the patient's best interests. When treatment is on offer, if the patient lacks the capacity to consent or refuse the treatment, decisions are made taking into account the benefits versus risks of the proposed treatment AND discussing with family members who are involved in the care of the patients. It is important to note that by law doctors are not obliged to provide futile treatment and patients/relatives cannot demand treatment that is not on offer. However, good medical practice dictates that such decisions should be made in conjunction with the family based on the patient's wishes.
2. Human Rights Act. The key sections relevant to DNR (or DNAR) include Article 2 (the right to life), Article 3 (the right to be free from inhuman or degrading treatment), Article 8 (the right to respect for privacy and family life), Article 10 (the right to hold opinions and receive information), and Article 14 (the right to be free from discriminatory practice).

3. UK law also dictates that a patient or relative cannot demand a treatment that is deemed inappropriate. The doctor or the hospital team is not obliged to provide a treatment that they deem to be harmful or futile. Patients have a right to refuse treatment. When a valid lasting power of attorney has been appointed by the person for health and life-sustaining treatment, they can consent, or in some circumstances refuse, but cannot demand a treatment deemed inappropriate.

With regard to advance directives or a Recommended Summary Plan for Emergency Care and Treatment (ReSPECT), these advance decisions to refuse treatment are documents in which a person states their wishes in advance as to whether to receive or not receive medical treatments. This may also include specific sections on CPR. An advance directive, when obtained correctly in a patient with capacity, is legally binding unless the patient has subsequently changed their decision.

Key Points

- Be empathetic to the friend as her mother is very sick.
- Be honest in explaining the seriousness of the situation.
- Explain that CPR can be futile and be aware of why it is not prudent to perform CPR in some patients.
- Express your knowledge of DNAR in simple language so that the friend can understand.

References

1. General Medical Council. Treatment and care towards the end of life: good practice in decision making. Available from: https://www.gmc-uk.org/ethical-guidance/ethical-guidance-for-doctors/treatment-and-care-towards-the-end-of-life.

2.	Resuscitation Council UK. Decisions relating to cardiopulmonary resuscitation (3rd edition – 1st revision). Guidance from the British Medical Association, Resuscitation Council UK, and the Royal College of Nursing. Available from: https://www.resus.org.uk/library/publications/publication-decisions-relating-cardiopulmonary.

Section**2**

General ethics

Section editor: Thanthullu Vasu

Introduction to general ethics

In the previous section, ethical dilemmas surrounding a clinical or medical aspect were discussed; in MMI stations, there can also be stations on general ethics. This type of scenario is non-clinical, in which the candidate's approach to honesty, probity and ethical approach is tested.

The GMC 'Ethical guidance' clearly stresses the need for a high level of professional conduct by a doctor; the candidate can use this guidance to support their answer.

Must do

To deal with a general ethical scenario, a candidate should:

- Always keep patient safety as the prime objective — the character of a doctor can affect patient safety in a different context.
- Take an empathetic approach towards the person in the dilemma, but make sure that patient safety is the key.
- Try to understand why the person in question is doing this; have they insight regarding their mistake?
- If they have insight that they are making a mistake, it is easier to proceed. If not, safety concerns arise, and help should be sought.
- Know whom to ask for help, for example, mentor, college tutor, senior colleague, etc. Do not try to solve a problem yourself, as it might not be practicable in many situations in real life; help should be sought when needed.
- Conclude by explaining their position/stance in this dilemma.

Common mistakes

Common mistakes made by candidates include:

- Being anxious and thinking that they need to solve the problem.
- Not understanding the person in their question approach and also their motivation.
- Being judgemental or critical about the person in question; in the other extreme, being too empathetic and saying it is OK to do. Both approaches can lead to problems, so it is important to be empathetic, but at the same time, critical of mistakes. It should be clearly explained that these can compromise patient safety.
- Not concluding the station or thanking the actor and examiners. The candidate should always conclude the session and thank the actor and examiner at the end.

We strongly suggest that the candidate practises a few general ethical dilemma questions with their friends or colleagues and structure their answers with clarity.

GMC 'Ethical guidance'

Always quote the ethical guidance published by the General Medical Council (GMC); this is available on their website: https://www.gmc-uk.org/ethical-guidance.

A candidate might not know all these guidances in full, but even if they quote these GMC documents/guidances they can add value to their answer in the ethical scenario. It is worth reading the summary of the 'Good medical practice' guideline of the GMC.

GMC guidance for medical students

GMC guidance for medical students ('Achieving good medical practice: guidance for medical students') is available online at: https://www.gmc-uk.org/education/standards-guidance-and-curricula/guidance/student-professionalism-and-ftp/achieving-good-medical-practice.

It is vital that candidates read the summary and guidelines and can quote this in the context of the general ethical dilemma. The GMC recognises that medical students are studying to join a trusted profession that will bring them into contact with patients and members of the public. It expects medical students to demonstrate a high standard of behaviour at all times, justifying the trust placed in them by the public as future members of the medical profession.

In Domain 4 (Maintaining trust) of this document, the GMC stresses the need for students to show respect to patients. When there is a mistake, doctors should be open and honest with patients and their families. The document clearly stresses the need to demonstrate honesty; it gives examples of various situations with regard to this. It is essential not to pass off the work of others as their own; this is plagiarism; even self-plagiarising their own previously assessed work is considered dishonest. It stresses the need to be open and truthful about the practical part of the medical course, in that the student should not claim to have done something, such as a practical procedure, if they have not. The GMC clarifies that the student should not say that they have attended teaching sessions if they have not done so; and it stresses not to ask another student to sign for them.

Being a reflective practitioner

The GMC stresses the need to be a reflective practitioner and gives guidance to medical students; this is available at: https://www.gmc-uk.org/education/standards-guidance-and-curricula/guidance/reflective-practice/the-reflective-practitioner---a-guide-for-medical-students.

It is essential that medical students take time to reflect on experiences that have made them think or question their ideas or values; this is important for their individual well-being and development as a professional. Whilst doing so, it is important to anonymise patient data or details that can identify them, to maintain patient confidentiality.

Question 26

Is it OK for doctors to strike?

Thanthullu Vasu

Question

The Doctors' Association has expressed its concern that the Government has not made efforts to increase the number of doctors in the National Health Service; it quotes that there is low morale and increased workload and that doctors' pay has not increased with the inflation rate. It has called for its members to strike for 2 days in the busy Christmas week.

The Government has replied that there is a 'record number of doctors' in the NHS and it has allocated huge sums of money to deal with the COVID pandemic. It has warned doctors not to strike as this will hinder patient care.

In the next station, the examiner will question the candidate's views with regard to this strike action by the Doctors' Association.

Themes for discussion (■ Table 2.1)

Table 2.1.	
Question themes	**What is expected from the candidate?**
1 The candidate greets the examiner and has good body language.	The candidate is presentable and uses good communication skills; always recommended in any station.
2 The examiner asks for the candidate's views on the strike problem.	The candidate gives a good opening statement showing that they understand the situation. They clearly state the problem, the ethical dilemmas, why it is important with regard to the medical profession, and how it can affect patient care.
3 The candidate understands the reasons for the strike and gives the arguments for the 'pro' stance.	The candidate clearly understands the pros of the strike action: • Doctors also have a right to strike like any other profession. • There is poor morale among healthcare professionals; they are not treated well for the job they do. • The COVID pandemic has brought more demands with fewer resources. • Underfunding in the NHS has been a longstanding problem. • Patient safety can be compromised by overworked, poorly paid, under-resourced staff.
4 The candidate gives the 'con' reasons for the doctors' strike in clear, simple language.	The candidate clearly understands the cons of the strike action: • Patient care can be significantly hindered due to the strike action. • Many patients have already waited for a long time, even many months or years, for their elective procedures; a strike will affect this and will lead to much longer waits for these patients.

Table 2.1.

Question themes	What is expected from the candidate?
	• Doctors have an ethical duty to help!
	• Harm to patients is a risk due to strike and this cannot be supported.
	• Emergency care, if affected, can lead to significant patient harm.
5 The candidate has a clear opinion and gives their judgement and opinion regarding the problem.	• The candidate lists both pros and cons in a schematic way; then concludes what they think should be done.
	• There is no fixed answer on whether they should support or oppose strike action, but the clarity in the answer and the supporting statements are marked in the MMI.
	• The candidate is not confused and gives a clear conclusion to the problem.
	• The candidate explains that they are not happy with the strike, but this is a last resort and empathises with the patient stance.
6 The examiner asks what is the Hippocratic Oath.	• The candidate has awareness of the Hippocratic Oath and why it is taken in medical school.
	• 'Do no harm' is the motto and patient care is the priority.
7 How could harm still be avoided if doctors go on strike?	• The candidate understands the workings of the healthcare system and gives simple practical solutions.
	• One of the ways to tackle this problem would be to continue carrying out emergency work and plan accordingly, such that urgent care is not affected.
	• Doctors can avoid elective work alone but look at ways to reinstate these patients and plan them effectively.
	• Adequate notice to the public can help them plan and understand the reasons for the strike.
	• Another solution would be to go on strike in batches, so that care is staggered but not stopped.

Table 2.1.

	Question themes	What is expected from the candidate?
8	What will be the public opinion if doctors go on strike? Will they support them?	• The candidate understands the frustration shared by the public and looks at ways to explain their position. • The candidate realises that strikes are undertaken only as a last resort after taking all interventions to meet their demand. • Public frustration can be avoided if emergency care is not affected, and an explanation of steps taken to avoid patient harm is given. • It is futile to strike without adequate explanation to the public and to take steps to prevent patient harm.
9	Striking during the Christmas period or holiday time can be detrimental.	The candidate has clarity in their answer; they understand that the timing of the strike can affect public and staff rotas in a significant way. Conversely, elective surgeries might be limited during holiday time and the candidate is aware of this.
10	Conclusion of the station.	The candidate concludes the session and thanks the examiner at the end. This gains the candidate extra bonus points.

Discussion

The candidate gives the pros and cons and their judgement in a balanced way with regard to the ethical scenario of a doctors' strike. Having a personal opinion is important, but the statements for and against it should be explained clearly.

The Hippocratic Oath is taken by new doctors, promising they will uphold professional ethical standards. It pledges to prescribe only beneficial treatments, according to the doctor's abilities and judgement; it refrains from doing harm; it also pledges to live an exemplary personal and professional life. Most modern schools have modified the original Greek version to suit recent times; 'First, do no harm' is a vital part of the Oath in most versions.

Key Points

- There are pros and cons to any ethical dilemma; the candidate must be aware of both.
- The candidate should be able to come to a clear conclusion and explain their reasoning behind this decision.
- Patient safety is quoted in this scenario; the candidate must be aware of ways to minimise harm due to the strike action.

References

1. General Medical Council. Good medical practice. Available from: https://www.gmc-uk.org/ethical-guidance/ethical-guidance-for-doctors/good-medical-practice.

Question 27

Problems with social media

Thanthullu Vasu

Question

Karina is a medical student who has an assignment to submit to her supervisor. The supervisor — Mr Roberts — has told Karina that he is off work after a back operation.

Karina is frustrated and tells her year group Facebook chat that Mr Roberts has not marked her assignment and is off sick with a back operation.

Mr Roberts is a private man and was very upset when he has enquiries from other students; he therefore complains to the medical school. Therefore, Karina has a meeting with the head of the medical school.

What are the issues of social media in this instance? The examiner will discuss these issues in the next station.

Themes for discussion (■ Table 2.2)

	Question themes	What is expected from the candidate?
	Table 2.2.	
1	The candidate greets the examiner, has good body language, and speaks coherently and clearly.	The candidate gives a good opening statement when asked about the problem. They empathise, realising the problem, and could mention: 'I am very sorry to hear this story!' 'It is very sad...'
2	The candidate is aware of the problems related to social media.	The candidate discusses the issues of social media clearly and in simple language. They explain it in the context of the given example in the question.
3	Confidentiality and privacy.	The candidate gives an assurance to the examiner that they understand the need to maintain confidentiality and privacy. It is a mistake to have mentioned Mr Roberts in social media without his permission. Social media can create problems and doctors should be conscious and fully aware before posting any message or Tweet.
4	Issues of social media.	The candidate understands that when using social media, the message could be spread widely and there is no control. Once a message is posted, there is difficulty in retracting it. A doctor has a responsibility to maintain confidentiality.
5	What went wrong in this example?	The candidate explains the problems from Karina's and Mr Roberts's aspects and explains the need for confidentiality.

Table 2.2.

Question themes	What is expected from the candidate?
6 Give two practical and positive effects of social media in healthcare.	The candidate gives examples of benefits in healthcare, such as health education and promoting public health. It can be helped to steer policy discussions in healthcare delivery. It can help to establish regional or national professional networks. It can facilitate patients' access to information about their health and services. Giving general health information with anonymity (maintaining patient confidentiality) is important in these scenarios. Examples such as education on the benefits of vaccination, preventing infection, and promoting good physical or mental health can be used.
7 Will you use social media to communicate with patients?	The candidate understands the role of social media, its benefits and, at the same time, the need to maintain patient confidentiality. The candidate can opine either supporting or being against social media, but the key is to explain the limitations and care taken to maintain confidentiality.
8 What will you do if you get a Facebook friend request from a patient?	The candidate understands the need for confidentiality and maintaining professionalism. This could lead to problems, as social media is not restricted or private and the candidate realises the seriousness of this problem.
9 Do you know of any guidelines regarding social media use for doctors?	The candidate should be aware of the General Medical Council's 'Ethical guidance' document entitled 'Doctors' use of social media, 2013'.
10 Concludes the session.	The candidate concludes the session and thanks the examiner.

Discussion

It is important to realise that the standards expected from doctors do not change because they are communicating through social media rather than through a traditional face-to-face approach. In fact, they must be more careful with the new challenges that can compromise patient confidentiality. The same situation applies to colleagues in healthcare services.

The UK General Medical Council notes that many improper disclosures of patient information are unintentional. Using social media has blurred the boundaries between public and private lives, but a doctor must always keep in mind that online information can be easily accessed by others; any posted message cannot be retracted easily.

The GMC also states that a doctor must maintain a professional boundary between themselves and their patient. If a patient contacts them through a private profile, the doctor should clearly mention that they cannot mix social and professional relationships and direct them to their professional profile.

The GMC has strict guidance that the doctor must treat their colleagues fairly and with respect. Online postings have the same laws of copyright and defamation as written or verbal communications, whether they are made in a personal or professional capacity.

Key Points

- Be aware of the risks of social media.
- Maintaining confidentiality is important, whether it is a patient or a colleague.
- The candidate should be aware of the GMC guidance on social media.
- A doctor must maintain a professional boundary between themselves and their patient.

References

1. General Medical Council. Doctors' use of social media. Available from: https://www.gmc-uk.org/ethical-guidance/ethical-guidance-for-doctors/doctors-use-of-social-media.

Question 28

Posting photographs of patients or specimens on a public forum

Gokul Parameswaran

Question

A patient's health information is very sensitive and confidential, with huge resources being invested to keeping these data secure. However, clinical photographs are often published on public platforms (e.g. textbooks, journals, social media, etc.) to improve medical education, allow greater clinician collaboration and empower patients to better understand therapeutic options.

Whilst clinical photographs have been used for these purposes for decades, the growth of the internet has meant that these images can now be viewed by virtually anyone in the world. This raises questions of patient confidentiality and consent that will be discussed in the next station.

Themes for discussion (■ Table 2.3)

Table 2.3.

Question themes	What is expected from the candidate?
1 The candidate greets the examiner and has good body language.	The candidate is presentable and uses good communication skills; always recommended in any station.
2 Should we take clinical photographs?	The candidate gives a good opening statement showing that they understand the situation.
3 The candidate explains the pros of clinical photographs, i.e. why photographs of patients/specimens are needed.	The candidate clearly understands the pros of clinical photographs: • Integral to training students, thereby having a great benefit to the medical community and therefore society. • Can help patients give more informed consent to particular therapies (e.g. in plastic surgery). • Sharing scans or other patient-related data on public forums encourages international clinical collaboration. This may help to improve patient outcomes.
4 The candidate explains the cons of clinical photographs, i.e. why photographs of patients/specimens are not needed.	The candidate clearly understands the cons of clinical photographs: • Patient confidentiality is compromised so clear consent will be needed prior to posting. If possible, it is important to post photographs in such a way that the anonymity of the person in the photo is maintained. • Although photographs are key to medical education, they might not benefit the patient at an individual level. • Despite initial consent, once posted, the photographs cannot be 'taken back', meaning they could be used in ways in which the patient does not feel comfortable.

Table 2.3.

Question themes	What is expected from the candidate?
5 Do you know what is patient consent? Patients have a right to choose how their data are used.	The candidate should understand the principles of patient consent and autonomy. Clinical photographs should only be shared if explicit permission is granted by the patient after being informed of the exact reasons why the information is wished to be shared.
6 How could harm be avoided when taking clinical photographs? The candidate understands and explains what could be done.	There are various possible answers: • Developing other software to create artificial images that exemplify clinical findings, reducing the need for actual clinical photographs in medical education. • Trying to minimise postings on fully public platforms, e.g. only post images on sites that require a login, etc. • Explicitly obtaining patient consent prior to posting the image. Patients should be able to revoke consent at any stage, which would mean their image is removed.
7 The candidate has a clear opinion/conclusion and explains their reasons.	In this station, the candidate should consider either side of the argument and try to cohesively present their thoughts. They should emphasise the importance of consent, as well as ways to minimise posting clinical photographs on public forums.
8 Judgement and clarity.	The candidate has clarity in their answer and can explain the pros and cons, concluding clearly. A clear presentation, smiling throughout and avoiding repetition — these steps can increase the scores in this station. Showing empathy for patients who have to compromise their confidentiality can gain the candidate extra points.
9 Conclusion.	The candidate concludes the session and thanks the examiner at the end. This might gain the candidate extra bonus points.

Discussion

The key to this question is the conflict between breaching patient confidentiality and the potential benefits of sharing clinical photographs on public forums. The candidate should clearly understand that sharing clinical photographs without patient consent is unacceptable and they could face serious consequences from the GMC for doing so.

However, to answer this question comprehensively, it is important that the candidate acknowledges the potential advantages of sharing clinical photographs with the medical profession, other patients, and society. When doing this, you should place emphasis on the importance of conserving patient dignity and maintaining confidentiality.

Key Points

- There are pros and cons to any ethical dilemma; the candidate must be aware of both.
- The candidate should be able to clearly come to a conclusion and explain their reasoning.
- The candidate should understand the importance of patient confidentiality and balance it with the potential benefits of breaking confidentiality and be aware that they should try and minimise breaches in patient confidentiality.

References

1. General Medical Council. Doctors' use of social media. Available from: https://www.gmc-uk.org/ethical-guidance/ethical-guidance-for-doctors/doctors-use-of-social-media.

Question 29

Communicating with patients on social media

Gokul Parameswaran

Question

Social media has become an almost universal means of communication all over the world. Occasionally, patients who have known their doctor for a long time may try to add and communicate with their doctor on social media. Whilst the GMC does not explicitly prohibit all interactions between patients and doctors on social media, the 2013 guidelines on 'Maintaining a Boundary Between You and the Patient' state that 'you must consider the potential risks involved in using social media and the effect that inappropriate use could have on your patient's trust in you'.

In this station, we can consider the complex issues that can be raised by communicating with a patient on social media.

Themes for discussion (■ Table 2.4)

Table 2.4.

	Question themes	What is expected from the candidate?
1	The candidate greets the examiner and has good body language.	The candidate is presentable and uses good communication skills; always recommended in any station.
2	Explanation of the scenario.	The candidate gives a good opening statement showing that they understand the situation.
3	The candidate volunteers pros for communicating with patients on social media.	The candidate clearly understands the pros: • Most patients have access to social media and might feel it to be a more convenient form of communication. • It is the choice of the doctor and patient to decide what forms of communication work best between them. • Doctors volunteer information about themselves in a consultation anyway (e.g. if they are married, where they went on holiday, etc.), so this is no different.
4	The candidate volunteers cons for communicating with patients on social media.	The candidate clearly understands the cons: • May blur the line between professional and personal life. • In a face-to-face consultation, we can control what patients learn; this might be difficult if delivered via online or social media. • You may become personally involved in a patient's life making aspects of your job more difficult (e.g. discussing palliative treatment options with a patient).

Table 2.4.

Question themes	What is expected from the candidate?
5 Shows awareness of current GMC guidelines about the use of social media.	Whilst the GMC does not explicitly prohibit all contact between doctors and patients on social media, the 'Doctors' use of social media' does state that 'if a patient contacts you about their care or other professional matter through your private profile, you should indicate that you cannot mix social and professional relationships and, when appropriate direct them to your professional profile'. This clarifies that we should not discuss a patient's clinical care with them on social media platforms.
6 Understands what is meant by professionalism and how it can be harmed by communicating with patients on social media.	The candidate should understand the concept of professionalism. The ability of doctors to look and behave in a way that is expected of them, even in times of stress, is important to medicine. The candidate should appreciate that this may become impaired by interacting with patients on social media.
7 Understands possible solutions and presents them in a clear, simple language.	A few ways are possible to answer this question with available solutions. However, they should all incorporate the key point that social media interactions between doctors and patients can impair the doctor-patient relationship and so should be done carefully.
8 Judgement and clarity.	The candidate has clarity in their answer and can explain the pros and cons, concluding clearly. A clear presentation, smiling throughout and avoiding repetition — these steps can increase the scores in this station.
9 Conclusion.	The candidate concludes the session and thanks the examiner at the end. This might gain the candidate extra bonus points.

Discussion

The key to answering this question is understanding the concept of professionalism. It is important to understand that the information on many people's social media site is highly personal, including photographs, comments or viewpoints, and therefore blurs the line between what is part of a doctor's professional life and what is part of their personal life. Therefore, to tackle this station, it is important that these issues are appreciated and an answer that addresses them directly is given.

Key Points

- There are pros and cons to any ethical dilemma; the candidate must be aware of both.
- The candidate should be aware of the current GMC ethical guidelines with regard to social media use.
- The candidate should understand the concept of professionalism in medicine and appreciate how communicating with their patients on social media may threaten this.

References

1. General Medical Council. Doctors' use of social media. Available from: https://www.gmc-uk.org/ethical-guidance/ethical-guidance-for-doctors/doctors-use-of-social-media.

Question 30

Should the healthcare system fund weight loss surgery?

Gokul Parameswaran

Question

The rates of obesity have drastically risen in the UK over the last 50 years, causing a huge strain on NHS resources. Whilst some people argue that the NHS should continue to fund weight loss surgeries, others argue against it. The examiner will explore this ethical dilemma and your views on this problem in the next station.

Themes for discussion (■ Table 2.5)

Table 2.5.	
Question themes	**What is expected from the candidate?**
1 The candidate greets the examiner and has good body language.	The candidate is presentable and uses good communication skills; always recommended in any station.

Table 2.5.

	Question themes	What is expected from the candidate?
2	Should the NHS fund weight loss surgeries?	The candidate gives a good opening statement showing that they understand the situation.
3	The candidate volunteers cons for weight loss surgery, i.e. why we should not fund surgery?	The candidate clearly understands the cons of offering surgery: • Expensive treatment option. • Many patients regain weight after surgery. • Obesity could be considered as 'self-inflicted' as an individual's lifestyle directly causes them to gain weight. • Cheaper treatment options are available including lifestyle regimes, certain drugs, etc.
4	The candidate volunteers pros for surgery, i.e. why we should fund surgery?	The candidate clearly understands the pros of offering surgery: • Obesity is closely linked to socioeconomic and genetic factors meaning it may not be a 'choice' for everyone. • Treating obesity reduces the chances of developing other health problems (e.g. cardiovascular disease, type 2 diabetes, etc.), which could cost the NHS more than the surgery in the long term. • Other 'self-inflicted' problems are treated on the NHS including health problems arising from excessive drinking or smoking, as well as injuries from extreme sports; obesity is more genetic in aetiology and these patients should be offered treatment. • Rationing one type of patient is against the principle of Aneurin Bevan's National Health Service, which gives free treatment for all.

Table 2.5.

	Question themes	What is expected from the candidate?
5	Do you know what justice is? Treating all patients equally.	The candidate understands the ethical principle of justice. As per this principle, it is important to treat all patients equally and fairly. This means that we should not discriminate against patients who are obese, but should also ensure that resources are not allotted disproportionately to patients who are obese alone.
6	The candidate has a clear opinion/conclusion and explains their reasons.	The candidate can choose a few paths, but judgement should consider the principle of justice. The key principle is the best allocation of resources to benefit the most people. They should acknowledge the flaws in the argument that, as obesity is 'self-inflicted', patients should not have weight loss surgery.
		If the candidate chooses to say weight loss surgery should not be allowed, they should focus on how it is ineffective in helping patients to lose weight and how those resources may be better spent on developing other weight loss strategies.
7	Judgement and clarity.	The candidate has clarity in their answer and can explain the pros and cons, concluding clearly. A clear presentation, smiling throughout and avoiding repetition — these steps can increase the scores in this station.
8	Conclusion.	The candidate concludes the session and thanks the examiner at the end. This gains the candidate extra bonus points.

Discussion

The key to this question is understanding the principle of justice. You should clearly acknowledge that, whilst obesity is influenced by an individual's lifestyle choices, their ability to make these choices is different for different people. Therefore, it is critical to state that it is not in line with the NHS principle of equality to treat patients who are obese differently. This means that the focus of your answer to this question should be on whether you believe weight loss surgery is the best allocation of resources to reduce the overall prevalence of obesity in the UK.

Rates of obesity have drastically risen in the UK over the last 50 years, causing a huge strain on NHS resources. Individuals who are obese are predisposed to experience many physical and mental health problems including, but not limited to, heart disease, diabetes, depression, and insomnia. Currently, aside from lifestyle modifications, one of the primary strategies for treating obesity is weight loss surgery. Despite this option being much more expensive than lifestyle modifications, research has shown that it is often not effective in the long term as patients regain weight over time. Others also argue as, ultimately, it is an individual's choice to lead a particular lifestyle; obesity is self-inflicted and so is not the NHS's responsibility to treat.

However, others believe that this argument is flawed, as obesity has huge socioeconomic and genetic components, calling into question how much of a 'choice' people make. In addition to this, proponents of surgery argue that even if weight-reducing surgery is sometimes ineffective and expensive, it can improve the health of an individual by a sufficient margin that it reduces the overall cost of their care (i.e. patients are less likely to develop other diseases related to obesity, reducing the overall burden on the NHS). The conflicts between personal choice, the responsibilities of the NHS, and the relative value of therapeutic options can be explored in this station.

Key Points

- There are pros and cons to any ethical dilemma; the candidate must be aware of both.
- The candidate should be able to clearly come to a conclusion and explain their reasoning.
- Understand the principle of justice and explain why we should not discriminate against patients with perceived 'self-inflicted' health problems.
- Argue whether you believe weight loss surgery is the most effective allocation of resources to reduce the overall prevalence of obesity.

References

1.   General Medical Council. Good medical practice. Available from: https://www.gmc-uk.org/ethical-guidance/ethical-guidance-for-doctors/good-medical-practice.

Question 31

Should the NHS fund smoking cessation treatments?

Thiagarajan Sridhar

Question

In the next station, the examiner will discuss whether the NHS should fund smoking cessation treatments. Ethical principles underlying this dilemma will be explored.

Themes for discussion (■ Table 2.6)

Table 2.6.	
Question themes	**What is expected from the candidate?**
1 The candidate greets the examiner and has good body language.	The candidate is presentable and uses good communication skills; always recommended in any station.

Table 2.6.

	Question themes	What is expected from the candidate?
2	The candidate explains the pros of funding smoking cessation.	The candidate lists points to support funding smoking cessation: • Support for the patient. • Decreases the chance of developing smoking-related diseases. • Improves general health. • Overall, reduces the burden on the NHS in the long run.
3	The candidate also explains the cons of funding smoking cessation.	The NHS should not fund smoking cessation because: • Expensive and a burden on the taxpayer. • Patients have a choice and they can make their own decisions. • Patients spend money on cigarettes so they should be able to fund smoking cessation medications themselves. • No emphasis on other problems such as alcohol cessation. • Legislation can ban cigarettes. • It removes funding from other needed NHS areas, as money will be diverted rather than created.
4	The candidate has a clear opinion about the problem.	The candidate can select any one of the options, either supporting or against funding. The candidate should be able to clearly explain the reasons and rationale for their opinion. They should exhibit a good understanding of this complex issue and how NHS funding works.
5	What are the harms of smoking?	The candidate should be able to discuss general issues with smoking and mention smoking-related diseases, COPD, cancer, cardiovascular issues, etc.

Table 2.6.

Question themes	What is expected from the candidate?
6 What are the public health impacts due to smoking?	The candidate should be able to describe the burden on the nation's health. Increased illness, reduced productivity, and more financial burden on state spending on smoking cessation programmes and also screening programmes. The candidate can also discuss the harmful effects of passive smoking.
7 Do you think tobacco companies should be funding smoking cessation?	Supporting comments — profit making, and shareholder interests can give some money back to society, so they should be legislated to fund.
	Opposing comments — business interests are separate. People would have invested in the company for income, pensions, etc. They are already being taxed, so any additional funding should be voluntary rather than compulsory.
8 Conclusion.	The candidate has clarity in their answer and can explain the pros and cons, concluding clearly. A clear presentation, smiling throughout and avoiding repetition — these steps can increase the scores in this station. The candidate thanks the examiner at the end.

Discussion

This is an important issue in understanding the impact on public health and how much the state can support personal habits. The candidate should be able to discuss the pros and cons and should be able to give a balanced view. They should be aware of wider health economics and the preventive aspects of healthcare.

The candidates should appreciate the wider impact of medical professionals in dealing with different aspects of healthcare, including prevention, health education and treatment.

This station is also a great example of how various organisations can work together to improve the health of patients and how the NHS plays a central role in coordinating this.

Key Points

- There are pros and cons to any argument; the candidate has to be aware of both.
- The candidate should be able to clearly come to a conclusion and explain their reasoning.
- They should understand the role of public health and preventive aspects of healthcare.
- They should be confident in dealing with difficult debatable topics in a balanced way.

References

1. NHS UK. NHS stop smoking services help you quit. Available from: https://www.nhs.uk/live-well/quit-smoking/nhs-stop-smoking-services-help-you-quit.
2. NHS UK. Better Health, Let's do this - Quit smoking. Available from: https://www.nhs.uk/better-health/quit-smoking.

Question32

Should the NHS/social care fund holidays for patients with depression?

Balamurugan Nambi

Question

In patients with depression, medications have limited benefits and they can have significant side effects. Some research has shown that prescribing holidays might be better than medication for these patients. Would you support funding holidays through the NHS or social care? The examiner will explore this ethical dilemma and your views on this problem in the next station.

Themes for discussion (■ Table 2.7)

Table 2.7.	
Question themes	**What is expected from the candidate?**
1 The candidate greets the examiner and has good body language.	The candidate is presentable and uses good communication skills; always recommended in any station.

Table 2.7.

	Question themes	What is expected from the candidate?
2	Should the NHS or social care fund holidays for patients with depression?	The candidate gives a good opening statement showing that they understand the situation.
3	The candidate explains the benefits of funding holidays for patients with depression.	The candidate clearly understands the benefits of prescribing holidays: • Medications have limited benefits. • Medications are costly as they need to be taken for a long time, maybe the rest of the patient's life. • Medications can lead to side effects, which can again cost the taxpayer money via the NHS. • Holidays improve mood significantly. • Holidays to warmer destinations will improve the serotoninergic hormones that improve well-being. • Funding trips to some European destinations can be cheaper than medication costs.
4	The candidate gives reasons why holidays are not the right choice.	The candidate clearly understands the cons of offering holidays on prescription: • Medical management money should not be wasted on holidays. • A holiday for 4-5 days can bring happiness, but that is not a cure for mental illness. • Medical ethics pillar of 'justice' — is this money well spent? We need to consider those patients with other illnesses who need NHS funding, rather than spending it on holidays. • Rationing one type of patient is against the principles of Aneurin Bevan's National Health Service, which gives free treatment for all.

Table 2.7.

	Question themes	What is expected from the candidate?
5	Do you know what justice is? Treating all patients equally.	The candidate understands the ethical principle of justice. As per this principle, it is important to treat all patients equally and fairly. This means that we should not discriminate against patients who are mentally ill but should also ensure that resources are not allotted disproportionately to these patients alone.
6	The candidate has a clear opinion/conclusion and explains the reasons.	The candidate can choose two opposite paths, but their judgement should consider the principle of justice. The key principle is the best allocation of resources to benefit the most people. They should acknowledge that patients with depression can benefit from holidays, but having a clear conclusion is vital.
7	Judgement and clarity.	The candidate has clarity in their answer and can explain the pros and cons, concluding clearly. A clear presentation, smiling throughout and avoiding repetition — these steps can increase the scores in this station.
8	Conclusion.	The candidate concludes the session and thanks the examiner at the end. This gains the candidate extra bonus points.

Discussion

The key to this question is understanding the principle of justice. NHS funding is for all illnesses and the ethical dilemma is to argue if it is okay to spend on patients with depression alone. Funding is for medical pathways, and we could argue whether it is right to be spent on holidays.

Half of all mental health problems have been established by the age of 14, rising to 75% by age 24. Nearly two million adults were in contact with specialist mental health and learning disability services at some point in 2014/2015, although we know little about the quality of their care and there remains an extensive unmet need for mental healthcare. Poor mental health carries an economic and social cost of £105 billion a year in England. Analysis commissioned by NHS England found that the national cost of dedicated mental health support and services across government departments in England totals £34 billion each year. The NHS in England planned to spend £12.2 billion on mental health in 2018/2019. That is roughly £1 in every £10 spent by the Department of Health and Social Care.

Mental illness management requires the development of new ways to improve the quality and productivity of services. Experts observed positive results among a group of 3380 working men and women aged 45-52, when they provided 10 extra days of paid leave; this decreased the likelihood of depression by 29% for American women. However, research is not yet fully supportive of this. Another German study of 40 middle managers (July 2018) showed that even a short vacation could reduce overall stress levels.

Holidays can make patients feel healthier and happier, and they can reduce stress levels, make them resilient and connect them with others in a positive way. It also provides an opportunity to relax, recover from the demands of work, and spend time with family and friends.

The argument for paid vacation leave can be argued based on human rights: according to the United Nations' Universal Declaration of Human Rights: 'Everyone has the right to rest and leisure, including reasonable limitation of working hours and periodic holidays with pay'.

Key Points

- There are pros and cons to any ethical dilemma; the candidate must be aware of both.
- The candidate should be able to clearly come to a conclusion and explain their reasoning.
- It is important to understand the principle of justice and explain why we should not discriminate against patients with mental illness, but at the same time look at the benefits of holidays.

References

1. Kim D. Does paid vacation leave protect against depression among working Americans? A national longitudinal fixed effects analysis. *Scand J Work Environ Health* 2019; 45(1): 22-32.

2. Blank C, Gatterer K, Leichtfried V, *et al.* Short vacation improves stress-level and well-being in German-speaking middle-managers – a randomized controlled trial. *Int J Environ Res Public Health* 2018; 15(1): 130.

3. World Travel & Tourism Council. 9 reasons travel is good for your mental health. Available from: https://travelhub.wttc.org/blog/9-reasons-travel-is-good-for-your-mental-health.

4. NHS UK. The five year forward view for mental health. Available from: https://www.england.nhs.uk/wp-content/uploads/2016/02/Mental-Health-Taskforce-FYFV-final.pdf.

Question 33

A parent requesting circumcision for a child

Thiagarajan Sridhar

Question

The National Health Service does not fund elective circumcision without a medical indication. A father requests circumcision for his child, who is your patient, for religious reasons. The next station will focus on this ethical dilemma; the examiner will ask questions on this scenario.

Themes for discussion (■ Table 2.8)

Table 2.8.	
Question themes	**What is expected from the candidate?**
1 The candidate greets the examiner and has good body language.	The candidate is presentable and uses good communication skills; always recommended in any station.

Table 2.8.

Question themes	What is expected from the candidate?
2 The candidate understands the ethical dilemma.	The candidate gives a good opening statement showing that they understand the situation.
3 The candidate understands the rationale of the request from the parent.	The candidate understands and appreciates the reasons for this request: • The parent is within his rights to discuss this with a medical professional. • The parent has religious reasons to believe that this will be in their child's best interests. • The candidate is empathetic to the needs of the parent rather than dismissing the parent's concerns.
4 The candidate explains the legal, ethical and practical aspects of such a request.	The candidate explains the legal and ethical position of the National Health Service about circumcision: • It is not funded by the NHS. • It is only carried out for medical reasons such as phimosis, infection, etc. • There are ethical dilemmas in the parent's request versus the child's understanding. • It must be privately funded if needed, and legally allowed if needed. • It needs aseptic precautions for the surgery.
5 The candidate is sensitive to the issue and the parent's needs.	The candidate should be able to discuss this sensitive matter without bias. The candidate should not be patronising to the parent. The candidate should, at the same time, be clear about what the NHS can and cannot offer.

Table 2.8.

	Question themes	What is expected from the candidate?
6	What is your opinion about non-therapeutic male circumcision?	The candidate can have a personal view but should know both the pros and cons of the position. For: • Respects religious sentiments. • Therapeutic benefits shown in some studies. • Prevents parents from going to unscrupulous non-medical people who might offer this procedure that can be dangerous to the child's health. • Risks of infection. Against: • Not possible to offer all treatment options on the NHS. • Benefits are unclear to be offered routinely for non-medical reasons. • Consent for an invasive procedure (this is not illegal) that a child might regret after reaching adulthood.
7	Judgement and clarity.	The candidate has clarity in their answer and can explain the pros and cons, concluding clearly. A clear presentation, smiling throughout and avoiding repetition — these steps can increase the scores in this station. The candidate shows empathy for the needs of the patient/parent.
8	Conclusion.	The candidate concludes the session and thanks the examiner at the end. This gains the candidate extra bonus points.

Discussion

This question throws up many legal and ethical challenges. The candidate should be sensitive to everyone's needs, but also understand and appreciate the limitations of NHS resources to offer unproven procedures.

Doctors should be clear when there is no consensus about a particular treatment if they are not illegal. They should be able to confidently discuss the reasons with the parents. They should always have the child's best interests in their mind.

GMC's guidance

If patients (or those with parental responsibility for them) ask for a procedure, such as circumcision of male children, for mainly religious or cultural reasons, you should discuss with them the benefits, risks and side effects of the procedure. You should only provide procedures, that patients have requested, when you have the requisite knowledge, skills and experience to do so safely and where you have assessed this to be of overall benefit to the patient. If the patient is a child, you should usually provide a procedure or treatment that you assess to be in their best interests. In all circumstances, you will also need the patient's or parental consent (see the GMC's 'Personal beliefs and medical practice').

Key Points

- There are pros and cons to any ethical dilemma; the candidate has to be aware of both.
- The candidate should be able to clearly explain their reasoning.
- The candidate should quote the General Medical Council's 'Good medical practice' document or the American Medical Council's or a similar body's code of ethics to show that they are aware of the ethics behind the scenario.
- They should be sensitive to the patient's requests and beliefs.

References

1. British Medical Association. Non-therapeutic male circumcision (NTMC) of children – practical guidance for doctors. Available from: https://www.bma.org.uk/media/1847/bma-non-therapeutic-male-circumcision-of-children-guidance-2019.pdf.

2. General Medical Council. 0-18 years: guidance for all doctors. Available from: https://www.gmc-uk.org/ethical-guidance/ethical-guidance-for-doctors/0-18-years.

3. British Association of Paediatric Surgeons. Circumcision (child) parent leaflet. Available from: http://www.baps.org.uk/resources/documents/circumcision.

4. General Medical Council. Personal beliefs and medical practice. Available from: https://www.gmc-uk.org/ethical-guidance/ethical-guidance-for-doctors/personal-beliefs-and-medical-practice.

Question 34

Patient confidentiality and misattributed paternity

Vijaianitha Nallendran

Question

You are a GP and have referred a pregnant patient and her partner to the genetic counselling clinic. The couple undergoes genetic testing as their fetus has been found to have an autosomal recessive condition. The pregnant lady has tested positive to be the carrier of the recessive gene. However, her partner has tested negative for the condition. The conclusion of the result is that the partner is not the biological father of the fetus.

The next station will discuss the ethical dilemmas surrounding confidentiality issues and your opinion on this situation.

Themes for discussion (▓ Table 2.9)

Table 2.9.

Question themes	What is expected from the candidate?
1 The candidate greets the examiner and has good body language.	The candidate is presentable and uses good communication skills; always recommended in any station.
2 Is it right for doctors to disclose the information to the partner?	The candidate gives a good opening statement showing that they understand the situation.
3 The candidate volunteers the cons of disclosing the information.	The candidate clearly understands the cons of disclosing information: • It breaches the duty of confidentiality to the mother and her right to privacy. • Trust is an essential part of the doctor-patient relationship and confidentiality is central to this. • Women may avoid attending the clinic and receiving appropriate care. • The patient and the overall public trust in doctors will be reduced if confidentiality is breached. • It breaches the duty of non-maleficence to at least one parent and may potentially disrupt family harmony. • Misattributed paternity is an incidental finding, and it could be argued that there is therefore no duty to inform. • Women are more socially disadvantaged and can experience more economic and social implications if the truth is informed.

Table 2.9.

	Question themes	What is expected from the candidate?
4	The candidate also explains the pros of disclosing the information.	The candidate clearly understands the pros of disclosing the information: • The partner has a right to know about his misattributed paternity and exercise his autonomy. • This will give him the knowledge that any of his future children are not at risk of inheriting the genetic condition. • This will prevent him from making decisions such as avoiding having any future children. • This will avoid performing unnecessary interventions such as amniocentesis in future pregnancies. • There is a claim that it is paternalistic of doctors to not disclose information based on their value judgement on what is best for the family. • This information is important for the child.
5	What actions does the doctor need to take in this situation?	• The Committee on Assessing Genetic Risks of the Institute of Medicine (1994) recommends disclosing it to the woman. • The woman can be persuaded to disclose the information to the partner. • Misattributed paternity continues to be a highly divisive issue in clinical ethics. • Several different approaches may be ethically defensible. • A decision about disclosure should be made in the context of a particular child and in the context of the couple and their relationship — a context-specific moral judgement should be made. • A care-based perspective rather than a rights-based perspective needs to be taken. • Ethics of care is grounded in voice and relationships giving importance to listening carefully to patients' wishes and listening with respect. • An MDT approach is valuable in making such decisions.

Table 2.9.

	Question themes	What is expected from the candidate?
6	Do you know the situations when confidentiality can be overridden?	The candidate understands the GMC recommendations.
		Doctors may disclose personal information without breaching duties of confidentiality when the following circumstances apply:
		• The disclosure is of overall benefit to a patient who lacks the capacity to consent.
		• Disclosure is required by law.
		• Disclosure has been approved under a statutory process that sets aside the common law duty of confidentiality.
		• Disclosure can be justified in the public/individual interest.
7	What factors need to be taken into consideration if disclosing personal information without consent?	• Potential harm or distress to the patient from disclosure.
		• Potential harm to trust in doctors generally.
		• Potential harm to others if the information is not disclosed.
		• Potential benefits to individuals/society from the release of information.
		• Nature of the information that is being disclosed and views expressed by the patient.
		• Whether harm can be avoided, or benefits gained without breaching patient privacy or with minimal intrusion.
8	Whom can you ask for advice in the trust?	• Caldicott guardian.
		• Trust legal advisers.
		• Senior clinicians in the case of junior doctors.

Table 2.9.

	Question themes	What is expected from the candidate?
9	Judgement and clarity.	The candidate has clarity in their answer and can explain the pros and cons, concluding clearly. A clear presentation, smiling throughout and avoiding repetition — these steps can increase the scores in this station.
10	Conclusion.	The candidate concludes the session and thanks the examiner at the end. This might gain the candidate extra bonus points.

Discussion

Please make sure that you can explain the pros and cons and are confident in choosing one side and explaining the reasons for this stance. Explaining ethical dilemmas is key in this station.

Misattributed paternity continues to be a highly divisive issue in clinical ethics.

Whilst general guidelines ought to be considered, context-specific moral judgements should not be avoided. A decision about disclosure should be made in the context of a particular child and in the context of the couple and their relationship — a context-specific moral judgement should be made.

A care-based perspective rather than a rights-based perspective needs to be taken. More than imposed standards of justice, the ethics of care are grounded in voice and relationships, recognising the importance of a patient being listened to carefully and heard with respect. The ethics of care has the potential to both inform and advise the timing and content of genetic disclosure. A blind standard of physician disclosure should not be seen as best practice. Instead, relationally informed and patient-empowered disclosure should be seen as the best approach.

Key Points

- There are pros and cons to any ethical dilemma; the candidate has to be aware of both.
- The candidate should be able to clearly come to a conclusion and explain their reasoning.
- A care-based perspective rather than a rights-based perspective might be used in this scenario.
- The candidate should be aware of the situations when confidentiality can be broken and can quote the GMC guidance regarding this.

References

1. General Medical Council. Disclosures for the protection of patient and others. Available from: https://www.gmc-uk.org/ethical-guidance/ethical-guidance-for-doctors/confidentiality/disclosures-for-the-protection-of-patients-and-others.

2. Howe E. Ethical issues when non-paternity is an incidental finding. *Int J Pregn Chi Birth* 2021; 7(1): 1-4.

3. The American College of Obstetricians and Gynecologists. Ethical issues in genetic testing. Committee opinion. Ethical issues in genetic testing. ACOG Committee Opinion No. 410. American College of Obstetricians and Gynecologists. *Obstet Gynecol* 2008; 111: 1495-502.

Question 35

Probity issues: a student asking for an illness note

James Francis

Question

One of your patients is a university student; he missed an important class at university and asks you to give him an illness note to show his tutor. You find no reasons for his illness or his absence. What would you do now? How would you respond to your patient?

Themes for discussion (■ Table 2.10)

Table 2.10.	
Question themes	**What is expected from the candidate?**
1 The candidate greets the examiner and has good body language.	The candidate is presentable and uses good communication skills; always recommended in any station.

Table 2.10.

	Question themes	What is expected from the candidate?
		This is a complex scenario; the candidate understands this complexity but stays calm and has a good approach.
2	The examiner asks the candidate to describe the scenario.	The candidate introduces the situation and lists the problems clearly.
		They clearly state that it is wrong to issue an illness/sick note in the absence of any evidence of illness. The candidate explains that they are not happy to issue a sick note in this situation.
3	The candidate clarifies that it is clearly WRONG to issue a sickness note without a reason.	The candidate understands the issues and clearly acknowledges that issuing a sickness note in the absence of any illness is a probity issue and brings the doctor's professional integrity into question.
		The candidate explains that maintaining integrity is vital for the doctor's profession and discusses the need for this.
4	The examiner asks what the reasoning is behind the doctor's action (in this case, non-issuance of illness note).	The candidate understands the problems of this immoral action: • The doctor's probity is in question. • It is ethically wrong to provide a false certificate. • It is a lie! • You are supporting a fraudulent action of the student. • You are encouraging the behaviour. • It is against the Hippocratic Oath taken by the doctor.

Table 2.10.

	Question themes	What is expected from the candidate?
5	The candidate voluntarily quotes the GMC guidance on maintaining integrity.	The candidate explains and quotes the GMC's guidance, 'Good medical practice'; Domain 4 deals with maintaining integrity.
		If the candidate does not volunteer an answer, the examiner can ask if the candidate is aware of any guidance.
6	The examiner asks what the candidate will do in this situation.	The candidate clearly says that it is WRONG to issue a false certificate or note. They will explain the reason to the student and stress the need to be honest and discuss this with their mentor/teacher.
7	The candidate is empathetic and supportive but, at the same time, clearly and firmly explains that this is wrong.	The candidate can take an empathetic approach to the patient and acknowledge the difficulty that the patient finds himself/herself in.
		The candidate may want to explore the exact reason why the patient missed the class, despite knowing that it was important to attend.
		It will be useful to know if this situation arose due to any circumstances relating to an underlying illness or to any other external cause or factors.
8	The examiner asks what other advice the candidate will give to the patient.	The candidate continues the discussion in an empathetic way.
		It may be useful to explore the outcome for the patient due to their non-attendance and whether they have missed any such classes or deadlines in the past.
		The patient must be encouraged to meet their tutor/mentor and explain the reasons for missing the class in an honest manner and work with the tutor to avoid any such occurrences in the future.

Table 2.10.

	Question themes	What is expected from the candidate?
9	Conclusion.	The candidate summarises the situation clearly; the candidate understands the need for integrity and probity. The candidate concludes the session by saying thank you to the examiner.

Discussion

This is a complex scenario, but the candidate has to clearly explain that it is wrong to give a false note or certificate. The probity of the doctor is in question and the candidate should be aware that the GMC takes this seriously. Society has high expectations for the professionalism of doctors, and they should do their best to keep up with these expectations.

Key Points

- Always introduce yourself to the examiner, thank them and appropriately close the session.
- You should be aware of the importance of maintaining integrity and honesty as a doctor.
- You should clearly mention that it is wrong to issue a sick note in the absence of any evidence of illness.
- Maintain respect and be supportive and empathetic to your patient, but at the same time, express the fact that honesty is the most important principle.

References

1. British Medical Association. Issuing fit notes. Available from: https://www.bma.org.uk/advice-and-support/gp-practices/gp-service-provision/issuing-fit-notes.

2. Department for Work & Pensions. Getting the most out of the fit note: guidance for healthcare professionals. Available from: https://www.gov.uk/government/publications/fit-note-guidance-for-healthcare-professionals/getting-the-most-out-of-the-fit-note-guidance-for-healthcare-professionals.

3. General Medical Council. Good medical practice. Domain 4: Maintaining trust. Available from: https://www.gmc-uk.org/ethical-guidance/ethical-guidance-for-doctors/good-medical-practice/Domain-4---maintaining-trust#paragraph-65.

4. General Medical Council. Achieving good medical practice: guidance for medical students. Available from: https://www.gmc-uk.org/education/standards-guidance-and-curricula/guidance/student-professionalism-and-ftp/achieving-good-medical-practice.

5. American Medical Association. Code of Medical Ethics overview. Available from: https://www.ama-assn.org/delivering-care/ethics/code-medical-ethics-overview.

6. Canadian Medical Association. CMA Code of Ethics and Professionalism. Available from: https://policybase.cma.ca/viewer?file=%2Fmedia%2FPolicyPDF%2FPD19-03S.pdf#page=1.

7. Australian Medical Association. Code of Ethics 2004. Revised 2016. Available from: https://www.ama.com.au/articles/code-ethics-2004-editorially-revised-2006-revised-2016.

Question 36

A friend who is cheating as they have learning difficulties

Gokul Parameswaran

Question

Your friend receives extra time for medical school exams for their learning difficulties. One day, after a party, they disclose to you that they have no learning difficulties and are cheating the system. How will you approach this scenario?

Themes for discussion (■ Table 2.11)

Table 2.11.	
Question themes	**What is expected from the candidate?**
1 The candidate greets the examiner and has good body language.	The candidate is presentable and uses good communication skills; always recommended in any station.

Table 2.11.

Question themes	What is expected from the candidate?
2 Explanation of the scenario.	The candidate gives a good opening statement showing that they understand the situation.
3 The candidate explains why they should NOT escalate or notify the medical school.	The candidate is aware of reasons not to notify the medical school: • You have a commitment to your friend so you should value your relationship with them and help them. • Your friend has placed trust in you and told you their secret. • If you escalate or notify the mentor or medical school, your friendship is in question. • The proof is not adequate, as the friend might retract the statement later.
4 The candidate explains why they SHOULD escalate or notify their mentor or responsible person in the medical school.	The candidate is aware of the reasons to notify the medical school: • Unfair on other medical students as your friend is cheating the system to gain advantages that no one else has. • It's unclear if they would pass if they did exams fairly. This may cause them to be an incompetent doctor in the future. • May encourage further dishonesty in their career; could possibly undermine the trust in the medical profession. • By doing nothing in this scenario, you would facilitate their dishonest actions. • The extra time was allotted to students with learning difficulties; this unfair action is an injustice to such students.

Table 2.11.

Question themes	What is expected from the candidate?
5 The candidate has a clear opinion on this issue and explains the reasons.	For this scenario, although the candidate should present both sides of the scenario, they need to be aware it is not acceptable to ignore their friend's statement as it is against the student code of conduct and is unfair to the rest of the student body.
6 Clearly lay out the next steps of action to be taken.	The candidate should clearly explain to their friend why what they are doing is not acceptable and should tell them that they will notify the medical school about this.

They can be supportive of their friend but being honest is essential. However, it is important for the candidate to demonstrate empathy. |
| 7 Judgement and clarity. | The candidate has clarity in their answer and can explain the pros and cons, concluding clearly. A clear presentation, smiling throughout and avoiding repetition — these steps can increase the scores in this station. |
| 8 Conclusion. | The candidate concludes the session and thanks the examiner at the end. This gains the candidate extra bonus points. |

Discussion

Learning difficulties refer to a broad spectrum of conditions including dyslexia, attention deficit hyperactive disorders (ADHDs), and dyspraxia. To give those individuals diagnosed with these conditions a fair opportunity to complete their medical school exams, these students are given extra time. However, as these conditions are diagnosed by self-reported symptoms and cognitive tests, it is possible to obtain a diagnosis without truly experiencing the condition. In this scenario, the central conflict arises from the trust the friend had placed in the candidate by telling them this secret and in the wider responsibility the candidate has to the student body as well as the medical school to notify them of the friend's statement.

The dilemma in this question is to balance the trust the friend had placed in the candidate by telling them about their secret with the wider responsibility to the medical school and society. Whilst the candidate should not be aggressive towards their friend, they should also recognise the consequences of the friend's action on the system; by cheating in their exam, the friend is worsening the quality of medical education, has an unfair advantage over other students and has compromised their integrity, which is one of the most important traits of a doctor. Therefore, if the candidate did not notify the medical school of this statement, they would be helping facilitate their friend's cheating. This means that even if your friend protests, the candidate should explain why what they are doing is unacceptable and that they will notify the medical school.

Key Points

- The candidate should be able to conclude that they will notify the medical school.
- They should understand that the friend's cheating is disadvantaging the rest of the year, calling into question their integrity and this could worsen the overall quality of doctors.
- Express empathy towards the friend but the candidate should be firm in telling them that they will notify the medical school about the cheating.

References

1. General Medical Council. Good medical practice. Available from: https://www.gmc-uk.org/ethical-guidance/ethical-guidance-for-doctors/good-medical-practice.

Question37

A patient failing to disclose information to their landlord

Kodaganallur Parthasarathi Krishnan

Question

Your landlord rents the next-door flat to a new tenant. He tells you that the new tenant has passed all the checks and he is happy about it. You find out that this tenant is one of your patients who has drug dependency issues along with significant financial difficulties. What will you do now? Will you disclose this to the landlord?

Themes for discussion (■ Table 2.12)

Table 2.12.	
Question themes	**What is expected from the candidate?**
1 The candidate greets the examiner, has good body language and speaks coherently.	The candidate is presentable and uses good communication skills; always recommended in any station.

Table 2.12.

Question themes	What is expected from the candidate?
	This is a complex scenario; the candidate understands this complexity but stays calm and has a good approach to the answer.
2 The examiner asks the candidate to describe the scenario.	The candidate is expected to verbalise the contents of this station showing a good understanding and giving importance to these issues: • The new tenant is a patient and this raises confidentiality issues. • This person has a drug dependency and financial issues. • A doctor is expected to be truthful and honest. • Maintaining your loyalty to your landlord and the effect of this on society.
3 The examiner asks how the candidate is going to proceed with this situation.	The candidate explains that maintaining integrity is vital for a doctor's profession. They begin by answering they will approach the patient (new tenant) and discuss these issues with them and ask if they have disclosed these to the landlord.
4 The new tenant is not showing any sign of acceptance of the claims and shows his anger to the candidate.	The candidate is expected to say that they will remain calm and composed. It is important that their character is displayed by the attitude they show and therefore maintain a quiet demeanour. They try to explain the morality of the profession and the need for doctors to exhibit a high level of professionalism that is expected by the public. Being open and honest is a key feature to ensure that the doctor is a safe and reliable person.
5 The tenant shows his displeasure and asks you to keep quiet as he is your patient.	The candidate explains and quotes the GMC guidance, 'Good medical practice'; Domain 4 deals with maintaining integrity.

Table 2.12.

Question themes	What is expected from the candidate?
6 The candidate is empathetic and supportive but, at the same time, explains clearly and firmly that this is wrong.	The candidate can take an empathetic approach but knows the balance and explains the need to discuss this with the patient: • The candidate says that this is WRONG. • They support the patient in rectifying/correcting the mistake. • They encourage the patient to disclose their problems. • They advise them not to repeat such mistakes in future. • They subsequently check that the tenant has had a discussion with the landlord.
7 The examiner asks what the candidate will do if the patient does not listen or accept the comments.	The candidate clarifies that they will be firm in telling the tenant that this is wrong: • The candidate explains that if the patient does not listen, they will inform the landlord. • The GMC expects doctors to be open and honest and to disclose the facts. • Confidentiality breaches are accountable by the GMC, but it is wise to encourage the patient to disclose it themselves, explaining in an empathetic manner the need for and importance of honesty.
8 Conclusion.	The candidate summarises the situation clearly; the candidate understands the need for integrity and probity. The candidate concludes the session by saying thank you to the examiner.

Discussion

This is a very important question in the domain of probity/integrity of doctors; one such question will definitely come up in the MMI as this is taken seriously by medical schools and the GMC.

The UK General Medical Council (GMC) regulates the profession, and they have published a very important guidance, 'Good medical practice'; this guidance deals with the professionalism of doctors. It has four domains: Domain 1 on knowledge, skills and performance; Domain 2 on safety and quality; Domain 3 on communication partnership and teamwork; and Domain 4 on maintaining trust. Domain 4 deals with showing respect and treating patients fairly; it is important for doctors to act with honesty and integrity. This guidance clarifies that doctors must make sure that their conduct justifies their patients' trust in them and the public's trust in the profession.

One of the key aspects of the MMI is to select the right candidate for medical school in a stringent manner so that these candidates display the highest personal qualities that indicate they will become good doctors. It becomes the duty of the candidate in the MMI to express and show this to the examiners in this short duration; the candidate should be ready to express their high levels of integrity and honesty in these challenging scenario questions.

The GMC also has similar guidance for medical students, and it is worth quoting this in the station to make sure that the candidate is aware of this (see 'Achieving good medical practice: guidance for medical students').

The American Medical Association adopted the AMA Code of Medical Ethics in 1847; it has 11 chapters, of which the ninth chapter deals with professional self-regulation. It necessitates that doctors hold high standards of conduct.

The Canadian Medical Association Code of Ethics defines that an honest physician is forthright, respects the truth, and does their best to seek, preserve, and communicate that truth sensitively and respectfully. This is displayed in the section answers within this book (note the words — respect truth; do best to seek, preserve and communicate truth; sensitive and respectful).

Similar guidelines are also produced by the Australian Medical Association. Section 3.1 describes the necessity for professional conduct by physicians. It clearly explains that doctors must recognise that their personal conduct may affect their reputation and that of their profession.

Depending on your country and the medical council/association, it is appropriate to quote this code of ethics to add value to your answer.

Key Points

- Always introduce yourself to the examiner and thank them, and appropriately close the session.
- You should be aware of the importance for a doctor to maintain integrity and honesty.
- You should clearly mention that the action of this patient was wrong.
- You must take responsibility for clearly mentioning it, correcting and checking that it has been corrected.
- If not, you should take the responsibility of notifying the affected party.
- The candidate should quote the General Medical Council's 'Good medical practice' document or the American Medical Council's or a similar body's code of ethics to show that they are aware of the ethics behind the scenario.
- Maintain respect and be supportive of the patient, but at the same time, express the idea that honesty is the most important principle.

References

1. General Medical Council. Good medical practice. Domain 4: Maintaining trust. Available from: https://www.gmc-uk.org/ethical-guidance/ethical-guidance-for-doctors/good-medical-practice/domain-4---maintaining-trust#paragraph-65.

2. General Medical Council. Achieving good medical practice: guidance for medical students. Available from: https://www.gmc-uk.org/education/standards-guidance-and-curricula/guidance/student-professionalism-and-ftp/achieving-good-medical-practice.

3. American Medical Association. Code of Medical Ethics overview. Available from: https://www.ama-assn.org/delivering-care/ethics/code-medical-ethics-overview.

4. Canadian Medical Association. Code of ethics and professionalism. Available from: https://policybase.cma.ca/viewer?file=%2Fmedia%2FPolicyPDF%2FPD19–03S.pdf#page=1.

5. Australian Medical Association. Code of Ethics 2004. Revised 2016. Available from: https://www.ama.com.au/articles/code-ethics-2004-editorially-revised-2006-revised-2016.

Question38

A friend asking you to sign for their attendance

Gokul Parameswaran

Question

You are a medical school student; you have mandatory lessons on ethical issues. One of your friends finds the topic boring although it is mandatory. He asks you to sign in his attendance stating that he has got another project to do. What will you do?

The examiner will discuss the ethical aspects of probity in this situation.

Themes for discussion (■ Table 2.13)

Table 2.13.	
Question themes	**What is expected from the candidate?**
1 The candidate greets the examiner and has good body language.	The candidate is presentable and uses good communication skills; always recommended in any station.

Table 2.13.

	Question themes	What is expected from the candidate?
2	Explanation of scenario.	The candidate gives a good opening statement showing that they understand the situation.
3	Why should you sign for his attendance? The candidate explains the possible reasons.	The candidate gives possible reasons why he could sign the attendance for his friend: • The candidate has a commitment to their friend and should value the relationship with them and help them with this task. • They may be overwhelmed by other academic work or personal circumstances meaning that they cannot attend; he quotes that he has another important project to do. • He might catch up with the ethical topic or the candidate could detail him later.
4	The candidate gives reasons why they should NOT sign the attendance and explain why it is wrong.	The candidate explains reasons why they should NOT agree: • Sessions are compulsory for a reason and would compromise a wider responsibility to medicine. • Your friend would be compromising their integrity and in facilitating them, you would be doing the same. • This would be unfair to other students who have attended the session. • It may encourage them not to attend other mandatory sessions in the future. • The probity of the friend and the candidate is in question; the GMC takes probity as a serious issue.
5	The candidate has a clear opinion/conclusion and explains the reasons.	For this scenario, although the candidate should present both sides of the scenario, they need to be aware that it is not acceptable to sign attendance for anybody else. The sessions are compulsory for a reason, with teaching on ethics being a GMC requirement.

Table 2.13.

	Question themes	What is expected from the candidate?
6	Showing empathy to the friend, whilst being clear of the responsibilities.	Whilst it is sufficient to present both sides for this station, to achieve the highest marks it is important to understand why the friend did not want to attend the teaching. For example, they may have other academic or personal issues preventing them from attending. In this case, the candidate could help them get in touch with the medical school to make other arrangements.
7	Transparency — explain the consequences of not attending the mandatory teaching.	Whilst it is important not to be confrontational, it is also key that the friend attends the teaching. Therefore, the candidate should clearly tell the friend that if they simply miss the teaching, then they will notify the medical school.
8	Judgement and clarity.	The candidate has clarity in their answer and can explain the pros and cons, concluding clearly. A clear presentation, smiling throughout and avoiding repetition — these steps can increase the scores in this station. There is empathy towards the friend. Make it clear that they would explore why the friend did not want to attend the session.
9	Conclusion.	The candidate concludes the session and thanks the examiner at the end. This gains the candidate extra bonus points.

Discussion

Medical school can be an extremely stressful time when each student must balance their academic, extracurricular, and personal commitments. It can often be tempting to not attend certain teaching sessions to focus on other responsibilities that appear more pressing. However, mandatory sessions, especially on topics such as ethics, are compulsory for a reason and so must be attended and not skipped. This scenario tests the candidate's ability to balance their sympathy for a friend with a wider responsibility to the medical profession in general.

The central conflict in this question is balancing the trust the friend has placed in the candidate by asking them to sign for their attendance with their wider responsibility to the medical profession. Whilst they should state potential reasons why they may want to sign in on their behalf, the candidate should be clear in saying that they will not sign in a friend to a mandatory session. By signing, they would be compromising their own integrity, as well as encouraging their friend not to attend other compulsory sessions in the future. However, they should be aware that their friend may have other reasons for not wanting to attend the session. Therefore, the candidate should try and explore these potential reasons so that they can explain the importance of attending the teaching or help the friend access any additional support they need if they are struggling with academic or other personal issues.

Key Points

- There are pros and cons to any ethical dilemma; the candidate must be aware of both.
- The candidate should be able to conclude that they will not sign on behalf of their friend.
- Ethics teaching is compulsory for a reason and is viewed by the GMC as being necessary to becoming a doctor in the UK. Therefore, it cannot simply be skipped.
- The candidate should express empathy towards their friend to help them to overcome any other issues stopping them from attending the ethics teaching session.

References

1. General Medical Council. Good medical practice. Available from: https://www.gmc-uk.org/ethical-guidance/ethical-guidance-for-doctors/good-medical-practice.

Section**3**

Communication — medical scenarios

Section editor: Shreya Shyam

Introduction to communication

If knowledge is power, communication is the king.

Medical school applicants often fall into a common trap of simply memorising knowledge and regurgitating it in the interviews; what they often overlook is the communication skills that bring meaning to the knowledge they gain:

The ability to comfort a crying patient cannot be lifted from the page to the person.

Therefore, this section covers the key points and guidance for communicating in an interview setting. The skills you will hone are transferable to clinical and non-clinical situations encountered in your career and life.

Step 1: 'Who am I?'

When you begin the interview role-play station, you are performing a part. Just like the actor, you will be given a prompt with information on the situation as well as the role of your character, for example, 'junior doctor', 'medical student', etc.

In the pressure of an interview setting, it is easy to forget or ignore these details. In fact, this 'role' determines how you should respond. A simple example is a situation in which a patient approaches you for advice. A medical student's role would be to comfort the patient and direct them towards a more experienced professional, whereas the role of a general practitioner/family doctor would be to effectively communicate advice to the patient.

Therefore, when beginning the role play, greet the role player with, 'Hello, my name is [ ] and I am a [given role].'

Step 2: 'Who are they?'

Most candidates miss this step! Many interviewees launch into tackling the situation without introducing themselves or even confirming the identity of the person they are talking to. Although this step may seem trivial in an interview, in a clinical context it is essential to confirm a person's identity before further consultation. This is to establish their trust and to have the correct conversation with the correct person, an important safety practice. Therefore, after introducing yourself, ask the person to state their name and date of birth (or another identity), confirm that these match the prompt, and then continue.

Step 3: 'Why are they here?'

Patient-centred care is the mantra of the century, a shift from the paternalistic care of the past. One key feature of patient-centred care is giving the patient the chance to express their feelings, concerns and reasons for approaching the clinician. In the interview, a good way of prompting an actor to communicate is by asking, 'Why have you come in today?' or 'How may I help you?'. It is better to cue the actor to set the scene than for the candidate to act based on the prompt alone.

Step 4: 'Actions speak louder than words'

Verbal communication is the tip of the iceberg in the skills of any professional. A clinician's body language, especially when they are listening to the patient, can play a huge role in the patient-clinician relationship. During the role-play setting, the 'actor' could perform in many ways: bursting into tears, shouting angrily, or giving no emotional response. It is important that, no matter how the situation varies, the candidate remains calm and empathetic. Ways in which the candidate can present themselves include maintaining eye contact, nodding, giving pauses whenever necessary and responding to the actor. Most importantly, they must always show compassion, e.g. by offering tissues, apologising, holding hands, etc. Under no circumstance should a candidate escalate their emotions or manner to match that of the actor.

Step 5: 'What, So what, Now what'

After the candidate has given time for the actor to explain the situation, it is useful for them to summarise the situation into a few points, to ensure they are on the same page as the actor. This is the 'What'.

Then comes the 'So what'. It is the role of the candidate to clarify the consequences of the situation and clear the actor's doubts. Rather than assuming the level of knowledge of a patient, a good clinician will first listen to the patient's understanding of the situation before filling in the gaps. It is important for the candidate to be calm and use clear language when clarifying doubts.

Finally, the 'Now what'. The candidate should give appropriate advice based on what steps need to be taken forward with the person. The example interview questions in this chapter will provide templates for the type of steps needed to be taken in different situations; candidates can also prepare by reading GMC guidelines and watching online role-play situations.

Step 6: The three tells

The first tell: Tell what you are going to tell.
The second tell: Tell.
The third tell: Tell what you told.

In a clinical setting, perhaps the third tell is the most important, as the consultation is only as valuable as the understanding the patient gains from the meeting. Towards the end of the station, the candidate should ask the actor for feedback and recap what has been discussed, clarifying any doubts as needed. An essential question is, 'Is there anything else that I can do for you today?'.

Finally, thank the actor and the examiner for their time.

Note

Use the following questions as a framework for the role-play station. In the following prompts, filter the information that is relevant to your role, and do not become distracted by unnecessary details.

Practice makes perfect.

Question 39

Delivering a diagnosis: showing empathy

Balaji Varadhan

Question

You are a junior doctor working on a care ward for older patients. During your daily ward rounds, you have been assigned the task of delivering and discussing a new diagnosis of Alzheimer's disease with a patient's wife. The patient has been in your ward for a couple of weeks. He has been struggling with a gradual loss of memory.

Themes for discussion (■ Table 3.1)

Table 3.1.	
Question themes	**What is expected from the candidate?**
1 The candidate greets the examiner.	Good body language and a presentable manner.

Table 3.1.

	Question themes	What is expected from the candidate?
2	The candidate greets the patient's wife and checks their identity.	'Hello, my name is Dr X and I am a junior doctor on this ward.'
		'Can you please state your name, how you are related to the patient, and confirm their details?'
		'Before we proceed with this consultation, would you like a friend, family member or a member of staff to be present?'
3	The candidate explains the results.	'Do you know why your husband is in the hospital and what is your current understanding of his condition?'
		'Your husband has a condition called Alzheimer's disease.'
4	Alzheimer's dementia.	'Are you familiar with the word dementia? What does it mean to you?'
		'Dementia is a group of symptoms associated with a decline of brain function. One common cause of dementia is Alzheimer's disease, with which your husband has been diagnosed.'
		'Dementia can have an impact on your husband's memory, mental skills, language and movement.'
		'As a result, dementia can affect your husband's ability to carry out daily activities independently. It is recommended that in future consultations your husband is accompanied by yourself and/or other family members.'
		'Interventions will be necessary to maintain your husband's quality of life; this may put more responsibility on you and other family members.'

Table 3.1.

	Question themes	What is expected from the candidate?
5	Communication.	The candidate must speak slowly and clearly, taking regular pauses to ask the patient's wife if they understand the information.
6	Treatment.	'We will arrange a meeting with a specialist in order to discuss future treatment options.' (As a junior doctor, you may not have the necessary knowledge to advise on the treatment options.)
7	Role player asks about discharge planning.	'Your husband will be declared 'fit for discharge' by a clinician when he no longer requires medical care on the ward. He will be assisted to return home.' 'We understand that you may have concerns about how to care for your husband once he has been discharged. We will talk you through the support available and answer any questions you have.' 'Please don't worry, we will be there for support every step of the way.'
8	Family asks for details on the support available.	'I can offer you a leaflet with information on Alzheimer's disease and guidance on how to care for your husband.' 'We will contact your GP surgery to find a local support group for patients living with dementia, and their carers.' 'If you have any further questions or concerns, you can approach your local GP for advice, or alternatively call this helpline.'

	Question themes	What is expected from the candidate?
9	Conclusion.	The candidate summarises what has been covered in the communication station.
		'Is there anything else I can do to help?'
		Finish by thanking the actor and examiner.

Table 3.1.

Role play for the actor

The actor's role is to act as the patient's wife. They will appear anxious about the Alzheimer's diagnosis, and if the candidate does not reassure them, they will show distress. The patient's wife will have many questions about the impact of Alzheimer's on the patient and the rest of the family. They will be worried about the patient being discharged from the hospital and will be unsure how to care for the patient whilst also balancing their role as the main income earner. The actor would use phrases such as 'I do not know how we'll cope now' and 'I'm going to lose my career'.

The role player will become more and more distressed unless the candidate reassures them and provides easily understandable advice.

Discussion

The UK has an ageing demographic, resulting in age-related conditions such as Alzheimer's disease, becoming a greater challenge for people and the NHS. Therefore, the role-play situation discussed above is likely to arise in the careers of most medical professionals. A clinician has the important role of comforting the patient and their family members, answering pressing questions, and referring patients/family members to the best sources of support.

The personal skills that the examiner is looking for in the candidate include showing empathy, listening, and the ability to communicate. These should be used in combination with knowledge about Alzheimer's disease and the sources of support available through the NHS.

Role-play stations may often be about specific conditions, e.g. heart disease, obesity, Alzheimer's, etc. A candidate should have basic knowledge of common conditions such as those studied in A-level biology. NHS websites and NHS choices are useful sources for learning about causes, symptoms and treatment. A candidate should also keep up to date on public health crises reported by the news.

The General Medical Council (GMC) states that doctors must treat patients and those close to them with dignity, respect and compassion, especially when they are facing difficult situations and decisions about care. They must respect their privacy and right to confidentiality.

The patient's wife will have many questions about the impact of the condition on the patient and the family. The candidate can categorise the effects using the biopsychosocial model that could provide more structure to their explanation.

If you do not know the answer, please tell the person that you will find the answer and get back to them as soon as possible.

Key Points

- Empathy is key: a compassionate candidate who does not know all the information is more suitable than a candidate who emotionlessly delivers facts to the patient.
- A good candidate is one who listens to the patient's wife and tailors the response based on how much she already knows and their key concerns.
- Always conclude the role play by summarising and asking if there is anything else the person needs to know.

References

1.   General Medical Council. Good medical practice. Available from: https://www.gmc-uk.org/ethical-guidance/ethical-guidance-for-doctors/good-medical-practice.

2.   General Medical Council. Equalities and human rights. In: Treatment and care towards the end of life: good practice in decision making. Available from: https://www.gmc-uk.org/ethical-guidance/ethical-guidance-for-doctors/treatment-and-care-towards-the-end-of-life/principles.

Question 40

Breaking bad news: terminal illness

Balaji Varadhan

Question

You are a junior doctor working on the ward. Your registrar has been called away to A&E urgently and the ward nurse has requested you to see a patient who has been waiting for his biopsy results. The biopsy confirms metastatic gastric cancer, which is terminal; he is not suitable for any curative cancer treatment. You must explain this to the patient. In this station, the examiner will observe how you communicate with the patient.

Themes for discussion (■ Table 3.2)

Table 3.2.	
Question themes	**What is expected from the candidate?**
1 The candidate greets the examiner.	Good body language and a presentable manner.

Table 3.2.

	Question themes	What is expected from the candidate?
2	The candidate greets the patient and checks the identity of the patient.	'Hello, my name is Dr X and I am a junior doctor on this ward.'
		'Can you please state your name and date of birth?'
		'Before we proceed with this consultation, would you like a friend, family member or a member of staff to be present?'
3	The candidate explains the results.	'Why are you in the hospital today? What is your current understanding of your condition?'
		'Unfortunately, I have some bad news; your biopsy test result shows that you have gastric cancer or stomach cancer and it has spread.' Give time for the patient to reflect, be empathetic, then add 'I am sorry again, but let me explain what this is.'
		'What is your understanding of the word cancer?'
		'Cancer is a condition in which cells divide uncontrollably, forming tumours and damaging the healthy tissue around them. Gastric cancer is cancer found in the stomach and it can cause symptoms affecting digestion, e.g. reflux, nausea and weight loss.'
		'The word metastatic means that the cancer has spread from the stomach to other parts of the body.'
		'Unfortunately, for your type of cancer there is no treatment that will cure your condition. However, we can discuss treatment options for managing your symptoms and supporting your quality of life.'
		The candidate gives time for the patient to take in the message and come to terms with their situation. If the role player reacts with tears, they could provide some tissues that might be placed at the station.
		If the role player becomes angry, the candidate will be calm and say sorry for the bad news.

Table 3.2.

	Question themes	What is expected from the candidate?
4	Being empathetic.	The candidate shows empathy by giving the patient time to digest the information, listening to the patient, and responding to the patient with verbal and body language. 'Would you like me to call a friend, family or a member of staff to be with you?' 'Would you like some water?' 'Do you understand the diagnosis? Is there anything you want me to go over or any questions you want me to address?'
5	Allow for denial.	The patient may be in distress. It is important for the candidate to acknowledge the patient's emotions without interrupting or criticising them. 'I understand that this must be very difficult to hear. Whatever questions and concerns you have, I am here to help or assist you.'
6	Symptom control.	'We will arrange a meeting with a specialist in order to discuss future treatment options for controlling symptoms.' (As a junior doctor, you may not have the necessary knowledge to advise on the treatment options.) 'I can offer you a leaflet with information on gastric cancer and the ways we can help you.' 'We will contact your GP surgery to find a local support group for patients living with gastric cancer.' 'If you have any further questions or concerns, you can approach your local GP for advice, or alternatively call this helpline.'

	Question themes	What is expected from the candidate?
7	Conclusion.	The candidate summarises what has been covered in the communication station.
		'Is there anything else I can do for you?'
		Finally, the candidate thanks the role player and the examiner.

Table 3.2.

Role play for the actor

The actor is instructed to act as a patient who has been waiting for biopsy results. The patient is irritable and anxious due to the wait, and they will repeatedly interrupt and talk over the candidate. The patient will be agitated by the diagnosis and will repeatedly ask the candidate to explain the information again. When told that their cancer cannot be cured, the patient will remain in denial and will reject the prognosis. It is important for the candidate to understand the patient's emotions and act in a compassionate and supportive manner.

Discussion

A diagnosis of cancer is life-changing! Each person's response to the news is different and can range from grief, to rage, to complete denial. A candidate's role in this situation is to first give the patient a pause after the delivery, in order for them to register the information. Then, as the patient's response unfolds, the candidate must remain compassionate and understanding, giving the patient a chance to voice their concerns and questions.

Understanding the distinction between sympathy and empathy is a key skill of a good clinician. Sympathy is 'feeling sorry' for an individual, it makes assumptions about the patient's feelings, and evokes pity in the clinician, which can seem condescending and be harmful to the patient. An example of a phrase that demonstrates sympathy is: 'I'm sorry, I know you must be feeling upset right now'.

Empathy is an active process, it involves listening to a patient and understanding why they feel how they feel. Empathy is the ability to share someone else's feelings. An example is: 'I understand that you are worried because you are the main earner of your family'. A good candidate is one who listens to a patient to understand them, rather than making assumptions. Empathy is a more effective way to connect with those going through significant emotional pain.

Key Points

- Deliver a warning shot before giving the patient the diagnosis.
- Listen to the patient and show empathy as opposed to sympathy.
- Always conclude the role play by summarising and asking if there is anything else the person needs to know.
- Even for conditions that we cannot cure, we can still care.

References

1. Parvardhan C. Breaking bad news. *BMJ* 2005; 37: 1131.
2. Kisling J. The difference between empathy and sympathy. Available from: https://www.psychmc.com/articles/empathy-vs-sympathy.

Question 41

An angry relative: their mother was not treated appropriately

Priya Gauthama

Question

You are a junior doctor working in a GP surgery. You are meeting Ms Meena Patel, the daughter of an 80-year-old lady named Mrs Roma Patel, a patient at the practice. Meena is very angry that her mother was not treated properly in the GP surgery last time and she still has an ongoing cough. This is a role-play scenario; you must communicate with Meena and address her questions. The examiner will observe your communication with Meena.

Themes for discussion (■ Table 3.3)

Table 3.3.	
Question themes	**What is expected from the candidate?**
1 The candidate introduces themselves.	The candidate has good body language and a presentable manner. The candidate understands the complex situation but stays calm and has a confident approach.

Table 3.3.

Question themes	What is expected from the candidate?
2 The candidate confirms that they are speaking to the right person — with their name and confirms that her mother is a patient.	'Hello, my name is Dr X and I am a junior doctor on this ward.'
	'Can you please state your name, how you are related to the patient, and confirm their details?'
	'Before we proceed with this consultation, would you like a chaperone or another family member to be present?'
	In real life, you might check the address and date of birth of the patient also.
3 The candidate starts with 'Sorry'.	'I am very sorry for any discomfort your mother has experienced, as well as any frustration or anger you feel as a result.'
	'Can you talk me through the situation and how you feel at the moment?'
	The candidate remains calm and composed; the candidate is empathetic and apologetic. These are displayed in their words (saying sorry, I understand your frustration, etc.) and their body language. Keeping eye contact, staying at the same level and listening to the angry patient are all important active actions here. Despite Meena being angry, the candidate is supportive and compassionate.
4 Actor continues to be angry.	The candidate remains calm and composed, reiterating their apology whilst showing empathy.
	'I apologise; I can understand why this situation may make you feel this way, and I will do my best to help you.'

Table 3.3.

	Question themes	What is expected from the candidate?
5	Meena Patel is worried that the delay has compromised her mother's healthcare.	'When your mother previously came to the surgery for consultation, she was checked by a clinician and given the appropriate advice and treatment based on their observation.' 'I understand that you are not satisfied with the care that was given; however, I can assure you that we are doing our best to provide the correct treatment for your mother.'
6	Meena says that her mother is struggling to breathe now.	'I will arrange for you and your mother to meet a specialist, who will examine your mother and determine the best possible treatment plan for her.' (The candidate understands that as a junior doctor they do not have the knowledge to discuss treatment options.) 'The specialist will examine your mother before making the treatment plan. Examples of investigations could include a chest X-ray and blood tests to rule out a chest infection. The specialist will explain these tests in detail to you and your mother before they are carried out.'
7	Meena Patel is still not convinced with the answers given by the candidate and she wants to complain.	'I am sorry that you are upset and I can talk you through our GP surgery complaints procedure. I can also give you this leaflet that talks you through the process of registering a complaint.' The candidate can mention the Patient Advice and Liaison Service (PALS). 'If you would like, I can request a senior member of the staff to come and talk to you and your mother in order to address any questions and concerns.'

Table 3.3.

Question themes	What is expected from the candidate?
8 Conclusion.	The candidate thanks the relative for listening and conveys apologies again.
	'Is there anything else that I can do for you today?'
	'I will make all the necessary arrangements and keep you updated.'
	The candidate concludes the session.

Role play for the actor

The actor was told to act as Ms Meena Patel, the daughter of the patient. She will show anger and ask the doctor for an explanation as to why her mother was not treated properly when she came in with a cough. Mrs Patel was seen last time by a nurse and was sent home with some advice. She is still coughing and struggling to breathe now. Meena Patel feels that if her mother had been treated the first time properly by a doctor then she would have been better.

The actor was told to calm down only if the candidate apologises and says 'sorry'. She will repeatedly say, 'I am very upset' until the candidate apologises. Despite the candidate's efforts she will show interest in lodging a complaint, e.g. 'I want to complain as this has compromised my mother's health'.

Discussion

In a clinical setting, we might face situations where a patient or their family member might get angry, distressed or challenging. Their illness or pain, fear, anxiety, communication or language difficulties, unrealistic expectations, alcohol or substance misuse, previous poor experience, lack of resources in the practice, long waiting times, lack of appointments, etc. could be reasons for this behaviour. Managing angry patients is an important skill to acquire when you are training to be a doctor. Key skills include: identifying the problem, staying calm with active listening and not taking anger personally. Reassure the patient and acknowledge their grievances. Understanding their source of anger will help you to find the correct solution.

You could use ICE communication techniques for this scenario: Ideas/Concerns/Expectations.

The Patient Advice and Liaison Service (PALS) offers confidential advice, support and information on health-related matters to the public. PALS provides help in many forms, including information on health-related questions as well as support and advice on resolving problems encountered regarding the NHS. PALS also helps to improve the NHS by listening to patient concerns and suggestions.

If a patient is not happy with an NHS service, they can make a complaint. Usually, a patient first complains to the person or organisation providing the service, such as the GP, dentist, hospital or pharmacist. If necessary, the complaint can be escalated to the commissioner of that service, either NHS England or the area clinical commissioning group (CCG). In general, NHS England commissions most primary care services, such as GP and dental services. CCGs oversee the commissioning of secondary care, such as hospital care and some community services. CCGs have changed recently to different systems called Integrated Care Systems (ICS); these are partnerships of organisations that come together to plan and deliver joined-up health and care services.

Being a doctor is humbling and most rewarding; seeing a patient in their moments of great vulnerability, pain and fear, when they are more prone to be angry and frustrated, witnessing the full spectrum of their emotions and supporting them by listening to them, places a doctor in a unique and privileged position. Being empathetic is the most important quality of a doctor.

Key Points

- An empathetic approach and saying 'sorry' are vital in these situations.
- It is important to listen to the reasons of the patient behind their frustration. Hearing their side of the story will help to improve the patient-clinician relationship and will lead to successful communication.
- Always conclude the session in a patient role play by asking if there is anything else that the patient wants to ask.

References

1. Mills R. Managing angry patients and relatives. Available from: https://www.bma.org.uk/advice-and-support/your-wellbeing/insight-and-advice/first-times-in-medicine/managing-angry-patients-and-relatives.

2. NHS UK. How to complain to the NHS. Available from: https://www.nhs.uk/using-the-nhs/about-the-nhs/how-to-complain-to-the-nhs.

Question 42

A blood sample is missing: inform the patient

Siva Thanthullu

Question

You are a junior doctor in a GP surgery. You took blood samples for Ms Owen yesterday; unfortunately, the sample went missing and the patient has attended the GP surgery today in an angry state. You are not sure how the sample went missing. You have to explain this to Ms Owen and convince her to have a repeat sample taken. You are the only available clinician in the GP surgery today.

Themes for discussion (■ Table 3.4)

Table 3.4.	
Question themes	**What is expected from the candidate?**
1 The candidate introduces themselves.	The candidate has good body language and a presentable manner. The candidate understands the complex situation but stays calm and has a confident approach.

Table 3.4.

	Question themes	What is expected from the candidate?
2	The candidate confirms that they are speaking to the right patient — with their name.	'Hello, my name is Dr X and I am a junior doctor in the GP surgery.' 'Can you please state your name and date of birth?' 'Before we proceed with this consultation, would you like a friend, family member or a member of staff to be present?'
3	The candidate starts with 'Sorry'.	'As you know Ms Owen, I took blood samples from you yesterday. Unfortunately, the samples have gone missing and could not be tested, I am very sorry for this inconvenience.' 'It is still very important for us to do the blood test and review the results; therefore, please will you allow me to take a repeat sample? I understand that this may be frustrating for you, and I once again apologise.'
4	Explanation of the situation.	'I can assure you that I did my very best to take care of the sample. I do not know yet how the sample went missing; however, I will bring the matter up with senior members of staff to try and better understand what happened.' 'I am sorry that this has happened, and I can understand your feelings of frustration.' The candidate explains that they did their best but conveys apologies. They should preferably use simple, non-medical language to explain to the actor.

Table 3.4.

Question themes	What is expected from the candidate?
5 The candidate says there is no guarantee that the repeat sample will stay safe, but that they will do their best to protect it.	'I understand that you are concerned that this sample may also go missing. I can assure you that I will address the missing sample with senior staff and reflect on any mistakes on my part. This will help me ensure that I take the appropriate steps to reduce the risk of the repeat sample also going missing.'
	The actor/role player will be upset and question how they can ensure it will be safely sent again; the candidate has to be calm and composed. They should be apologetic and convey their empathy at the same time.
6 The candidate explains that he/she is the only doctor and will try their best to make sure it reaches the laboratory safely; however, if Ms Owen needs, we can rearrange another appointment with a different clinician.	'I am sorry that the loss of the previous sample has reduced your trust in me. I will do my best to address and reflect on this mistake in order to reduce the risk of this sample going missing, as well as restore your trust in me.'
	'I am the only available clinician in the GP surgery today. I would greatly appreciate it if you allowed me to take a repeat blood sample, as it is important for us to ensure that you get your blood test results as soon as possible.'
	'I would understand if you still want another clinician to take your blood test; however, the appointment would need to be rescheduled and this could add further delay to getting you your blood test results.'
7 The candidate explains that they will take steps to prevent this from happening in the future.	The candidate tells the patient that they will inform the supervising senior clinician of the loss; they will present this in a team meeting and follow up on how to avoid these mistakes in the future.

Table 3.4.

	Question themes	What is expected from the candidate?
8	The candidate explains that Ms Owen has a right to complain.	'I am sorry that you are upset and I can explain about our GP surgery complaints procedure. I can also give you this leaflet that details the complaints process.'
9	Conclusion.	The candidate thanks the patient and conveys apologies again. 'Is there anything else that I can do for you today?'

Role play for the actor

The actor plays the role of Ms Owen, who had a blood sample taken from her yesterday. The process was quite taxing and painful for Ms Owen; therefore, she is very distressed about allowing a repeat sample to be taken. This distress results in Ms Owen being very angry; she will repeatedly accuse the candidate of purposefully losing the blood sample, and will be very distrustful about allowing the candidate to take a repeat sample. Ms Owen will insist on lodging a complaint at the end of the appointment.

Discussion

No system is fool-proof and, despite its various safety measures, the NHS is no exception. Therefore, a key skill of any clinician is to explain to the patient how and why a mistake has occurred, as well as provide the next steps that need to be undertaken. The main qualities an examiner will search for in a candidate are honesty, communication skills and composure.

In a role-play scenario such as this, a candidate should structure their answer based on the NHS duty of candour. First, they must tell the 'patient' or their 'relatives' what has gone wrong. Then they must apologise openly for the mistake. Following this, they must offer an appropriate remedy or form of support to counteract the effects of the mistake. Finally, the candidate must fully explain the short-term and long-term effects of the mistake that has occurred. An interview response that is structured in this way is likely to cover, in a clear and understandable manner, most of the questions and concerns that the 'patient' will have.

Finally, the role player may still be dissatisfied at the end of the station, despite the best efforts of the candidate. In this scenario, a candidate should calmly assure the role player that they will talk them through the local complaints procedure, and they may also offer a leaflet on the same.

Key Points

- Structure your answer based on the elements of the duty of candour. More information about this can be found in GMC guidance.
- Stay composed and compassionate no matter how angry the patient is.
- Offer an explanation of the local complaints procedure to the role player if they are still dissatisfied at the end of the station.

References

1. Mills R. Managing angry patients and relatives. Available from: https://www.bma.org.uk/advice-and-support/your-wellbeing/insight-and-advice/first-times-in-medicine/managing-angry-patients-and-relatives.

2. NHS UK. How to complain to the NHS. Available from: https://www.nhs.uk/using-the-nhs/about-the-nhs/how-to-complain-to-the-nhs.

Question 43

An angry patient: a long wait in A&E

Priya Gauthama

Question

You are a junior doctor in a hospital A&E department. You are seeing Kate, who is the mother of a 6-year-old boy, Thomas, with tummy pain. Kate is very angry and upset that Thomas is being seen very late and they have been waiting for nearly 3 hours.

This is a role-play scenario; you must talk to Kate and address her questions.

An examiner will observe and mark your communication skills in this station.

Themes for discussion (■ Table 3.5)

Table 3.5.

Question themes	What is expected from the candidate?
1 The candidate introduces themselves.	The candidate understands the complexity but stays calm and has a good approach. They should show empathy with their body language, and speak clearly but calmly.
2 The candidate confirms that they are speaking to the right patient — by their names, Thomas and Kate.	'Hello, my name is Dr X and I am a junior doctor on this ward.' 'Can you please state your name, how you are related to the patient, and confirm their details?' 'Before we proceed with this consultation, would you like a friend, family member or a member of staff to be present?' It is important that the candidate introduces themselves and checks that they are speaking to the correct patient. In real life, they might check with the date of birth and address also.
3 The candidate starts with 'Sorry'.	'I am very sorry for the delay in your son Thomas being seen. I can assure you that a senior member of staff will be with him as soon as possible.' It is important that the candidate conveys apologies for the delay in this station.
4 The mother is angry at this point.	The candidate remains calm and composed; the candidate is empathetic and apologetic. 'I understand your frustration, and I appreciate that Thomas must be getting quite restless as well. I will talk to a senior member of staff about the wait, and is there anything I can do to make the wait comfortable in the meantime?'

Table 3.5.

	Question themes	What is expected from the candidate?
		The candidate has good body language: keeping eye contact, staying on the same level and listening to the angry parent are all important active actions here.
		Despite the mother being angry, the candidate is supportive and compassionate.
5	The mother is worried that the delay has compromised Thomas's care.	'When you arrived at A&E, a nurse checked over Thomas and observed his condition to be stable, with no danger. Doctors provide care to patients based on clinical urgency.'
		'I understand that you are worried about your son; however, I can assure you that he is in the right place for his care.'
		'The team are doing their best to see him as soon as possible and to provide him with the correct treatment.'
6	Kate is still not convinced with the answers given by the candidate and she wants to complain.	'I am sorry that you are upset and I can talk you through our hospital complaints procedure. I can also give you this leaflet that talks you through the process of registering a complaint.'
		The candidate can mention the Patient Advice and Liaison Service (PALS).
		'If you would like, I can request a senior member of the staff to come and talk to you and your son in order to address any questions and concerns.'
7	Conclusion.	The candidate thanks the patient and his mother and conveys apologies again.
		'Is there anything else that I can do please?'

Role play for the actor

The actor is playing the role of Kate, the mother of the patient Thomas. She will be angry and asks the doctor for an explanation of why there was such a delay in seeing Thomas. The actor will repeatedly say, 'I am very upset' and calm down only if the candidate apologises and says 'sorry'.

Despite the candidate's efforts, the actor will still be dissatisfied at the end of the role play and will say: 'I want to complain as this delay has compromised Thomas's care'.

Discussion

This is a very important station as most MMIs have an angry or frustrated patient/parent/carer. This is to check whether the candidate can listen, communicate and show empathy. Saying 'sorry' is key. If the candidate can calm the patient and make them listen, it is a success for this station.

The scenario of this question is likely to occur in the children's A&E during the winter months, when common infections are prevalent. During the summer months, cuts, bruises and accidental injuries are common following active sports during a bright and sunny day. The NHS has a maximum waiting time of 4 hours across all hospital A&E departments. There is a target that 95% of patients attending A&E should be seen within 4 hours. Recent available data from January 2022 show that 74.3% of patients were seen within 4 hours in all A&E departments. The 95% standard was last met in July 2015.

It is important for candidates to put themselves in other people's shoes. Children's health is the most pressing concern for any parent, and they may feel helpless or frustrated if there is a delay in seeing a doctor. There may also be other factors affecting them, like worries about work or other children left at home. A good candidate listens to the causes behind the parent's concerns and responds with the appropriate support.

Managing angry patients is an important skill, and a good way to approach this is the ICE communication tool that ensures that people's voices and perspectives are heard. ICE stands for Ideas, Concerns and Expectations.

'Ideas' refers to people's beliefs. In this scenario the candidate should ask Kate her beliefs about the causes behind her son's pain, as well as her beliefs about why there has been a long wait. 'Concerns' is more specific and relates to what worries Kate the most; a good candidate will be able to identify this by listening to Kate and asking her open-ended questions. 'Expectations' is the course of action/intervention that Kate wants to happen, for example, she is likely to want her son to be seen quickly.

As a junior doctor, you may not be able to comply with every person's expectations, but it is vital to listen to people's perspectives in a calm and composed manner. You should aim to reassure any concerns and work towards their expectations as much as possible.

The UK General Medical Council's (GMC) 'Good medical practice' guidance (Domain 2: Safety and quality) clarifies the need to respond to concerns openly and safely. Domain 3 (Communication partnership and teamwork) stresses that doctors must listen to patients, take account of their views, and respond honestly to their questions. One of the key aspects of this station is to stay calm but show empathy at the same time. Listening is an active skill and needs to be developed; at the same time, most stations take 5-7 minutes, and the candidate must apologise and convince the patient of the task, i.e. explaining the reason for the delay but at the same time not compromising the safety of the patient. The American Medical Association's ethical guidelines have a similar code in the patient rights section.

Key Points

- An empathetic approach and saying 'sorry' is vital in these situations.
- Use the ICE technique to understand the patient's perspective.
- Listen to the patient; convey apologies. If the patient/relative calms down, it will lead to successful communication.
- Always conclude the session; if it is a patient role play, do not forget to ask if there is anything else that the patient wants to ask.

References

1. General Medical Council. Good medical practice. Domain 2: Safety and quality. Available from: https://www.gmc-uk.org/ethical-guidance/ethical-guidance-for-doctors/good-medical-practice/domain-2----safety-and-quality#paragraph-22.

2. General Medical Council. Good medical practice. Domain 3: Communication partnership and teamwork. Available from: https://www.gmc-uk.org/ethical-guidance/ethical-guidance-for-doctors/good-medical-practice/domain-3---communication-partnership-and-teamwork#paragraph-31.

3. American Medical Association. Ethics — patient rights. Available from: https://www.ama-assn.org/delivering-care/ethics/patient-rights.

4. NHS UK. A&E attendances and emergency admissions. Statistical Commentary. Available from: https://www.england.nhs.uk/statistics/wp-content/uploads/sites/2/2022/02/Statistical-commentary-January-2022-jf8.pdf.

5. Mills R. Managing angry patients and relatives. Available from: https://www.bma.org.uk/advice-and-support/your-wellbeing/insight-and-advice/first-times-in-medicine/managing-angry-patients-and-relatives.

6. NHS UK. How to complain to the NHS. Available from: https://www.nhs.uk/using-the-nhs/about-the-nhs/how-to-complain-to-the-nhs.

Question 44

A mother with anxiety about the COVID vaccine

Siva Thanthullu

Question

You are a junior doctor in a GP surgery; an anxious mother, Mrs Gill, has come to see you. Her 13-year-old daughter was sent home with a letter from her school explaining that she would be given the COVID-19 vaccine in 4 weeks' time.

The mother is very worried about side effects and feels that it is wrong for the school to compel her daughter to have the vaccine.

You will talk to Mrs Gill and an examiner will observe the station.

Themes for discussion (▇ Table 3.6)

Table 3.6.		
	Question themes	**What is expected from the candidate?**
1	The candidate introduces themselves.	The candidate understands the complexity but stays calm and has a good approach. They should show empathy with their body language and speak clearly but calmly.
2	The candidate confirms that they are speaking to the right patient confirming her name as Mrs Gill.	'Hello, my name is Dr X and I am a junior doctor on this ward.' 'Can you please state your name, and date of birth?'
3	The candidate asks the mother why she is worried.	The candidate allows the mother to talk and listens actively to understand the reasons behind her anxiety. 'I understand that you are anxious about your daughter receiving a COVID-19 vaccine.' 'May I ask which aspects of the vaccine concern you?'
4	Mrs Gill explains why she is worried and the candidate listens to her concerns.	Mrs Gill has read lots of information on social media and has heard information from her family that the COVID vaccine is dangerous. She believes that the vaccine contains a tracking device. Additionally, according to her cousin's friend, they became seriously ill with COVID after getting the vaccine, and they believe the vaccine is the cause.
5	The candidate summarises and reflects on the patient's concerns.	The candidate expresses understanding towards the parent's worries and is empathetic; they summarise their understanding of the mother's worries to ensure they are on the same page. 'I understand that you are worried about the vaccine because… (the vaccine can cause side effects, it contains a tracking device, doesn't understand how the vaccine works, etc.).'

Table 3.6.

	Question themes	What is expected from the candidate?
6	The candidate stays calm and tries to reassure the mother.	'There is much information about the COVID-19 vaccine on the news and social media, and I understand that it can be frightening and difficult to find out whether the information is fake or not.'
		'I know that what happened to your cousin's friend is very concerning and that as a mother you are worried about your daughter; however, with your permission I can give you some information about the COVID vaccine and explain why it cannot cause COVID or the side effects that you are worried about. The side effects are minimal and less risky compared with getting the disease if not vaccinated.'
7	The actor gets angry and says: 'You do not have a daughter, how could you understand!'	The candidate stays calm and is empathetic.
		'I'm sorry if I angered you Mrs Gill. I didn't mean to do so. I do not have a daughter, but I do understand what it feels like to have concerns about the COVID-19 vaccine. I know that there are lots of information about it everywhere and it is hard to know what to believe.'
		'With your permission I will share some information about the vaccine that is reliable as it has been confirmed through research.'
8	The candidate explains the benefits of the vaccine and the side effects.	The candidate thanks the parent and conveys apologies again.
		The candidate emphasizes that the COVID vaccine has been tested as safe and all research results prove its benefits.
		The candidate can explore the mother's understanding first:
		'What is your understanding until now of the COVID-19 vaccine?'

Table 3.6.

	Question themes	What is expected from the candidate?
		'The COVID-19 vaccine contains material from the virus; this material is a harmless protein that helps teach the body how to respond if it is infected by the actual virus. There is no risk of catching COVID-19 from the vaccination, and the vaccine will reduce the risk of developing COVID-19.'
		'There are some side effects of the vaccine; however, these are usually outweighed by the benefits. Serious side effects are rare, and I can assure you that we, as clinicians, would not vaccinate your daughter if there was a serious risk of harm.'
		'If you would like more reliable information about the vaccine and its benefits, I can offer you this leaflet.'
9	Don't I have the power to take care of my child? Where is the autonomy?	The candidate answers the question calmly, and has an understanding of autonomy. The candidate explains the ethical principles of the vaccine.
10	The candidate explains in clear, simple language, with empathy.	Clear communication, explaining the pros and cons, detailing the scientific basis in simple language. Obtains the confidence of the mother that the candidate has good scientific knowledge to support their views.
11	Conclusion.	The candidate thanks the patient and conveys apologies again.
		'Is there anything else that I can do please?'

Role play for the actor

The actor has been told to perform as Mrs Gill. She will be visibly distressed and worried about the effects of the COVID vaccination on their daughter. She will become more and more flustered unless the candidate is empathetic and reassures them.

Mrs Gill will be angry about her perceived lack of autonomy as a parent, with phrases such as: 'I am very unhappy; this is not right'. She will become angry and say: 'You do not have a daughter. How could you understand?'

Once the candidate has explained the COVID vaccine, Mrs Gill will be very curious about the benefits and especially the risks of the vaccine.

Discussion

The COVID-19 pandemic has been a life-changing experience for the world, and COVID-19 vaccination is certainly one of the most important medical innovations in the past decade. However, with the dawn of this vaccination came fearmongering and misinformation through the news and social media. This resulted in widespread reluctance to take the vaccine, and many still refuse it today.

The role of a clinician is not only to treat, but to communicate. When faced with a person who is frightened or misinformed about a treatment or concept, a good way to approach them is the ICE communication tool that ensures that people's voices and perspectives are heard. ICE stands for Ideas, Concerns and Expectations.

'Ideas' refers to people's beliefs. In this scenario the candidate should ask Mrs Gill about her current understanding and beliefs about the COVID-19 vaccine and how it works. 'Concerns' relates to what worries Mrs Gill the most about the vaccine, as well as her concerns for the well-being of her daughter. 'Expectations' is the course of action/intervention that Mrs Gill wants to happen. For example, you may ask her: 'What were you hoping I could do for you today?'

As a junior doctor, you may not be able to comply with every person's expectations, but it is vital to listen to people's perspectives in a calm and composed manner. You should aim to reassure any concerns and work towards their expectations as much as possible.

Finally, a good candidate should be able to give Mrs Gill a brief, easily understandable explanation of the COVID-19 vaccine, as well as talk through its benefits and side effects. A good source of information is the NHS website, as this uses patient-friendly language that a candidate can utilise in their explanation.

Key Points

- Use the ICE communication tool when talking to a person who is frightened, confused or misinformed.
- Learn some basic information about recent medical innovations such as the COVID-19 vaccine through reliable sources such as the NHS website.
- Stay calm and composed; you need to instil confidence in the patient/relative.

References

1.	NHS UK. Coronavirus (COVID-19) vaccine. Available from: https://www.nhs.uk/conditions/coronavirus-covid-19/coronavirus-vaccination/coronavirus-vaccine.

Question 45

Patient concern: not meeting dietary requirements

Rupa Jayaraj

Question

You are a third-year medical student who has been placed on the general surgical ward for the last few weeks. You are practising taking histories from patients as medical school exams are coming up in the next few weeks. On asking about Mrs Williams' diet, she tells you that she is a vegetarian; however, she has been receiving meat in her meals. She has raised this issue before, but the meals continued to contain meat. Furthermore, she is too scared to raise the issue again as she is afraid of the head nurse and is worried that she might not get appropriate care if she raises concerns again.

This is a role-play station and you will be talking to the patient; the examiner will observe your communication skills.

Themes for discussion (▓ Table 3.7)

Table 3.7.

Question themes	What is expected from the candidate?
1 The candidate introduces themselves.	This is a complex scenario; the candidate understands this complexity but stays calm and has a good approach. They should show empathy with their body language, and speak clearly but calmly.
2 The candidate confirms the correct patient.	'Hello, my name is Dr X and I am a junior doctor on this ward.'
	'Can you please state your name and date of birth?'
3 The candidate apologises; the keyword is sorry.	'I am very sorry that your dietary needs were not met. I understand that being a vegetarian is an important lifestyle choice for you and it was not right that you were given the wrong food.'
	'I am also sorry that despite you raising the issue it was not taken into account. Your concerns are of the utmost importance to us, so I can assure you that the matter will be taken into account now.'
4 The candidate asks the patient to discuss the situation more.	The candidate tries to console the patient, letting her speak as much as possible.
	'On behalf of the team, I apologise for this mistake, and I can assure you that the situation was not your fault.'
	The candidate maintains eye contact, nods their head and acknowledges the patient's problem.
5 The actor starts to get frustrated and shouts at the candidate.	Here, it is vital that the candidate remains as calm as possible and does not change their demeanour. 'I can understand why you are frustrated, and once again I apologise and assure you that we will do our best to fix this mistake.'

Table 3.7.

	Question themes	What is expected from the candidate?
6	The candidate offers a solution.	'I can assure you that patient well-being is our utmost priority. I do not know how the wrong food was provided; however, I will bring the matter up with senior members of staff to try and better understand what happened, as well as record the mistake in the hospital incident reporting system.'
		'I understand that you are concerned that your concerns may again be ignored. As a team we will reflect on the mistake. This will help us ensure that we take the appropriate steps to reduce the risk of the same mistake happening in the future.'
7	The candidate explores the patient's feelings towards the head sister.	'You told me that you are scared of the head nurse. Could you please tell me a bit more about why you are afraid and whether anything has happened in the past?'
		The candidate explores this to find out if there is a harmful relationship between the patient and the head nurse. The patient says that the head nurse has been very rude and abrupt with her.
		'With your permission I can talk to senior staff who will bring this matter up with the head nurse.'
		Mrs Williams may be initially afraid about getting the head nurse involved. It is the role of the candidate to comfort her.
8	The patient wants to complain.	'I am sorry that you are upset and I can talk to you about our hospital complaints procedure. I can also give you this leaflet that talks you through the process of registering a complaint.'

Table 3.7.	
Question themes	**What is expected from the candidate?**
	The candidate can mention the Patient Advice and Liaison Service (PALS).
	'If you would like, I can request a senior member of staff to come and talk to you in order to address any questions and concerns.'
9 Conclusion.	The candidate thanks the patient and conveys apologies again.
	'Is there anything else that I can do for you today?'

Role play for actor

The actor is playing the role of Mrs Williams. Mrs Williams will be very anxious and initially reserved in her communication with the candidate, due to her previous experience with the head sister. Mrs Williams is a strict vegetarian; therefore, when recounting her past experience, she may become very distressed and tearful, with this escalating into her lashing out. Mrs Williams will be keen on complaining but afraid of getting the Head Sister involved; it is the role of the candidate to reason with Mrs Williams and assuage her fears.

Discussion

As detailed in the GMC guidelines, a good clinician should, 'treat patients and those close to them with dignity, respect and compassion'. Unfortunately, as was shown in events such as the mid-Staffordshire scandal (2005-2009), the level of patient care can become compromised. Additionally, the Francis Report, which explored the aforementioned mid-

Staffordshire scandal, showed that a bullying culture and intimidation culture in the NHS workplace could prevent reporting of adverse staff behaviour, resulting in poorer patient outcomes.

This role-play situation explores a candidate's ability to recognise that a patient has been mistreated, and take the appropriate steps to support the patient, as well as escalate the situation to the appropriate staff members. It is key that the candidate recognises their own limitations as a third-year medical student, such that they do not offer themselves to challenge the head nurse, instead of offering to speak to senior staff and report the incident in the hospital incident reporting system.

Key Points

- When approaching a frightened patient, give them time and space to feel comfortable and speak freely.
- Recognise the limitations of your role: a medical student should always escalate any issues and concerns.
- Make patients aware of their right to complain, and talk them through the procedure if necessary.

References

1. General Medical Council. Equalities and human rights. In: Treatment and care towards the end of life: good practice in decision making, pp. 7-9. Available from: https://www.gmc-uk.org/ethical-guidance/ethical-guidance-for-doctors/treatment-and-care-towards-the-end-of-life/principles.

2. NHS UK. Employers. Bullying in healthcare. Available from: https://www.nhsemployers.org/articles/bullying-healthcare.

Question 46

Eliciting a history from a patient

Rupa Jayaraj

Question

You are a second-year medical student gaining work experience in a GP surgery. Your supervising doctor has asked you to take a history from one of the patients inside room 10. They mention that the patient's presenting complaint is a fever. Please take a concise history from this patient and the examiner will observe and assess your communication skills.

Themes for discussion (■ Table 3.8)

Table 3.8.	
Question themes	**What is expected from the candidate?**
1 The candidate introduces themselves.	'Hello, my name is X and I am a second-year medical student posted for clinical learning in this GP surgery. Can I talk to you before you see the GP please?'
	'Can you please state your name, and date of birth?'
	'May I take your medical history by asking some questions?'

Table 3.8.

	Question themes	What is expected from the candidate?
2	Presenting complaint.	The candidate starts with an open question such as: 'Please can you tell me why you have come in today?'
		Here, the candidate shows active listening skills and demonstrates non-verbal cues to acknowledge the patient.
3	History of presenting complaint.	Once the patient has spoken, the candidate asks more specific questions:
		For example, they may use the SOCRATES acronym (more information below).
		'May I ask how long you have had this condition and when it started?'
		'In what parts of your body do you feel pain? Is this pain constant or does it come and go?'
		'Does this condition affect any of your daily activities such as work or hobbies?'
		The candidate also asks for red flag symptoms such as blood in stool, urine, coughing or vomiting blood.
		The candidate asks for a travel history in recent times given that the fever could have an infectious cause.
		They ask for a contact history, regarding any infection in contacts, and ask about the history of COVID in contacts.

Table 3.8.

	Question themes	What is expected from the candidate?
4	Past medical history.	The candidate asks about the patient's past medical history. This can include any previous operations, hospitalisation or details of GP visits. 'May I ask if you have previously been to the hospital? If so, then for what reasons?' 'For what reasons do you normally come to see the GP?' 'Do you have any other illness please?' If the actor offers some information regarding their past illness, the candidate asks for more details regarding the illness and finds out if it is well controlled.
5	Drug history.	The candidate asks about the patient's medications. 'Can you please tell me about any medication that you currently take or that you have taken in the past?' It is important to check for allergies, dosing and any over-the-counter drugs or herbal remedies.
6	Family history.	The candidate enquires about family history: 'Do you know of anyone in your family with a chronic illness such as diabetes, heart disease, etc.?' 'At the moment is anyone else in the house ill with a fever?'

Table 3.8.

	Question themes	What is expected from the candidate?
7	Social history.	The candidate asks about diet and lifestyle, smoking and alcohol consumption.
		'How would you describe your diet? How often do you eat vegetables and fruits?'
		'How would you describe your exercise levels? On average how much time do you spend a week being active?'
		The candidate asks about recent travel (food poisoning can cause fever). They also ask about vaccinations/immunisations.
8	The patient is anxious and worried; the candidate reassures them.	'The medical team are doing their best to help you, and I am sure my senior GP will get back to you soon.' The candidate does NOT promise them that they will get better but emphasises that the team is there for them and that they are getting the best care.
9	Conclusion.	The candidate thanks the patient for their time.
		'I will make sure the GP will get back to you with a treatment plan soon.'
		'Is there anything else that I can do for you today?'

Discussion

The ability of a clinician to take a patient's history is an important skill; indeed medical history is a powerful tool for forming diagnoses. The key skills that an examiner is searching for in the candidate include communication skills, an organised approach to asking questions, and particularly the ability to listen and gather the most important information from the patient's account.

As stated in the table above, SOCRATES is an acronym used by clinicians to structure their questions about a patient's medical history:

- The first 'S' stands for site: 'Where in your body do you feel pain/the symptoms?'
- The 'O' is for Onset: 'Did the symptoms start suddenly or gradually over time?'
- 'C' is Character: 'Is the pain sharp or dull, is it constant or throbbing?'
- 'R' is Radiation: 'Does the pain from your arm spread to any other parts of your body?'
- 'A' is Associated symptoms: 'Do you have any nausea or vomiting?'
- T: Time/duration: 'When did the symptoms start and how long have you had them?'
- E: Exacerbating/relieving factors: 'Do any activities or medications make the symptoms better or worse?'
- S: Severity: 'On a scale of 1-10, how bad are the symptoms?'

Key Points

- Gain a person's consent to take their history at the beginning of the session.
- You can use the acronym SOCRATES to structure your questions about a patient's history.
- You need a structure to ask questions in history taking.
- Listen out for any significant details in a patient's account that may require further exploration.

References

1. Jefferies C. The SOCRATES acronym in history taking. Available from: https://geekymedics.com/the-socrates-acronym-in-history-taking.

Question 47

Dealing with an intoxicated colleague

Rupa Jayaraj

Question

You are an FY1 doctor working on the renal ward. It is 8:30 a.m. and the registrar, Dr Smith, has still not arrived for the handover. Finally, you see him coming in lazily at 9:05 a.m. and suspect that something is not right. On speaking to him, you notice a strong smell of alcohol on his breath and can see drink stains on his shirt. This is a role-play station; please speak to your registrar colleague. An examiner will observe your communication skills in this station.

Themes for discussion (■ Table 3.9)

Table 3.9.	
Question themes	**What is expected from the candidate?**
1 The candidate speaks to their colleague professionally.	'Hello Dr Smith, my name is [candidate's name] and I am an FY1 doctor working on this renal ward. Please may I talk to you?'
	The candidate is professional and calm and takes the opportunity to speak to him in a small room, privately.

Table 3.9.

	Question themes	What is expected from the candidate?
2	The candidate asks how his colleague is and explains his worry about alcohol intake.	'Dr Smith, there is a smell of alcohol coming from you and stains on your shirt. Is there anything you want to tell me? I am worried about you.' This is done in a compassionate manner, without being too direct.
3	Dr Smith denies drinking any alcohol and gets angry.	Here, the candidate should remain calm and composed. They should not raise their voice or become flustered. The examiners will assess how the candidate deals with problems under stress/pressure. 'I am sorry that you are angry Dr Smith, and I am not accusing you of anything, I am just worried about your well-being.'
4	Dr Smith is about to walk away towards the patients in the ward.	The candidate should aim to stop Dr Smith from walking away as his presence in the ward could compromise patient care. 'Dr Smith, we, your colleagues, are here for you and want to help you, but we need you to be honest about what is going on. I know that you care about your patients, and you know that if you meet them and provide care for them in this state they could be at risk. Please can you tell me about what is going on and why you smell of alcohol?' The candidate should aim to use a compassionate and empathetic approach wherever possible. However, if Dr Smith is riled up and becomes verbally abusive, the candidate can mention calling for help, or calling security, depending on the circumstance.

Table 3.9.

	Question themes	What is expected from the candidate?
5	Dr Smith starts to listen and opens up.	Dr Smith has recently separated from his wife and is using alcohol as a coping mechanism.
		The candidate demonstrates compassion and empathetic listening skills: 'I am sorry that you've been feeling this way Dr Smith; we are all here for you'.
		'If you want to talk more about how you're feeling, we can have a catch-up over coffee whenever you are free.'
6	Dr Smith is convinced that the candidate will report his behaviour to the consultant.	'I know your patients matter to you Dr Smith, so you understand that it is not in their best interest for them to meet you in this state.'
		'Will you come with me to talk to the consultant doctor about what is going on? I assure you that we all understand how you are feeling and that the staff will support you.'
		'I would also recommend that you talk to the hospital about receiving support for your alcohol coping mechanism. There are Alcoholics Anonymous support groups that may help you meet other people who are feeling the same way you are.'
		The candidate remains professional and offers to call a taxi for Dr Smith to go home.
7	Conclusion.	The candidate has been empathetic with the colleague throughout the conversation, but always considers patient safety as a key issue. They conclude the station by accepting that the registrar will move out of the patient area and agree to liaise with a consultant or senior staff to look at the way forward to rectify the situation.

Role play for the actor

The actor is playing the role of Dr Smith. Dr Smith will be intoxicated, and his speech will be slightly slurred and at some points incoherent. At first, Dr Smith will be very reserved and unwilling to talk to the candidate, instead insisting that he will go to see the patients. When the candidate prevents Dr Smith from going to the patients, he may become angry and start shouting. If the candidate is compassionate and a good listener, Dr Smith will reveal the cause of his drinking and be more open to receiving support.

Discussion

This hypothetical situation is commonly presented in the interview setting, due to its ability to test a candidate's ability to reason with a colleague in a high-pressure situation.

There is a risk of the candidate veering towards one of two extremes. On the one hand, they may be extremely compassionate to Dr Smith verging on lenient, allowing him to continue to the ward and meet the patients. On the other hand, the candidate may rigidly follow the strict guidelines and challenge Dr Smith without exploring the situation and the reasons behind his drinking. A good candidate is level-headed; they will compassionately listen to Dr Smith, whilst gently but firmly preventing him from meeting the patients and encouraging him to seek support.

The key ethical principles at play in this situation are non-maleficence and the duty of candour.

Non-maleficence: a patient who is seen by an intoxicated doctor may be at risk of harm, either due to the care provided or due to a breakdown in the patient-clinician relationship. Therefore, under no circumstances should the candidate allow Dr Smith to continue into the ward and meet the patients.

Duty of candour: Dr Smith has a duty to be honest and open about when things go wrong. In this case, he must address his intoxication in the workplace. The candidate should encourage Dr Smith himself to be honest and open to a senior member of staff, e.g. a consultant doctor on the ward.

However, if Dr Smith cannot be persuaded to be candid about his situation, the candidate must address it with the appropriate senior staff.

Key Points

- A good candidate will keep patient safety as their priority while also try to empathise and understand why their colleague is acting a certain way.
- Under no circumstances should the care provided to a patient be compromised.
- Wherever possible, a candidate should first persuade the colleague to be honest and progress the situation, but if this fails then it is the candidate's role to talk to senior staff.

References

1. General Medical Council. A colleague's fitness to practise. Available from: https://www.gmc-uk.org/ethical-guidance/learning-materials/a-colleagues-fitness-to-practise.

2. General Medical Council. The professional duty of candour. Available from: https://www.gmc-uk.org/ethical-guidance/ethical-guidance-for-doctors/candour---openness-and-honesty-when-things-go-wrong/the-professional-duty-of-candour.

Question 48

Breaking bad news: explaining postoperative complications

Selvakumar Panchatsharam

Question

You are a surgeon; you are going to talk to a patient, Mrs Jones, on whom you performed a hip replacement surgery yesterday. Mrs Jones is recovering in the ward and is in some physical pain due to the surgery. You must inform them that she has developed nerve damage during surgery, which will cause leg weakness that could last for a long time.

An examiner will observe your communication skills in this station.

Themes for discussion (■ Table 3.10)

Table 3.10.		
	Question themes	**What is expected from the candidate?**
1	The candidate introduces themselves and confirms that they are speaking to the correct patient (Mrs Jones).	'Hello, my name is Dr X and I am the surgeon who performed hip surgery on you yesterday.' 'Can you please state your name, and date of birth?'

Table 3.10.

Question themes	What is expected from the candidate?
	The candidate has good body language. They sit down at eye level with the actor, making eye contact, and leaning forward slightly.
2 Setting the agenda for the difficult conversation.	'I am here to talk to you about yesterday's operation. Before we start, would you like any friends, family or other members of staff to be present?'
3 The candidate breaks the bad news and apologises.	'Unfortunately, I am sorry that I have some bad news for you. Whilst performing your complex hip operation yesterday, one of the nerves in your leg was damaged. I am very sorry.'
	Pause and allow the patient to understand the information and express their emotions. The clear opening sentence gives a warning that an error has happened and allows the patient to prepare for the conversation. It gets the attention needed from the patient.
	'This nerve damage could result in longer-term weakness of the leg. We will need to do more tests to identify the level of damage and decide what measures can be offered. Once again, I apologise that this occurred.'
	The key is to say 'sorry' and be honest and open about the error that has happened.
4 Mrs Jones is angry at this point and accuses the candidate of carelessness.	'I understand this is very distressing for you. I can assure you that the mistake was not deliberate and that your care is our utmost priority.'
	Despite Mrs Jones being angry, the candidate is calm and composed. They show empathy for the patient.

Table 3.10.

	Question themes	What is expected from the candidate?
5	Mrs Jones asks how the mistake could have happened.	'During the surgery, I and our team of doctors and nurses took as much care as possible. Unfortunately, nerve damage is a rare but recognised complication during the surgery.'
		'I understand that this is very distressing for you and I am sorry for this.'
6	Mrs Jones asks what can be done about this.	'I can assure you that we are taking this matter seriously.'
		'Are you in any physical distress and experiencing pain or numbness in your leg? We will attend to any symptoms first and try our best to make you comfortable.'
		'We will actively follow up with you and address your progress through regular consultations to assess your progress.'
		'I will request some investigations to assess the extent of the damage and also refer you to a specialist to see if there are any measures that we can take in the recovery.'
		The candidate reassures Mrs Jones but does not offer false hopes. They are honest about the potential long-term impact of nerve damage.
		'I understand that you have questions about why this complication occurred and may be concerned about the quality of care we provide. The surgical team and I are going to complete a serious incident form that will be reported to the hospital risk management team who will perform an independent root cause analysis to look for any lessons to be learnt from this incident. Once this is completed, we will contact you, and we as a team will learn from any mistakes we made.'

	Question themes	What is expected from the candidate?
	Table 3.10.	
7	The patient says that she wants to complain.	'I am sorry that you are upset, and I can talk you through our hospital complaints procedure. I can also give you this leaflet that talks you through the process of registering a complaint.'
		The candidate can mention the Patient Advice and Liaison Service (PALS).
		'If you would like, I can request a senior member of staff to come and talk to you in order to address any questions and concerns.'
		Acknowledge that the patient has a right to complain and direct them to the pathway.
8	Conclusion.	The candidate thanks the patient for their time.
		Concludes by saying 'sorry' again and that they will make all the necessary arrangements.
		Gives the opportunity for further questions if any.
		'Once again I am sorry, and is there anything else that I can do for you today?'

Role play for the actor

The actor is given the role of Mrs Jones, who underwent a hip replacement surgery yesterday. Mrs Jones is now recovering in the ward and is in some pain after surgery. She becomes very distressed when she is told about the nerve damage and is worried about any future consequences. She is also impatient to know how the incident happened and accuses the doctor of carelessness. Mrs Jones wants to complain about this incident as it could be life-changing for her.

Discussion

Whilst serious errors such as nerve damage are quite rare, medical errors are inevitable in clinical practice; they can potentially lead to physical harm and emotional distress. Therefore, it is a key skill for clinicians to inform a patient when a mistake has been made, discuss the short-term and long-term impact as well as form an action plan for mitigating the impact.

Although a clinician may be anxious about breaking bad news, trust and honesty underpin the doctor-patient relationship. One of the pillars of the GMC's 'Good medical practice' guidance is probity, and every doctor has a professional duty of candour.

This scenario includes a complex interplay of multiple themes discussed elsewhere including:

1. Breaking bad news — appropriate setting, pacing the interview, warning shot, pause and proceed, active listening acknowledging the patient's emotions and feelings, and showing empathy.
2. Explaining medical error — saying 'sorry', with openness and honesty.
3. Duty of candour and probity.
4. Handling complaints.

In this scenario the candidate can use the following framework described by R. Buckman to effectively communicate and handle the situation — the CONES protocol:

- C: Context. Physical context is important, your body language, shaking hands, appearing relaxed and calm.
- O: Opening remark. To set the scene use phrases such as 'I'd like to talk to you about...' It is also worth giving a warning shot of what is to come. Saying 'sorry' is paramount.
- N: Narrative. Explaining events in a logical way, pausing to respond to a patient's emotions. Answer questions honestly and truthfully. When you are not sure do not hesitate to say that you do not know but will find out and get back to them. Also, accept and convey that the outlook could be bad.

- E: Emotions. Showing an empathetic response, identifying the patient's emotions, identifying the cause of the emotion (as in this case it is obvious), and responding in a way to show that you are acknowledging their emotions.
- S: Strategy and Summary. 'The front-burner' strategy, making the patient realise that this is a priority for you, and your care for the patient continues and does not stop. Also, it is important to mention follow-up actions on your part offering a chance to answer any further queries.

Key Points

- Patients must be informed about the exact nature and scale of the error.
- Address immediate distress and possible implications and long-term effects.
- Explain how the mistake came about and what steps are being put in place to prevent the same error from happening again.
- Explain that the mistake is being investigated and express regret that such an event has occurred.
- Put aside some time to address the patient's anxiety, express regret and show humility.
- Form an action plan with the patient and prioritise the patient's needs.

References

1. Buckman R. Disclosing error: the CONES protocol. In: Buckman R. *Practical plans for difficult conversations in medicine.* Baltimore: Johns Hopkins University Press; 2010.

2. MacDonald E. Overall plan of management of difficult conversations. In: Macdonald E. *Difficult Conversations in Medicine.* Oxford, United Kingdom: Oxford University Press; 2004.

Question 49

Explaining to a patient that you gave a wrong diagnosis

Rupa Jayaraj

Question

You are a junior doctor working on the cancer ward. A patient, Mr Khan, came to the outpatient clinic a week ago with a lump in his armpit. Upon initial investigations, this was deemed a benign lump. However, in the medical notes it was described as 'malignant'. After seeing this, you spoke to the patient and broke the bad news to them that they had a cancerous lesion.

However, after speaking with your senior consultant today, she tells you that the lump is benign and that all the investigations have proved this. A meeting with the multidisciplinary team also confirms this. Mr Khan is not aware of the misdiagnosis. You must speak to Mr Khan and explain this error. An examiner will observe your communication skills in this station.

Themes for discussion (■ Table 3.11)

Table 3.11.		
	Question themes	**What is expected from the candidate?**
1	The candidate introduces themselves.	'Hello, my name is [name] and I am a junior doctor working on this ward. You may remember that we met recently to discuss the diagnosis of the lump in your armpit.'
		'Can you please confirm your name, and date of birth?'
		The candidate should show empathy with their body language, and also speak clearly but calmly.
2	The candidate asks for consent to talk with Mr Khan about their diagnosis.	'As you may recall, we met previously to discuss the lump in your armpit. Is it OK to discuss the diagnosis with you?'
		'Before we begin, would you like any friends, family members or staff present?'
3	The candidate apologises; the keyword is 'sorry'.	'First of all, I would like to apologise and tell you that I gave you misinformation about your diagnosis the last time we met. Your armpit lump is not cancerous. All investigations show that it is benign. I am sorry about this. I have checked all information and discussed it with my senior consultant before I came here.'
		'I understand that this information may come as a shock to you. I am sorry; I understand that the false diagnosis could have caused you a lot of emotional distress.'
4	Mr Khan is upset as he had told all his family and friends and was not able to sleep properly this week.	'I can understand why you are upset, and I am sorry that you have felt distressed the past week.'
		'This mistake was made by the team. Whilst the investigations show the lump to be benign, it was incorrectly described as cancerous in the patient notes. I was misled by the clinical documentation. I am sorry.'

Table 3.11.

	Question themes	What is expected from the candidate?
		'I can assure you that we as a team will not leave this matter unaddressed. We will report it to the hospital incident reporting system and reflect on our own actions to ensure that we do not make a similar mistake in the future.'
		The candidate should maintain eye contact and show active listening. They should also allow time for pauses so that Mr Khan has time to process the information.
5	The candidate offers Mr Khan to speak with the consultant later if he wishes.	'Do you have any more questions for me now? I can arrange a meeting with a consultant so that you can talk in more detail and address any concerns.'
6	Mr Khan asks the candidate to promise him it is not cancer.	The candidate does not promise, but goes on to explain that from all the investigations and discussions with the team, they are confident it is not cancer.
7	Mr Khan wants to complain as he is 'upset going through a terrible time in the last week'.	'I am sorry that you are upset, and I can talk you through our hospital complaints procedure. I can also give you this leaflet that talks you through the process of registering a complaint.'
		The candidate can mention the Patient Advice and Liaison Service (PALS).
		'If you would like, I can request a senior member of staff to come and talk to you in order to address any questions and concerns.'
		The candidate explains that this will be discussed in the team/audit meeting, and steps will be taken to ensure that such an error does not happen again.
8	The candidate asks Mr Khan if he is OK. Once again, they apologise and conclude the session.	The candidate thanks the patient for their time. 'Once again I am sorry, and is there anything else that I can do for you today?'

Role play for the actor

The actor is playing the role of the patient Mr Khan. Mr Khan is visibly distressed at the beginning of the role play; it is evident that the misdiagnosis has taken an emotional toll on him. When told the correct diagnosis, Mr Khan is initially unable to process the information and remains in disbelief. Mr Khan then becomes upset and angry about the false information he was given and wishes to lodge a complaint at the end of the role play.

Discussion

A candidate may make the mistake of viewing this role-play situation in a light-hearted manner. After all, many patients given a cancer diagnosis would hope that it was, in fact, mistakenly given. However, it is easy to underestimate the emotional toll that a false diagnosis can take on a patient, no matter the nature of the true diagnosis. A good candidate will show empathy and use active listening skills to understand and address Mr Khan's emotions, without discounting them.

A medical error, such as delivering a false diagnosis, is a situation that can damage the patient-clinician relationship. In order for a clinician to restore the patient's trust, an apology alone is not sufficient. In addition, a clinician should describe how they and/or the medical team are going to reflect and better themselves, such that a similar mistake is not repeated in the future. A good way of doing this is by mentioning the concept of the hospital incidence reporting system and the appraisal process, which are methods by which clinicians work on continuing professional development.

Key Points

- Listen to the patient in order to understand their views and emotions.
- Do not just tell the patient that you will 'do better'. Tell them how you will work towards reflecting and making this positive change.
- Make the patient aware of their right to complain and offer to talk them through the hospital complaints procedure.

References

1.   General Medical Council. Continuing professional development. Available from: https://www.gmc-uk.org/education/standards-guidance-and-curricula/guidance/continuing-professional-development.

Question 50

A patient taking herbal medicines

Vijaianitha Nallendran

Question

You are a doctor in a GP surgery. You are about to meet Ms Patel who is 58 years old and experiencing postmenopausal bleeding. On questioning she informs you that she has been experiencing menopausal symptoms in the form of hot flushes and night sweats. She says she has been taking St John's wort for the last few years and it has been helping her with the symptoms.

You as a clinician realise that her postmenopausal bleeding could be caused by herbal medicine and that the patient should no longer take her medication. You also realise during the conversation that Ms Patel does not have a good command of English and you have to keep repeating yourself during the consultation.

This is a role-play scenario; you must explain to Ms Patel and convince her to stop taking the herbal medicine as it is the cause of her postmenopausal bleeding. You are the only available clinician in the GP surgery today. An examiner will observe to assess your communication skills in this station.

Themes for discussion (■ Table 3.12)

Table 3.12.	
Question themes	**What is expected from the candidate?**
1 The candidate introduces themselves and confirms the identity of the patient.	'Hello, my name is Dr X and I am a doctor at this GP surgery.' 'Can you please state your name, and date of birth?'
2 The candidate should make sure that the patient is able to understand them. They ask whether they would need the help of an interpreter to improve communication. Ms Patel does not want an interpreter.	GMC recommendation: 'You must give the patient the information they want or need to know in a way that they can understand. You should make sure that arrangements are made, wherever possible, to meet a patient's language and communication needs.' 'Ms Patel, do you need an interpreter to translate what I am saying?' Ms Patel states that she does not want a translator. 'OK Ms Patel, I will begin the consultation now. Please let me know at any point if you are unsure about what I am saying and want me to speak slower or repeat myself.'
3 The candidate takes a good history and communicates well.	The candidate can listen to the patient with empathy regarding her menopausal symptoms. Listening without interruption, probing questions when needed and the ability to empathise are the qualities that will score points for the candidate.
4 The candidate gives clear information on the evidence regarding St John's wort.	'I understand that St John's wort has been making you feel better; however, this can be the cause for your postmenopausal bleeding.' 'When you buy St John's wort over the counter, it can vary in dose, the strength of the effect and how long the relief lasts. Without a doctor or pharmacist to monitor the type and dose of the medicine, there is a greater risk of side effects such as postmenopausal bleeding, as you are experiencing.'

Table 3.12.

Question themes	What is expected from the candidate?
5 Ms Patel becomes angry when told to stop taking St John's wort. She says that her menopausal bleeding is affecting her family life and she is in distress.	The candidate stays calm and listens to the concerns and distress of Ms Patel. They actively listen and, when she finishes talking, tell her the need to stop taking herbal medicine. 'Herbal medicine could be the cause of your bleeding and it is wise to stop and assess.' 'I can understand your distress and am sorry for this. But you need to listen to how we can help you now. We are suggesting this in your best interest.'
6 The candidate is able to listen with empathy regarding the patient's concerns and acknowledges their concern.	It is important to develop a relationship with the patient. For this, actively listening to the patient's views and being empathetic to the patient's concerns is important. The GMC recommendations regarding communication: • You must listen to patients, take account of their views, and respond honestly to their questions. • You must work in partnership with patients, sharing with them the information they will need to make decisions about their care, including: their condition, its likely progression, and the options for treatment, including associated risks and uncertainties.
7 The candidate can give alternative treatment recommendations.	It is an added advantage if the candidate has knowledge about hormone replacement therapy and can help to counsel the patient appropriately. If the candidate does not have the correct knowledge, they need to inform the patient that they are unable to advise alternatives, but would however be able to give them further information once they speak to senior staff. This should score them more marks.

Table 3.12.

	Question themes	What is expected from the candidate?
		The GMC recommendations: • You must keep your professional knowledge and skills up to date. • You must be honest and trustworthy in all your communication with patients and colleagues. This means that you must make clear the limits of your knowledge and ensure that any information that you give is accurate.
8	The candidate is able to provide information regarding websites that might empower the patient with the knowledge to make the right decisions.	If the candidate recommends to the patient information leaflets and websites to provide her with more information to make decisions, this should score more points.
9	The candidate refers the patient to specialist clinics such as a gynaecology clinic or postmenopausal bleed clinic.	The candidate should refer the patient via the appropriate channels to the postmenopausal bleeding clinic to investigate and manage their condition.
10	Conclusion.	The candidate confirms that the patient has understood everything and makes sure that the patient does not have any further questions.
11	Global impression about the candidate's communication skills.	The candidate's ability to develop a good rapport with the patient and their ability to convince the patient to stop taking the medication should score them points.

Role play for the actor

The actor was told to act as Ms Patel. She had to show that she did not have a good grasp of English knowledge and had to ask the doctor to repeat the conversations again and again until the doctor asked whether they would need help from an interpreter. She will decline the need for an interpreter.

The actor was asked to become extremely upset when the doctor asked them to stop taking the herbal medicine that is helping her be able to carry on with her life without major problems. She was instructed to give information about the menopausal symptoms that were significantly affecting her quality of life, when asked specifically by the candidate.

She is really concerned that she had a terrible time when she had hot flushes. She was very irritable, unable to sleep, had mood swings and had terrible fights with her husband.

Discussion

This is an important station and most MMIs have an angry or unsatisfied patient. The aim of this station is to check whether the candidate can listen, communicate and show empathy. If the candidate can convince the patient to follow their advice and make them stop taking the medication, it is a success for this station.

The UK General Medical Council's (GMC) 'Good medical practice' guidance, Domain 3 (Communication partnership and teamwork) stresses that doctors must listen to patients, take account of their views, and respond honestly to their questions. The GMC guidance for medical students also promotes the same messages, but gives advice to inform supervisors involved in the care.

Listening is an active skill and needs to be developed; at the same time, most stations last for 5-7 minutes, and the candidate must impart appropriate knowledge, develop a relationship and convince the patient for the task, i.e. stop the medication. Practising repeatedly with mock actors can give confidence to the candidate to face real MMI scenarios.

As a medical student, the GMC expects that they not only learn the scientific and clinical aspects but have the professional skills and identity that will help them provide a high standard of care to their patients. Having good communication skills helps to develop a good partnership with patients.

Key Points

- In a patient role-play scenario, it is important to introduce yourself and confirm that you are speaking to the right patient.
- Checking the need for additional support such as interpreters will score points.
- It is important to listen to the patient and be empathetic towards their concerns and explain and convince them to stop taking medications. It is important to treat them with respect whatever their life choices and beliefs.
- It is important to empower patients with knowledge by providing them with information leaflets and important websites.
- Always conclude the session; if it is a patient role play, do not forget to ask if there is anything else that the patient wants.

References

1. General Medical Council. Good medical practice. Domain 3: Communication partnership and teamwork. Available from: https://www.gmc-uk.org/ethical-guidance/ethical-guidance-for-doctors/good-medical-practice/domain-3---communication-partnership-and-teamwork#paragraph-31.

2. General Medical Council. Achieving good medical practice: guidance for medical students. Domain 4: Maintaining trust. Available from: https://www.gmc-uk.org/education/standards-guidance-and-curricula/guidance/student-professionalism-and-ftp/achieving-good-medical-practice/domain-4-maintaining-trust#act-with-honesty-and-integrity.

Question 51

An anxious mother: her child is in pain

Priya Gauthama

Question

You are a junior doctor working in a GP surgery. You are seeing a 10-year-old boy, Jack. His mother, Karen, is very anxious and worried about Jack's headache.

This is a role-play scenario; you must talk to Karen and address her questions and worries. An examiner will be observing and assessing your communication skills.

Themes for discussion (■ Table 3.13)

Table 3.13.	
Question themes	**What is expected from the candidate?**
1 The candidate introduces themselves.	The candidate understands the complexity but stays calm and has a good approach. They should show empathy with their body language, and speak clearly but calmly.

Table 3.13.

	Question themes	What is expected from the candidate?
2	The candidate confirms that they are speaking to the right patient — the mother Karen (about her child Jack).	It is important that the candidate introduces themselves and checks that they are speaking to the correct patient. In real life, they might check the date of birth and address also.
3	Karen is worried that Jack's headache has been there for a while and not getting better.	Listen calmly to Karen to obtain more details on the headache. Reassure her, saying that headaches can be common at his age. Ask the following: Jack's vision, whether it has been tested recently, does he have any medical problems, whether he is on any regular medication, any vomiting, if anyone in the family is experiencing migraines, etc.
4	Additional questions from the candidate.	The candidate should ask if there are any issues in the school with his friends or any recent bereavement in the family and check about any triggers for his headaches, any fears or worries. Check whether he drinks enough water, eats on time, takes good physical exercise and sleeps well. Is Karen giving her son any painkillers for his headache relief?
		It is vital to take a history whilst being empathetic and giving confidence to the mother that her worries are being taken seriously.
5	Karen is still worried about his pain and concerned something could be wrong with his brain and asks for investigations such as an MRI of the brain.	Reassurance is the key here. Try to explain that the examination is normal.
		The candidate could insist on following simple strategies and review this after a week. In the meantime, Karen will maintain a headache diary. The candidate explains that they have discussed Jack with senior consultants or paediatricians and they have advised and been reassured that everything is normal and that clinical management guidelines have been followed.
		If Karen is not convinced with the answer, the candidate can explain the option of referral to hospital doctors for further assessment and investigation.

Table 3.13.

	Question themes	What is expected from the candidate?
6	Now, Karen slowly opens up about her own significant anxiety whenever Jack gets ill.	If the candidate asks empathetically, Karen will explain that she is experiencing anxiety. Listen to her concerns and worries; if she is in tears, offer her tissues and wait for her to settle. 'I am sorry to hear about your health.' 'Have you mentioned this to your GP?' 'I suggest that you get support for your condition.' 'I can write to your GP who can make all the necessary arrangements to help with your anxiety.'
7	Karen asks again whether there is anything serious.	The candidate reassures her and says that all protocols and guidelines have been followed. Jack has received the best care and he has no serious problems.
8	The candidate provides a plan for follow-up.	The candidate explains that Jack will be followed up in the outpatient clinic to make sure that the symptoms are settled. If not, appropriate investigations or treatment can be planned.
9	Global impression of the communication.	The candidate listens to the mother and allays her anxiety. They have been confident and empathetic at the same time.
10	Conclusion.	The candidate concludes the session by asking, 'Is there anything else that I can do please?'

Role play for the actor

The actor was told to act as Karen. She had to be anxious and explain her worries about her son Jack's headache. She will explain her constant worries about Jack's pain. She will be asked to be nervous. Karen has been asked to open up to her own anxiety at the end.

Discussion

Parental anxiety is the term for anxiety related to a parent. It is a constant worry about their child's health and well-being, performance at school, and social activities. Most people will be anxious about their child's well-being. However, it can become worse in some and the parents will explain their constant worry about their child, not getting enough sleep by thinking about their children, having persistent thoughts that something could happen to their child, and excessive thoughts over minor illnesses relating to their children. It is a known fact that parental anxiety can have an impact on their relationship with their children, increasing their anxiety and fear as well.

A child with anxiety can experience a pounding heartbeat, breathing issues or chest pain, headaches, feeling dizzy, and sweating.

Key Points

- An empathetic approach and active listening to concerns are vital in these situations.
- Provide reassurance to the parent whilst making sure the patient is followed up.
- Explore illness/medical issues in the family affecting the children and offer professional help to the parents if needed.

References

1.   Katz B. Child Mind Institute. How to avoid passing anxiety on to your kids? Available from: https://childmind.org/article/how-to-avoid-passing-anxiety-on-to-your-kids.

Question 52

Anxiety for a blood test

Siva Thanthullu

Question

You are a junior doctor in a GP surgery; the supervising GP is busy and asks you to talk to an anxious patient, Alex, who is refusing to have a blood test. Alex has come in for a routine blood test but is very anxious. You need to find out the reasons for this and allay his anxiety. The examiner will observe your communication skills in this station.

Themes for discussion (■ Table 3.14)

Table 3.14.

	Question themes	What is expected from the candidate?
1	The candidate introduces themselves.	The candidate understands the complexity but stays calm and has a good approach. They should show empathy with their body language, and speak clearly but calmly.

Table 3.14.

Question themes	What is expected from the candidate?
	As Alex is anxious, the candidate allows the patient to talk and actively listens and finds the reasons for their anxiety.
2 The candidate confirms that they are speaking to the right patient, Alex.	It is important that the candidate introduces themselves and checks that they are speaking to the correct patient. In real life, they might check the date of birth and address also.
	The candidate checks the reasons for Alex's visit to the GP surgery, and having a blood test.
3 The candidate tries to talk to Alex and find the reason for the anxiety.	'Hi Alex, do you mind if I ask you why you are not keen to have your blood test today?'
	'Do you want to tell me how you feel about having your blood tests today please?'
	After gentle questioning, the role player says that he is upset and does not want any blood tests. He further informs that he does not like needles.
4 Empathetic approach from the candidate.	'We are here to help you. Is there anything we can do to help you Alex?'
	'We will not do anything without your permission, please be reassured.'
	The candidate has an empathetic approach, with convincing body language in a confident manner, and gains a rapport with Alex to open up about his issues.

Table 3.14.

Question themes	What is expected from the candidate?
5 The candidate reflects that they understand Alex's feelings.	'I appreciate your feelings, Alex.' 'I totally understand that the needles and blood test can be stressful.' The candidate is calm and composed; they show that they understand the feelings of the role player.
6 Once the role player is convinced that the candidate has an empathetic approach and is supportive, he opens up saying 'My brother had a blood test and was found to have cancer!'	The role player only opens up if the candidate has the right empathetic approach. Once Alex opens up regarding his fear, the candidate immediately responds by explaining Alex's feelings. The candidate says sorry for Alex's feelings and is supportive and empathetic. 'I am sorry to hear this. Is your brother OK now?' If Alex is in tears at this time, the candidate could offer tissues to help console him.
7 The candidate tries to find out what happened with his brother; this could help in further consultation.	The candidate finds out how his brother is now. When asked gently, the role player says that his brother is having treatment with chemotherapy and radiotherapy in the hospital. 'I hope that your brother gets well soon; please take care.'
8 The candidate explains the need for the blood test; stresses the importance given the history.	'I know that you have come for a routine blood test. It is important that you have this yearly check.' 'I hope everything will be fine, but given your brother's recent history, I want you to have this blood test to reassure yourself.'

Table 3.14.

	Question themes	What is expected from the candidate?
		The candidate stresses the need for a blood test, and explains in very simple language the procedure and the practicalities.
		If the candidate knows the name of Alex's brother, he could quote this in this conversation to create a closer rapport.
9	The candidate asks if there are any other worries and makes sure that there are none.	'Is there anything else that worries you Alex?' 'Are you happy to proceed with your blood test today please?' 'Is there anything else that is not clear with your blood test Alex?'
10	Conclusion.	The candidate thanks the patient and explains that the team is there to support Alex. The candidate concludes the session by asking, 'Is there anything else that I can do please?'

Role play for the actor

The actor was told to act as Alex, a patient who is very anxious. He opens up only when the candidate gives an empathetic, reassuring approach. Otherwise, he will just disclose that he does not want a blood test, is upset and does not like needles.

Once the candidate is supportive, Alex will open up to explain that his brother had a blood test and was found to have cancer. Alex is worried about having a blood test due to this, in case he is also found to have cancer. Alex's brother is progressing well with the treatment and is having chemotherapy and radiotherapy. If the candidate demonstrates an empathetic approach,

Alex will agree to have a blood test.

Discussion

Anxiety is a normal reaction to uncertainty and the unknown; patients coming to the hospital or having medical interventions can be anxious. Effective communication with active listening can help this distress in patients.

It is important to be honest and keep the conversation in simple understandable language. Asking what concerns the patient has and helping them open up to their issues can help doctors to understand the reasons for their anxiety. Staying calm and having an empathetic approach helps in these situations.

Relatives of patients diagnosed with cancer can experience anxiety and depression due to stress reactions. Communication within the family and explaining the medical process can help family members.

Key Points

- An empathetic approach and active listening to concerns are important.
- The key is to help the patient open up about their issues or reasons for anxiety.
- Explain the need for a blood test and stress the importance given the family history mentioned by the patient.

References

1.   Edwards B, Clarke V. The psychological impact of a cancer diagnosis on families: the influence of family functioning and patients' illness characteristics on depression and anxiety. *Psycho-oncology* 2004; 13(8): 562-76.

Question 53

Vaccination in a teenager: an anxious parent

Subramanian Ganesan

Question

You are working as a junior doctor in a GP surgery. You are seeing Amanda, who is 13 years old along with her mother Rosie; they are worried about the letter received from the school nurse regarding teenage vaccination. Please talk to them to address their concerns. The examiner will observe your communication skills in this station.

Themes for discussion (■ Table 3.15)

Table 3.15.	
Question themes	**What is expected from the candidate?**
1 The candidate greets the examiner, has good body language and speaks coherently.	The candidate is presentable and uses good communication skills; always recommended in any station.

Table 3.15.

Question themes	What is expected from the candidate?
2 The candidate introduces himself to Amanda and Rosie.	The candidate introduces themselves, asks the name of the people and confirms that they are speaking to the correct people.
3 The candidate asks about the concerns of the patient and the mother.	'Tell me what brings you here today please?' 'I understand that you are worried by this letter regarding vaccination; can you explain what worries you, Rosie?' 'I am sorry to hear about your worries; we are here to help you. Let me start by asking what worries you Rosie and Amanda?'
4 The candidate actively listens to the mother and the patient.	If asked empathetically, the role player, mother Rosie, will explain that she is worried about the human papillomavirus (HPV) vaccine given to all teenagers. The candidate says sorry for their worries and asks Rosie specifically what worries her regarding the vaccine.
5 The mother Rosie says that she does not want her teenage daughter to have the vaccine; she finds no reason for her daughter to have it and is worried about the side effects.	'I understand your worries Rosie, but let me explain why Amanda needs this vaccine.' 'This is a national programme in which all teenagers get the vaccine.' 'Girls and boys aged 12-13 years routinely get this HPV vaccine in two doses to protect them against cancers caused by this virus including cancer in the cervix, mouth, throat, anal and genital areas.' 'The vaccine is safe and effective; a vaccine can only be used if scientific tests, called clinical trials, have shown that it is safe and effective, and that the benefits outweigh any risks.'

Table 3.15.	
Question themes	**What is expected from the candidate?**
	'The HPV vaccine is used worldwide, including the UK, Australia, USA, Canada and most western countries; more than 100 million people are vaccinated worldwide.'
	The candidate explains the scientific facts, whilst giving confidence in simple understandable language.
6 Amanda is worried about pain during vaccination.	'Amanda, it will hurt, but it is a very tiny needle. The school nurse will do it gently and one of your friends can stay next to you if you wish also.'
	'You need this vaccine to prevent some cancers. It is essential that you have this please.'
	'We will make sure that it is done gently and there will be someone to support you throughout the process.'
7 The candidate checks that both the teenager and mother are happy and reassured.	The candidate confirms that both Amanda and Rosie are happy and reassured.
	'Is there anything else that worries you? Anything else that you want to ask me please?'
8 Conclusion.	The candidate concludes and thanks both Rosie and Amanda; they promise to arrange the vaccination.
	'Is there anything else that I can do for you both today please?'

Discussion

The World Health Organization (WHO) says that the two public health interventions that have had the greatest impact on the world's health are clean water and vaccines. In the United Kingdom, 'Immunisation against infectious disease', also known as the 'Green Book', has the latest information on vaccines and vaccination procedures. The teenage vaccines are given as part of the national immunisation programme.

Vaccines for teenagers include:

- At the age of 12 to 13 years — the HPV vaccine is in two doses.
- At the age of 14 years — a 3-in-1 teenage booster; meningitis ACWY vaccine (against meningococcal A, C, W and Y strains).

The HPV vaccine helps to protect individuals against cancers caused by human papillomavirus that include cervical cancer, some mouth and throat cancers, and cancers of the anal and genital areas. In England, girls and boys are routinely offered the first HPV vaccine when they are in year 8 (12-13 years old). The second dose is offered after 6-24 months. It is important to have both doses for proper protection.

As with all vaccines, some people may have minor side effects, such as mild swelling, redness or tenderness where the injection is given. But usually, this settles down with cautious monitoring and judicial use of painkillers (paracetamol or ibuprofen). Sometimes a small painless lump develops, but this usually disappears in a few weeks. More serious effects are rare, but include fever, headache, dizziness, feeling sick and swollen glands.

Key Points

- Active listening to both the mother and patient is important; allay their anxiety with confidence and by using simple understandable language.
- Stress the importance of vaccination and explain that it is scientifically proven to be safe and effective.
- Before concluding, ask if there are any other concerns.

References

1. Public Health England. Immunisations for young people. Available from: https://www.gov.uk/government/publications/immunisations-for-young-people.

2. NHS UK. HPV vaccine overview. Available from: https://www.nhs.uk/conditions/vaccinations/hpv-human-papillomavirus-vaccine.

3. NHS UK. HPV vaccine safety. Available from: https://www.nhs.uk/conditions/vaccinations/hpv-vaccine-safety.

Section**4**

Communication — general scenarios

Section editor: Shreya Shyam

Introduction to non-medical communication

A good doctor should be a good communicator. In the medical communication role-play setting (which we have seen in Section 3), the candidate is given the role of a medical student or a clinician and must communicate with a patient. Example situations included: breaking bad news, explaining a clinical procedure, apologising for a mistake, etc.

One limitation of medical communication role plays is that the questions are often variations of the same concept and therefore it is possible for the candidate to memorise and deliver a formulaic answer.

Therefore, there is importance for non-medical communication stations. These stations have a variety of role-play situations ranging from apologising to an elderly neighbour for running over their cat, to teaching the role-play actor to tie their shoelaces. Due to the diversity of scenarios, there is no fixed approach a candidate can take, and the station tests the versatility and adaptability of the candidate's communication skills.

In particular, the situations in non-medical role-play situations are often complex; in real life, they would require a much longer time to resolve than the 5 minutes given in the interview station. It is easy for a candidate to become fixated on 'solving' the situation quickly within the given time frame, when the focus of the station is in fact for 'communicating' as effectively as possible in the available time. The example questions in this chapter illustrate some of the key communication skills looked for by the examiner in the candidate's performance.

Question 54

Damaged a friend's iPad

Hari Adharsh Prabhu

Question

You and your friend Jake are both second-year medical students. You have borrowed your friend's iPad device to complete a project. By accident, you knocked the device off the edge of a table and broke it. You have to tell your friend this bad news and calm him down. An examiner will observe to assess your communication skills.

Themes for discussion (■ Table 4.1)

Table 4.1.	
Question themes	**What is expected from the candidate?**
1 The candidate greets the examiner appropriately, and communicates effectively with positive body language.	The candidate introduces themselves, taking care to remember that they are talking to a friend who knows them.

Table 4.1.

Question themes	What is expected from the candidate?
	'Hi Jake, it's me [insert name].'
	Communication is clear and appropriately paced, with regular pauses integrated at appropriate times to allow the friend to process the conversation.
2 Role play starts. The candidate initiates the conversation with a pre-emptive phrase.	'Jake, is this an OK time for me to tell you something important?'
	The candidate pre-empts the bad news with an appropriate warning shot, such as 'I am very sorry, but I have some bad news to tell you'.
	Reducing the shock of the bad news is important, as this gives the friend time to mentally prepare themselves.
3 The candidate breaks the news appropriately, being apologetic, succinct, and clear in their communication.	The candidate breaks the news in a sensitive and succinct manner, assuming full responsibility for breaking the device.
	'I'm really sorry Jake; as you know, I borrowed your iPad to finish a project. By accident, I knocked the tablet off a table and broke it. It was completely my mistake, I'm really very sorry.'
4 The friend acts angrily; the candidate maintains an apologetic manner and stays composed.	The candidate profusely apologises, displaying empathy and open body language. Making eye contact and facing the friend is very important.
	The candidate regularly pauses and allows the friend to voice their thoughts and feelings.

Table 4.1.

Question themes	What is expected from the candidate?
5 The candidate displays active listening and tries to calm the friend down, offering reassurance and empathy.	The candidate listens to what the friend tells them and asks appropriate questions or makes suggestions based on what they have been told. 'I completely understand that the iPad will be expensive to replace; I remember how careful you always were with it. I will do my best to compensate you for it.' 'I understand why you feel angry; you trusted me to take care of the device, but instead I broke it by mistake. You are right to be upset, and I'll do my best to make this up to you.'
6 The actor is still angry as the device was a gift from his girlfriend and because he needs it for his university work.	'I will do my best to replace the device and make this up to you.' 'I know that the device was a gift from your girlfriend, and I will apologise to her as well. Jake, I know that you are angry, and you may not trust me anymore, but I'll do my best to make things right.'
The candidate offers a solution to the broken device.	'I know that you use the device for university work. I can lend you my laptop until I'm able to replace yours.' 'Is there anything in particular you want me to do that will work towards fixing this mistake?' The candidate should convince the friend that his emotion has been respected and that they understand the importance of the device, as it was gifted by someone very important.
7 The candidate explains how they will prevent this from happening again in the future.	'I think I've learnt that I am too clumsy and sometimes careless with expensive items. I will work towards being more careful in the future.'

Table 4.1.

	Question themes	What is expected from the candidate?
		The candidate says that they will take steps to ensure this does not occur again, such as by keeping fragile items away from the edge of the table in the future, or by taking greater care with valuable items.
		The candidate shows a desire to reflect on the situation and the mistake, by showing what they have learnt from the mistake.
8	Role play ends. Conclusion.	'I'm sorry again Jake. Thank you for talking things through with me and I'll definitely work to make this up to you.'
		The candidate draws the conversation to a close, by agreeing to an appropriate solution with the friend.
		'Is there anything else I can do for you right now?'
		The candidate thanks the examiner and the role player after the role play ends.

Role play for the actor

The actor was told to act as the candidate's friend Jake. Jake will talk about their daily life until the candidate appropriately attempts to take control of the conversation (such as by saying 'I have something important I want to talk to you about; would now be a good time?'). After the bad news is broken, Jake will become very angry and shout at the candidate, using phrases such as 'I thought I could trust you', and 'How could you be so careless?' Jake will only calm down if the candidate accepts full responsibility, apologises multiple times, and keeps calm without raising their voice.

Discussion

Many MMIs will have a role-play station in which the candidate must either break bad news or apologise for making a mistake. This station will assess interpersonal skills and the ability to empathise with others, so both verbal and non-verbal communication is of paramount importance.

Another key skill that the examiners will seek is the ability of the candidate to accept responsibility and say 'sorry'. Honesty and accepting responsibility are features of the 'duty of candour', which became a legal requirement for clinicians following the introduction of The Health and Social Care Act in 2008. The duty of candour dictates that every healthcare professional should be open and honest when things go wrong with the treatment or care that causes or could cause potential harm to the patient. Being honest and admitting to the mistake is very important in ensuring that a patient's trust in the medical profession is maintained, also allowing patients to make fully informed autonomous decisions about their healthcare. Although this role play is not in a clinical setting, medical students and doctors are expected to follow principles of morality and honesty in both their clinical and non-clinical lives.

During the conversation, the candidate can ask some open-ended questions to allow the friend to speak their mind. They should respond to their friend's concerns in a manner that shows they are listening and taking them seriously. This is active listening, an especially important skill to develop for MMIs. Offering solutions to the problem will help to ease the friend's anxieties and defuse the situation. Reflection is a key skill of a doctor, so in this station you should reflect on why the mistake occurred and explain to the friend what you will do to prevent a similar mistake in the future.

Key Points

- Introduce yourself to the examiner and role player with appropriate body language. First impressions are always important.
- Ensure you ask them if they are free to talk prior to breaking the bad news and use a pre-emptive phrase to reduce the shock of the bad news. Also, be succinct and honest when breaking bad news.
- Maintain an empathetic manner throughout. Communicate at the correct pace and volume, display open body language by facing towards the friend, and make eye contact to increase trust and rapport during the conversation.
- Allow the friend to dictate the pace of the discussion, regularly pausing to allow them to pose their opinions, and process the discussion so far.
- Listen actively and ask appropriate questions/use phrases to display your understanding of their emotions and thoughts.
- Offer solutions for the future and reassure them that you will take full responsibility for your actions, showing them what you have learnt and how you will prevent this from happening again.
- Conclude the station appropriately, by checking if there is anything else that you can do for the friend.

References

1. General Medical Council. Good medical practice. Domain 4: Maintaining trust. Available from: https://www.gmc-uk.org/ethical-guidance/ethical-guidance-for-pas-and-aas/good-medical-practice-interim-standards-for-physician-associates-and-anaesthesia-associates/domain-4--maintaining-trust.

2. Shekar V, Brennan PA. Duty of candour and keeping patients safe. *Surgery* (Oxford) 2020; 38(10): 637-41.

3. UK Legislation. Health and social care act 2008. Available from: https://www.legislation.gov.uk/ukpga/2008/14/contents.

Question 55

Checking on a friend whose mood has recently changed

Hari Adharsh Prabhu

Question

Your friend Mike, who is normally very studious and organised, has been acting differently lately. You are in the same team working on a group project at medical school. He seems very distant and withdrawn and is frequently late for meetings. His quality of work has also dropped. You suspect he is going through a difficult time, and you need to ask him to get support. How do you go about informing him?

An examiner will assess your communication skills in this station.

Themes for discussion (■ Table 4.2)

Table 4.2.

	Question themes	What is expected from the candidate?
1	The candidate greets the actor and examiner appropriately, communicating effectively with positive body language.	'Hi Mike, it's me [insert name].' Communication is clear and appropriately paced, with regular pauses integrated at appropriate times to allow the friend to contribute to the conversation.
2	Role play starts. The candidate initiates the conversation in a confidential setting.	'Mike, is this an OK time for me to talk to you about something important?' 'Can we please talk somewhere in private?' The candidate understands the importance of maintaining the confidentiality of sensitive information, and therefore conducting the discussion in a private setting. The candidate reassures Mike that they are only trying to help and that anything they talk about will be kept confidential.
3	The candidate gently brings attention to the changes in the friend's behaviour, using anecdotes from others.	The candidate initialises the conversation in a casual manner before highlighting the change in the friend's behaviour. 'Mike, we've been friends a while now, and you're always so punctual and hardworking. Recently, though, during our group project sessions, myself and the others have noticed that you seem to be more withdrawn and a bit different from normal. Is everything OK?' The candidate mentions that other colleagues have noticed these changes in order to make the message seem less personal and more objective; therefore, the friend is less likely to become agitated.

Table 4.2.

	Question themes	What is expected from the candidate?
4	The candidate discovers the underlying cause of the friend's deteriorating attitude to work.	The candidate asks open-ended questions to allow the friend to speak their mind and picks up on body language cues.
		'Has anything been going on lately?'
		'Anything you tell me is confidential. I'm only asking because you're my friend, and I care about you.'
		'I am here for you if you need me.'
		The candidate maintains a supportive and empathetic tone and does not jump to any conclusions about the friend and their situation.
		Mike reveals that he has recently started battling depression.
5	The candidate tries to determine other factors that could contribute to depression.	The candidate engages in a discussion to try to determine what is causing the depression.
		'I'm sorry to hear that you have been feeling that way. Did these feelings start recently or after any particular event?'
		This will inform what actions should be taken. It could be caused by physical (deteriorating health), psychological (negative thoughts), social (break-up, bereavement) or financial issues (struggling to afford medical school).
		Mike mentions 'family issues'.

Table 4.2.

	Question themes	What is expected from the candidate?
6	The candidate displays active listening.	The candidate listens to what the friend tells them and asks appropriate questions. The candidate shows an understanding of the importance of making the friend feel that their opinions and emotions have been respected. When the friend mentions 'family issues', the candidate should provide an empathetic response. 'Sorry to hear this Mike, is everything alright at home?' 'We all have trouble at home once in a while, I understand why you are feeling how you are, and I'm here for you.'
7	The candidate encourages Mike to seek help, acting with empathy and understanding.	'Have you talked to your GP or any other support advisers at uni?' 'I think it would be helpful for you to talk about what's going on with someone such as a counsellor or some other trained professional, who'll know how to best support you.' 'I understand that it can be difficult to talk about your home life and I really appreciate the fact that you opened up to me. A trained support worker would also be non-judgemental and give you a confidential space to talk and get support.'
8	Mike asks the candidate about the confidentiality of the conversation.	'Mike, I know that you've put a lot of trust in me by talking to me about what's going on, and I am really grateful for that.' 'This conversation is completely confidential, but as you know, I care about you and don't want you to get hurt.'

Table 4.2.

Question themes	What is expected from the candidate?
	'I really think you should seek support and talk to a trained professional who'll know how best to help you feel better. If you want, I can come along with you to give you support as well.'
	The candidate has to maintain confidentiality, but if the question comes up, they will explain that they might have to break confidentiality if there is a risk to Mike or his patients.
9 Conclusion.	'Thanks again for talking to me Mike. I'm here for you anytime you need me.'
	'Is there anything else you need help with or want to talk about today?'
	The candidate thanks the role player and the examiner.

Role play for the actor

The actor was told to act as the candidate's friend, Mike. Mike will not reveal any information until the candidate asks to speak to them in a confidential setting. Initially he will remain withdrawn and shy, until the candidate discusses their concerns directly with him. After this, Mike can become defensive, using phrases such as: 'I am trying my hardest; why can't you be more grateful?' until the candidate acts calmly and empathetically to gain their trust. Mike will reveal his depression and will mention 'family issues' if asked why he is struggling. Mike will remain reluctant to seek support until the candidate reassures him that the support services are confidential and will act in his best interest.

Discussion

Role-play questions such as these are common in medical school interviews because they are realistic and pose challenges that one may face as a medical student. The examiner will assess the candidate's empathy and ability to provide a non-judgemental and supportive response. The examiner will also assess communication and active listening skills.

It is important for the candidate to consider the many factors that could be affecting their friend's change in behaviour and communicate effectively with them. This is an essential aspect of good team working, which is a key skill that all doctors should have. The GMC's 'Good medical practice' guidance, Domain 3, explains about the importance of team working in further detail.

In a high-pressure environment such as medical school, it is possible for some students to experience anxiety or depression. Medical degrees are very demanding, and it is not uncommon for someone to be overwhelmed by seeing very sick patients or by the workload. Several studies have raised concerns about the prevalence of mental health conditions among medical students. There can be multiple reasons why someone will experience anxiety or depression and the most common reasons are:

- Deteriorating physical health (new disease diagnosis).
- Stress of university workload, exams (no work-life balance).
- Deteriorating mental well-being (excessive negative thinking, demotivation).
- Relationship issues, break-ups, or bereavements.
- Financial difficulties.

The candidate should signpost the actor to the appropriate sources of support. Examples include counsellors within the medical school, a GP or a telephone helpline. To learn more about this, a prospective candidate could refer to the GMC document 'Supporting students with mental health conditions' which gives an overview of mental health conditions faced by medical students and how to identify and support students who are struggling.

Finally, the candidate should maintain the confidentiality of their friend but make them aware that they may have to break confidentiality if the friend appears to be at risk, instead recommending that the friend seeks support from an appropriate source.

Key Points

- Ensure that you ask the friend if this is an appropriate time to discuss something important with them.
- Reassure them that anything you discuss is confidential and that you are only trying to help them.
- Look at them holistically and consider any physical or psychosocial factors that could be affecting them. This will affect how you respond to their specific issues.
- Show empathy, speak slowly and ask open questions that allow them to control the conversation.
- Encourage the friend to seek help from a qualified professional. Reassure them that you only want to help, and will provide a safe, confidential space to discuss any issues.

References

1. General Medical Council. Good medical practice. Domain 3: Communication partnership and teamwork. Available from: https://www.gmc-uk.org/ethical-guidance/ethical-guidance-for-doctors/good-medical-practice/domain-3---communication-partnership-and-teamwork#.

2. Dyrbye LN, Thomas MR, Shanafelt TD. Systematic review of depression, anxiety, and other indicators of psychological distress among U.S. and Canadian medical students. *Acad Med* 2006; 81(4): 354-73.

3. General Medical Council. Supporting students with mental health conditions. Available from: https://www.gmc-uk.org/-/media/documents/Supporting_students_with_mental_health_conditions_0816.pdf_53047904.pdf.

Question 56

Talking to a friend who is a drink-driver

Hari Adharsh Prabhu

Question

You are a student who works part time at a clothing shop. One of your colleagues, Shauna, has recently started coming into work both smelling of alcohol and appearing drunk. You do not know Shauna very well. Shauna is usually picked up by a friend after work; however, today it is clear that she is planning on driving home in an intoxicated state. How would you respond in this situation?

Themes for discussion (■ Table 4.3)

Table 4.3.	
Question themes	**What is expected from the candidate?**
1 The candidate greets the role player appropriately, and communicates effectively with positive body language.	The candidate approaches Shauna in a friendly manner, introduces themselves, and asks if they can talk with them in a private, confidential setting.

Table 4.3.

Question themes	What is expected from the candidate?
	'Hi there Shauna, my name is [insert name]. You've probably seen me working around the store?'
	'If it's alright with you, can we talk privately about something important?'
2 The candidate delicately asks Shauna about her drinking without challenging her outright.	The candidate initially tries to gently nudge Shauna into admitting her intoxication. A friendly manner is preferable to an accusatory tone.
	'Some of the other staff and I have recently noticed that you seem different from normal. Would you like to talk about anything confidential with me? I can be a pretty good listener.'
	If Shauna is reserved and does not respond, the candidate can encourage her further.
	'I know we aren't the closest, but I have heard from the others that you are a hard worker and a brilliant colleague. Recently though, we've noticed that you smell of alcohol and act like you've been drinking. Is there anything you want to talk about?'
3 Shauna opens up and talks about the reasons behind her drinking: her daughter has been recently diagnosed with late-stage cancer.	The candidate shows active listening, by giving Shauna time to talk, maintaining eye contact and responding to her with appropriate body language, e.g. offering to hold her hand, getting her tissues, etc.
	Once Shauna has finished voicing her feelings, the candidate shows empathy and tries to comfort her.
	'I'm really sorry about how you're feeling Shauna. I had no idea that you have been going through this at home.'

Table 4.3.

	Question themes	What is expected from the candidate?
		'Thank you for opening up to me. I understand that you're going through a difficult time, and it means a lot that you were able to open up to me.'
4	The candidate delicately brings up Shauna's drinking habits.	When Shauna seems comforted, the candidate gently brings up the topic of Shauna's drinking, in an empathetic and non-judgemental tone.
		'Did you begin drinking recently, after your daughter's diagnosis?'
		'How often do you drink during the day? Is there anything that makes you drink more or less often?'
		'How does alcohol make you feel? Does it help you to cope with your home situation?'
5	Does Shauna have insight into the problem?	The candidate can ask first whether Shauna realises that it is illegal to drink and drive.
		Is Shauna aware that she is putting herself at risk and putting others at risk by drink-driving?
		If she has insight, she needs access to the correct support and resources to overcome this problem.
		If she does not have insight, this problem can be bigger.
6	After talking to Shauna about her drinking, the candidate explains to her that driving whilst intoxicated could put her and others at risk.	'Shauna, I know that you normally get picked up by your friend when you drive home, but today it seems like you are going to drive?'
		The candidate explains that Shauna is putting herself and others at risk by driving while intoxicated.
	Shauna becomes angry and confronts the candidate.	'I'm sorry that you're angry but I'm telling you because I care about you. If you drive, you could be putting yourself and other people at risk.'

Table 4.3.

	Question themes	What is expected from the candidate?
7	The candidate offers support to Shauna regarding her drink-driving as well as her daughter's situation.	'I don't want you to put yourself or other people on the road at risk, so I'm happy to drive you home today or any other time when you aren't up to driving.'
		'I think that drinking might help you feel better about your situation at the moment; however, in the long term it won't make anything better.'
		'I think you should seek support from an Alcoholics Anonymous group where you can talk about how you are feeling with others in a confidential, non-judgemental setting.'
		'Your GP may have information about a local support group for relatives of patients with cancer. Perhaps you may benefit from talking to people who understand what you are going through and know how to help you.'
8	Conclusion.	'Thank you for opening up to me Shauna. Please find me anytime you need to talk and I'll do my best to support you in any way that I can.'
		The candidate thanks the role player and examiner at the end.

Role play for the actor

The actor will be playing the role of Shauna. Shauna will show signs of intoxication and will initially be reluctant to discuss this with the candidate. When the candidate gently encourages her to open up, she will reveal her daughter's cancer diagnosis as a trigger for her drinking, and she will become very emotional. When the candidate brings up the risks of Shauna driving in her intoxicated state, she will become angry and confrontational. If the candidate remains calm and offers Shauna ways of getting support, then she will become more reassured and more willing to avoid drink-driving.

Discussion

A role-play situation such as this can be emotionally challenging for the candidate. On the one hand, Shauna's home situation is unhappy, and the candidate may be driven by feelings of sympathy and sadness for her. Conversely, it is the candidate's duty to ensure that Shauna does not drive while intoxicated, which would endanger both her and others. The examiner will be assessing the candidate's ability to show empathy and compassion towards Shauna, whilst not allowing emotions to cloud their judgement.

A sign of a good clinician is the ability to show empathy as opposed to sympathy. Sympathy is 'feeling sorry' for an individual. It makes assumptions about the patient's feelings, and evokes pity in the clinician, which can seem condescending and be harmful to the patient. An example of a phrase that demonstrates sympathy is, 'I'm sorry, I know you must be feeling upset right now'. Empathy is an active process; it involves listening to a patient and understanding why they feel how they feel. An example is, 'I understand that you are worried because you are the main earner of your family'. A good candidate is one who listens to Shauna to understand them, rather than making assumptions.

When providing holistic care and support to an individual, it is important to take in all the factors that could be influencing their actions, in this case Shauna's drink-driving. These can generally be classified as physical, psychological and social factors. Repeated alcohol consumption could cause alcohol dependence and take a large physical toll on Shauna, making it difficult for her to break the addiction cycle. The psychological impact of her daughter's cancer diagnosis is a key trigger for Shauna's alcoholism. Social factors such as financial difficulties or a strained home setting could further impact the emotional, and therefore psychological, state of Shauna, further exacerbating the drinking. Addressing and providing support for the underlying causes of alcoholism, as opposed to simply reprimanding Shauna, would be the appropriate approach.

This station can appear in the medical communication section, where a patient reveals their drink-driving. It is your duty to explain the risks. Ethical issues of confidentiality can be discussed in this scenario, but patient and public safety is the priority. In this situation, the candidate explains that, whilst it is the duty of the doctor to care for the patient and maintain confidentiality, they must also protect and promote the health of the public. The candidate can quote Domain 2 of the GMC's 'Good medical practice' guidance.

Key Points

- A compassionate, empathetic manner is more likely to resonate with Shauna compared with an accusatory approach.
- It is important that, whilst you understand the complexity and emotions behind Shauna's situation, you insist that she must not drive whilst intoxicated.
- Communication is key. You should make sure you fully explain to Shauna the risks to herself and the public that are associated with driving whilst drunk.
- You should maintain an empathetic and reassuring manner and refer Shauna to the appropriate support services to address the underlying causes of her alcoholism as well as the alcoholism itself.

References

1. Kisling J. The difference between empathy and sympathy. Available from: https://www.psychmc.com/articles/empathy-vs-sympathy.
2. Becker HC. Alcohol dependence, withdrawal, and relapse. *Alcohol Res Health* 2008; 31(4): 348-61.
3. General Medical Council. Good medical practice. Domain 4: Maintaining trust. Available from: https://www.gmc-uk.org/ethical-guidance/ethical-guidance-for-doctors/good-medical-practice/domain-4---maintaining-trust.

Question 57

A friend who is googling symptoms and is getting anxious

James Francis

Question

You are a medical student. One of your friends, Bob, another student, has recently been feeling unwell. He searched for his symptoms on the internet and now believes that he needs emergency hospitalisation. You need to talk to him and reassure him.

An examiner will observe your communication skills in this station.

Themes for discussion (■ Table 4.4)

Table 4.4.		
	Question themes	**What is expected from the candidate?**
1	The candidate greets the role player, has good body language and speaks coherently.	'Hi Bob, it's me [insert name].'
		The candidate has a friendly approach with eye contact, open body language, etc.

Table 4.4.

	Question themes	What is expected from the candidate?
2	The candidate tries to gain an understanding of Bob's situation.	'I've heard from some of our friends that you haven't been feeling well recently. I'm really sorry to hear that.' 'Could you tell me how you've been feeling?' Bob explains that he has been having a sore throat and headaches, and has been very tired recently. After looking his symptoms up on the internet, he believes that he has the Ebola virus infection and that he must get emergency treatment. The candidate offers to listen to the colleague's symptoms and explore the reasoning in a sensitive and confidential way.
3	The candidate responds empathetically to Bob, whilst also explaining that looking up symptoms online is not very reliable.	'I'm sorry to hear that you've been feeling under the weather Bob. I understand that you must have also been anxious about your symptoms and the internet probably made you even more worried.' 'A lot of medical information that is out there on the web is not necessarily reliable. Anyone can put websites out there that contain misleading ideas, and this could have given you the wrong diagnosis.'
4	Bob becomes angry and accuses the candidate of being insensitive.	'I'm sorry if I offended you Bob. I understand that you were worried about your symptoms and that's why you googled them.' The candidate can draw on their own experiences to be more empathetic and reassure Bob. 'I've also looked up my symptoms before. I understand that when you are anxious, it can be reassuring to try and find advice online. However, from my own experiences, there is a lot of unreliable and false information online that can make you even more anxious.'

Table 4.4.

	Question themes	What is expected from the candidate?
5	The candidate explains why googling can be wrong.	The candidate understands the problems of this inappropriate action of googling one's own symptoms: • Googling one's own symptoms can increase pre-existing health anxiety. • Delaying seeking medical help can have detrimental effects, particularly if the symptoms are actually due to any underlying, undiagnosed medical condition. • The underlying anxiety and distress experienced by the friend can affect their studies and course work and may even have an impact on their ability to interact with patients in a safe and professional manner. • It is not professional, and the integrity of the friend is in question.
6	Bob becomes calmer and asks the candidate what they should do as they are still worried about their symptoms.	'The most reliable source of advice would be from your GP, as they are a trained medical professional, and they can also meet you in person.' 'In the meantime, you could ring the NHS 111 service for help and advice, or you could use the NHS website.' The candidate explains that not all online information is false, but that websites such as the NHS website that are peer reviewed and written by medical professionals are more reliable sources of information.
7	The candidate voluntarily quotes the GMC guidance on maintaining integrity.	The candidate explains and quotes the GMC guidance, 'Good medical practice'; Domain 4 deals with maintaining integrity. The GMC's 'Good medical practice' guidance also states that 'wherever possible you should avoid providing medical care to yourself or anyone with whom you have a close personal relationship'.

Table 4.4.		
	Question themes	**What is expected from the candidate?**
8	Conclusion.	'Thanks for talking to me about this Bob. I know you've been anxious about your symptoms, and I'm sure that your GP can give you a reliable diagnosis and recommend the appropriate treatment.'
		'Is there anything else you wish to discuss or ask me about?'

Role play for the actor

The actor is playing the role of Bob, who is the candidate's friend. Bob will be very anxious about his symptoms and will become irritable when the candidate suggests the unreliability of his online sources. When the candidate is empathetic and reassures Bob, he will become calmer and more open to the candidate's suggestions.

Discussion

Especially during the COVID-19 pandemic, there has been a widespread rise in unreliable medical information on the internet and social media. This information is usually not peer-reviewed or written by medical professionals; therefore, there is a risk of misleading details resulting in anxiety and fearmongering in the population. This role-play situation assesses the candidate's ability to reassure Bob in an empathetic and non-judgmental manner, as well as direct him towards the appropriate sources of advice.

Despite the fact that Bob is a medical student, it is understandable that when he himself is faced with symptoms, he becomes anxious and misled by online advice. A good candidate will try to explore the reasons behind Bob's anxiety and address these concerns. Drawing on one's own previous experiences of using online advice is a good way of showing empathy and reassuring Bob.

When directing Bob towards the appropriate sources of advice, the candidate should consider what determines the 'reliability' of online medical information. Good medical information is written by a trained medical professional, has been peer-reviewed, and very importantly is up to date. Examples of sources include the NICE guidelines, the NHS website, and NHS 111. Along with these sources, the candidate should importantly recommend that, if Bob is still worried, he can seek advice from his local GP who can examine him in person.

The UK General Medical Council (GMC) regulates the profession, and they have very important guidance, 'Good medical practice'; this guidance deals with the professionalism of doctors; It has four domains: Domain 1 on knowledge, skills and performance; Domain 2 on safety and quality; Domain 3 on communication partnership and teamwork; and Domain 4 on maintaining trust. Domain 4 deals with showing respect and treating patients fairly; it includes an important part covering the need for doctors to act with honesty and integrity. This guidance clarifies that doctors must make sure that their conduct justifies their patients' trust in them and the public's trust in the profession.

The American Medical Association adopted the AMA Code of Medical Ethics in 1847; it has 11 chapters, of which the ninth chapter deals with professional self-regulation. It necessitates doctors to hold high standards of conduct.

The Canadian Medical Association Code of Ethics defines that an honest physician is forthright, respects the truth, and does their best to seek, preserve, and communicate that truth sensitively and respectfully. This is displayed in the sections in the answers mentioned in this book (note the words — respect truth; do best to seek, preserve and communicate truth; sensitive and respectful).

Similar guidelines are also produced by the Australian Medical Association. Section 3.1 describes the necessity for professional conduct by physicians. It clearly explains that the doctor must recognise that personal conduct may affect their reputation and that of their profession.

Depending on your country and the medical council/association, it is appropriate to quote this code of ethics to add value to your answer.

Key Points

- Be compassionate and non-judgemental in your approach.
- Try to identify the factors affecting the role player's anxiety.
- Use your own experiences to reassure the role player and to show empathy.
- Direct the role player towards appropriate sources of advice such as the NICE guidelines and the NHS website.

References

1. General Medical Council. Guidance on assessing the seriousness of concerns relating to self-prescribing or prescribing to those in close personal relationships with doctors. Available from: https://www.gmc-uk.org/-/media/documents/11---guidance-on-assessing-the-seriousness-of-concerns-relating-to-prescribing_pdf-80650255.pdf.

2. NHS UK. Health A to Z. Available. Available from: https://www.nhs.uk/conditions.

3. NICE (National Institute for Health and Care Excellence). Conditions and diseases. Available from: https://www.nice.org.uk/guidance/conditions-and-diseases.

4. General Medical Council. Good medical practice. Domain 4: Maintaining trust. Available from: https://www.gmc-uk.org/ethical-guidance/ethical-guidance-for-doctors/good-medical-practice/domain-4---maintaining-trust#paragraph-65.

5. General Medical Council. Achieving good medical practice: guidance for medical students. Available from: https://www.gmc-uk.org/education/standards-guidance-and-curricula/guidance/student-professionalism-and-ftp/achieving-good-medical-practice.

6. American Medical Association. Code of Medical Ethics overview. Available from: https://www.ama-assn.org/delivering-care/ethics/code-medical-ethics-overview.

7. Canadian Medical Association. Code of ethics and professionalism. Available from: https://policybase.cma.ca/viewer?file=%2Fmedia%2FPolicyPDF%2FPD19–03S.pdf#page=1.

8. Australian Medical Association. Code of ethics 2004. Revised 2016. Available from: https://www.ama.com.au/articles/code-ethics-2004-editorially-revised-2006-revised-2016.

Question 58

Talking to a friend who has a phobia of flying in aeroplanes

Hari Adharsh Prabhu

Question

Your friend, Jody, needs to get on a flight next week, but as you book the tickets with her, she suddenly starts to panic and tells you that she does not want to go on a flight. You are in the middle of the shop. How do you talk to her in this situation?

An examiner will observe your communication skills in this station.

Themes for discussion (■ Table 4.5)

Table 4.5.		
	Question themes	**What is expected from the candidate?**
1	The candidate greets the role player appropriately, and communicates effectively with positive body language.	'Hi Jody, are you feeling OK? Talk to me about what's going on.' The candidate maintains eye contact and has open, friendly body language, giving appropriate regular pauses to allow the friend to talk.

Table 4.5.

Question themes	What is expected from the candidate?
2 The candidate encourages Jody to move to a more private location where they can talk confidentially.	The candidate understands the importance of maintaining the confidentiality of sensitive information, and therefore asks to conduct the discussion in a private setting, e.g. 'Why don't we move out of the shop over to a place where we can talk privately?'
3 Once in a confidential setting, the candidate begins to reassure Jody, whilst also trying to understand the situation.	'Are you feeling alright Jody? Can I get you a glass of water?' 'I'm here for you Jody when you're ready. Do you want to tell me what's going on and why you're upset?'
4 Jody insists that she does not want to go on the plane, but she does not explain why. The candidate must try to reassure her and understand the reasons for her fear.	The candidate asks the friend why she does not want to go on the plane and reassures her that they are there to support her. Good questions to ask are: • 'Have you had a bad experience on a flight in the past?' • 'Have you done something that helped you with flying in the past?' • 'Has something changed this time, that has made you anxious?' Jody reveals that their brother died very recently in a plane crash; therefore, she is worried about flying.
5 The candidate is supportive and empathetic when Jody reveals her loss.	The candidate maintains a supportive and empathetic tone throughout. 'I am really sorry for your loss Jody.' 'Thank you for telling me. I can only imagine how difficult that must have been for you.'

Table 4.5.

	Question themes	What is expected from the candidate?
6	The candidate displays active listening.	The candidate listens to what the friend tells them and asks appropriate questions or makes suggestions based on what they have been told. The candidate understands the importance of making the friend feel that their opinions and emotions have been respected.
7	The candidate suggests that the friend should seek professional support.	'I know that your loss must have been extremely difficult for you Jody. Have you talked about it with your GP or another professional? They can give you a safe and confidential setting to discuss how you're feeling without any judgement.' 'Your local GP could recommend a local support group for people who have recently experienced a loss. I know that you are going through a difficult time; maybe talking to other people with similar experiences could be useful.'
8	Jody agrees to seek support, but she is still afraid of flying. The candidate reassures her and offers alternative solutions.	'I understand that you are afraid Jody, and I want you to know that you are in control, and it is your decision to fly or not fly based on how you feel.' 'If you want, I can support you being next to you while flying but I will leave it to you to decide.' 'If you want, we can discuss alternatives to flying, and try to work together on anything else that might help.'
9	Conclusion.	'Thank you again for opening up to me Jody. I understand this was difficult and I really appreciate it.' 'Is there anything else you want me to do for you right now?' The candidate thanks the role player and the examiner.

Role play for the actor

The actor will play the role of the candidate's friend Jody. Jody will initially act scared and withdrawn, refusing to go on the flight. Jody will not reveal anything about her phobia in public until prompted by the candidate to go somewhere private. If the candidate does not offer, Jody will prompt the candidate.

When prompted by the candidate, Jody will reveal that her brother died in a plane crash and since then she has been scared of flying. She will agree to seek help if the candidate reassures her that if she seeks help, the professional will provide a confidential, safe space to discuss her issues without judgement.

Discussion

This station assesses the candidate's communication and empathy skills. A candidate must consider the many biopsychosocial factors that could affect an individual's life decisions or experiences. It is important that the candidate focuses mainly on the well-being of the friend and does not jump to conclusions. Active listening is very important here to ensure that the candidate builds a rapport with the friend and gains their trust in the conversation. This increases the likelihood of the friend being receptive to the advice and agreeing to seek help.

On a daily basis, clinicians care for and communicate with people who are in difficult situations. Doctors may encounter patients who are very nervous about surgery or adverse to taking certain drugs that could save their lives. Some patients also have a needle phobia and require support from their doctor. Identifying the root causes of a person's fear is vitally important, as doing so allows the doctor to alleviate their concerns and/or direct them to a professional who can best support them.

Key Points

- Confidentiality is important; ensure you conduct the conversation in a private setting and reassure the friend that you will maintain their trust.
- Show active listening in order to find reasons behind the friend's actions or behaviours.
- Do not make assumptions about a phobia; treat your friend with care and empathy.
- Recommend that the friend seeks help from an appropriate professional, e.g. GP or support group worker.

References

1. General Medical Council. Good medical practice. Domain 3: Communication partnership and teamwork. Available from: https://www.gmc-uk.org/ethical-guidance/ethical-guidance-for-doctors/good-medical-practice/domain-3---communication-partnership-and-teamwork.

Question 59

A friend's parents object to her having a pet

Hari Adharsh Prabhu

Question

You are talking to your best friend, Aminah. She is very upset because she wants a pet dog, but her parents are refusing. Your role is to talk to Aminah and try to help her reach a suitable solution. An examiner will observe your communication skills in this station.

Themes for discussion (■ Table 4.6)

Table 4.6.	
Question themes	**What is expected from the candidate?**
1 The candidate greets the actor appropriately and communicates effectively with positive body language.	'Hi Aminah, it's me [insert name]. How are you?' The candidate must use language that is friendly and appropriate to the situation.

Table 4.6.

Question themes	What is expected from the candidate?
	Communication is clear and appropriately paced, with regular pauses integrated at appropriate times to allow the actor to contribute to the conversation.
2 Aminah reveals the reason why she is upset and begins angrily talking about her parents. The candidate tries to calm her down.	'I'm sorry to hear that your parents don't want a dog, I know that you really like them.' The candidate shows empathy and acknowledges Aminah's feelings. 'I can understand why you're angry. Why don't we take a step back and talk about what exactly your parents said.'
3 The candidate acknowledges their friend's feelings but also tries to talk to her about her parent's point of view.	'You and I both love dogs and think they're great, but there are also a lot of downsides of having one that your parents might be worried about.' Examples of the parents' concerns the candidate could mention include: • Time commitment required to take the dog on walks every day. (Perhaps they are busy?) • Worried about extra costs of having a dog. • Worried about hygiene issues. • Possible fear of dogs (maybe they read something on the news).
4 Aminah becomes angry and states that the candidate is supporting her parents instead of her.	'I'm sorry that you feel that way. You're my friend and I didn't mean to hurt your feelings. I wanted to talk about how your parents might be feeling so we can understand their point of view.' The candidate remains calm and empathetic, and understands Aminah's feelings.

Table 4.6.

	Question themes	What is expected from the candidate?
5	The candidate brings the thoughts and concerns of the friend back to her parents.	The candidate can discuss the thoughts and concerns of the friend with the parents. The candidate can try to reach a compromise or agreement with the parents. For example, suggest that the family tries taking care of a friend's dog for a week and see how this goes. 'I know your parents well; shall I come and talk to them?' 'If you are happy with that, let's plan what we will say to them to convince them regarding having a pet.' 'We can tell them about the benefits of having a pet, including the effects on mood.'
6	The candidate offers appropriate solutions and compromises to Aminah.	'Why not ask your parents if it is the extra mess and work that is worrying them? If this is the worry, then you can offer to take responsibility for caring for the dog.' 'You told me the other day that you want to move out in the future. Maybe you can get a dog then?' 'It would be good if you sat down with your parents and had a talk about how you're feeling. Maybe you can all meet in the middle?'
7	Conclusion.	'Thanks for sharing this with me Aminah. I hope you and your parents can talk things through. Ask me if you need any help or if you want to talk more.' The candidate thanks the role player and the examiner.

Role play for the actor

The actor is playing the role of Aminah. Aminah is upset because she wants a dog, but her parents are not keen to get her one. She will become angry if it appears as though the candidate is sympathising with her parents, but will later calm down if the candidate remains empathetic and explains their approach.

Discussion

A role-play situation such as this investigates the mediation skills of the candidate, and their ability to remain impartial, whilst guiding and supporting others, a key skill of a good clinician. The role-play actor is playing the part of the candidate's friend; nevertheless, the candidate should consider not only her perspective but also that of her parents. This will show empathy and indicate that the candidate's emotions do not skew their decisions. A good candidate will also not worry about the final outcome of the conversation, instead focusing on keeping the conversation friendly and constructive, as well as encouraging open communication in this station.

Key Points

- Consider both the friend's and her parents' perspectives and remain impartial overall in your judgement.
- Encourage the friend and parents to put themselves in each other's shoes. This will help them understand the other person's perspectives and will help resolve the conflict.
- A compromise or solution should be reached that mitigates everyone's concerns and benefits everyone in some way.

References

1.   General Medical Council. Good medical practice. Domain 3: Communication partnership and teamwork. Available from: https://www.gmc-uk.org/ethical-guidance/ethical-guidance-for-doctors/good-medical-practice/domain-3---communication-partnership-and-teamwork.

Question 60

Communication with an individual who has a learning disability

Subramanian Ganesan

Question

You are volunteering in a care home. You have come across a young man, Mathew, who is 25 years old with a genetic condition called Down's syndrome that has caused a learning disability (intellectual disability). What are the issues you would expect to come across and how would you tackle the situation? In the next station, the examiner will discuss these issues and your opinion on this situation.

Themes for discussion (■ Table 4.7)

Table 4.7.	
Question themes	**What is expected from the candidate?**
1 The candidate greets the examiner and has good body language.	The candidate is presentable and uses good communication skills; always recommended in any station.

Table 4.7.

Question themes	What is expected from the candidate?
2 What are the challenges that people with learning difficulties will come across with their communication?	The candidate understands their difficulties and barriers: • Not able to tell someone how they feel. • Not being able to find the words they want to say. • Opening their mouth but no sounds/words jumbled. • Not getting the sounds right or words getting stuck. • Not able to hear or listen to the questions properly. • Not able to see, or able to understand, the signs and symbols or social cues around them. • Not able to understand the words, phrases or expressions used by others. • Not able to read or write down words to express their ideas. • Not able to join in a conversation. • They feel they are being ignored by others. • Upset if others do not understand or listen, making them feel unworthy of living, lack of confidence. • Take into account their physical disabilities that may constrain their communication ability. • Difficult in undertaking their daily activities such as shopping, medical appointments, etc.
3 How will you approach Mathew when you need to communicate with him?	• Understanding Mathew and his needs first. • Begin with empathy and a smile. • Express your empathetic emotions with appropriate body language. • Engagement/focus — show others that you are listening. • Maintain eye contact and facial expressions. • Wait for others to complete their conversation. • Ask open questions. • Choose the correct words to give a clear message. • Control your emotions. • LISTEN more than you speak.

Table 4.7.

	Question themes	What is expected from the candidate?
4	How would you help this person with a learning disability? What strategies would you follow?	• Face-to-face and one-to-one communication are the best way. • Quiet place with no distractions. • Good eye contact, facial expression, and the use of gestures. • Avoid jargon/long words or sentences. • Avoid words that they do not understand. • Go at their pace and follow their lead, build a rapport. • Do not rush and take your time, speak slowly. • Check with them that you are understood. • Watch them carefully for cues that are conveyed. • Make sure they understand the language you speak. • Ask their carer's help to assist you. • Use bigger text and bullet points if writing, and use simple colours. • Try drawing pictures, using photographs. • Use communication tools such as Makaton. • A person-centred approach based on their difficulties.
5	Do you know any communication tools or websites that are useful in such situations?	• British sign language. • Makaton sign language. • Alternative communication device — speech synthesiser. • Talking mats. • Communication books.
6	What different ways of communication do you know?	• Verbal communication — speaking. • Non-verbal — using expressions, eye contact and gestures. • Written communication — writing. • Visual — charts, pictures, etc.

Table 4.7.	
Question themes	**What is expected from the candidate?**
7 Conclusion.	The candidate concludes the session and thanks the examiner at the end. This gains the candidate extra bonus points.

Discussion

Communication is passing on information from one person to another using any means possible. Good communication is essential for doctors and their practice. It ensures the person is kept central to their decision making by including them in the conversation.

Effective communication should be clear, concise, and meet the needs of the person involved. It should be open, two-way, inclusive and patient-centric.

Approximately 1.5 million people in the UK have a learning disability. It is estimated that there are 286,000 children (180,000 boys and 106,000 girls) aged 0-17 years with a learning disability. Two-thirds of people with a learning disability have some form of communication difficulties and many of them would have had speech and language therapy intervention at a younger age.

There are many different types of sign language used around the world:

- British Sign Language (BSL) — this is used by deaf people in the UK and uses hand gestures, fingerspelling, lip patterns and facial expressions. A variation of BSL is called Sign Supported English (SSE) which uses BSL signs, but the structure and grammar are based on spoken English.
- Tactile signing — used by children who have both hearing loss and sight impairment, using touch medium.
- Makaton uses a combination of picture symbols and hand gestures that are similar to BSL and speech. It is used for children and adults with learning difficulties and communication issues.

321

Key Points

- Do not assume that a person with a learning disability cannot communicate.

- People with intellectual disabilities may understand more than they can demonstrate. Even if the person appears unresponsive, they may still understand.

- Communication is a mix of body language such as facial expressions, gestures, appropriate tone of voice and right words/phrases.

- The language and communication style should be tailored to individual needs.

- Although there are many barriers, overcome these by building rapport, working with the person and ensuring that they are included in your conversation. This will ensure that you are a good and effective communicator for people with intellectual disabilities.

References

1. Communicating with people with a learning disability – Mencap. Available from: https://www.mencap.org.uk/learning-disability-explained/communicating-people-learning-disability.

2. Royal College of Speech and Language Therapists. Giving voice. Available from: https://www.cppe.ac.uk/wizard/files/publications/leaflets/giving%20voice%20rcslp%20leaflet.pdf.

3. NHS UK. How to care for someone with communication difficulties. Available from: https://www.nhs.uk/conditions/social-care-and-support-guide/practical-tips-if-you-care-for-someone/how-to-care-for-someone-with-communication-difficulties.

4. Chew KL, Iacono T, Tracy J. Overcoming communication barriers – working with patients with intellectual disabilities. racgp.org.au. Available from: https://www.racgp.org.au/afp/2009/january-february/overcoming-communication-barriers. *Aust Fam Physician* 2009; 38(1-2): 10-4.

Question 61

Teaching an actor to tie shoelaces

Gamma Manohara Prasad

Question

The next station will assess your communication skills. You will be asked to teach an actor to tie their shoelaces. The actor will follow your instructions alone without using any prior knowledge. The station will assess how you can give instructions to another person and clearly convey your message.

The role player says: 'Hi. In this station, you are going to give me instructions on how to tie the laces on these shoes that I have on the table. I will do exactly what you tell me to do. Assume that I do not know how to tie them. You should be clear as I will follow your instructions'.

Themes for discussion (■ Table 4.8)

Table 4.8.

	Question themes	What is expected from the candidate?
1	The candidate greets the examiner and the actor, has good body language and speaks coherently.	'Hello, my name is [insert name]. May I ask your name please?' The candidate maintains good eye contact and confident body language.
2	The candidate clarifies the aim of the task at the start.	'My role is to explain to you how to tie shoelaces.' The candidate smiles at the examiner, to receive the question correctly and starts with an encouraging/positive statement. 'Sounds great, we can start whenever you are ready.'
3	The candidate clearly tells which hand (which side) of the actor to use.	Usually, confusion comes when describing whether to use the left or right hand; be aware that the examiner or role player is sitting just opposite to you and be clear.
4	The candidate talks through the task of tying the shoelaces.	The candidate is relaxed and gives clear, easily understandable instructions. They ensure that the instructions include sufficient detail. 'You begin by taking the string on your right side with your right hand...' 'Ensure that you continue holding the string in place.'
5	The candidate progresses to the stage of explaining how to make a loop with laces.	The candidate remains calm throughout, even if the actor is slow or makes mistakes.

Table 4.8.

	Question themes	What is expected from the candidate?
6	The actor is unsure how to tie the laces and does not fully follow one of the candidate's instructions.	The candidate remains calm and pleasant; they apologise for any mistake on their part. After asking the actor which part of the instruction was confusing, they try to rephrase the instruction in a clearer way.
		Even if the actor made a wrong move, be empathetic:
		'Sorry, can we undo that move; I am sorry I have not been clear. Let's start again from that step.'
7	The candidate remains motivational and friendly throughout the communication.	'You're doing great! Not too far left to go now.'
8	The role player asks questions that might be very simple.	The candidate responds to the questions in a pleasant manner, smiling throughout. They show by their body language that they are happy to answer the questions.
9	Aim of the task.	Some candidates can get upset if they are not progressing well; the aim is to assess your communication. Do not get frustrated if the role player cannot complete the task of tying shoelaces. If you have communicated well and stayed calm, that is more important.
10	The candidate thanks the actor and examiner and concludes the session.	Even if the task is not complete, thank the actor and apologise that you could not complete it.
		If completed, give the opportunity to ask questions:
		'Is there anything else that you want to ask me please?'
		'Are you happy with this task or is there anything that you want to ask?'
		'Thanks for doing it; we did it well.'

Discussion

Before any interview station, a candidate should reflect on its intended purpose and end goal. This communication station can be deliberately misleading; a candidate may become fixated on the outcome of tying the shoelaces. This in turn could result in them becoming caught up in small details of the method and becoming frustrated if the outcome is not achieved.

The true purpose of this station is to explore the verbal and non-verbal communication skills of the candidate and their ability to break down a task into easily understandable instructions. In a clinical setting, there is often an information asymmetry between the doctor and the patient, meaning that doctors must have the skill of communicating their medical knowledge in concise and clearly understandable terms.

A candidate can prepare for a communication station such as this by reading the GMC guidelines on effective communication. The guidelines can be accessed through the reference; however, some of the key concepts outlined include:

- Using patient-understandable language.
- Giving the patient opportunities to answer questions.
- Acknowledging the patient's feelings and considering their view when making decisions.

Key Points

- Remain calm and friendly throughout the station.
- The end goal is not tying the laces; it is communicating effectively.
- When the communication is not effective, ask the actor for feedback, reflect and change your approach accordingly.

References

1. Blomqvist A. The doctor as double agent: information asymmetry, health insurance, and medical care. *J Health Econ* 1991; 10(4): 411-32.

2. General Medical Council. Protecting children and young people: the responsibilities of all doctors. Available from: https://www.gmc-uk.org/ethical-guidance/ethical-guidance-for-doctors/protecting-children-and-young-people/communication-and-support.

Question 62

Picture-based communication station

Suresh Seetharaman

Question

This is a very common presentation in an MMI station. The candidate will be given a photograph or a picture and asked to describe it. It can be a simple photograph of day-to-day observance or even a drawing of a flower or object.

How to manage this task

All the principles of effective communication also apply in this scenario:

- Stay calm and talk throughout the station.
- Introduce yourself and greet the role player.
- Once a question is asked, reflect it back to confirm the task: 'you want me to describe the given photograph, thanks for asking me.'
- Take it slowly and in a relaxed manner; enjoy the task rather than becoming stressed to finish it.
- Try to exhibit good body language; smile and be pleasant.
- Create a structure to describe the picture: what it is, what is shown in it, describe the characters in the photograph, what the characters

are doing, colour structure, day or night — light features, how you enjoy seeing it, feelings of looking at the picture, etc.

- Expressing feelings based on what the photograph or picture portrays might help.
- What do you like in the photograph and what do you not like?
- What would be the idea that the artist is conveying through that photograph or drawing?
- Conclude the answer.
- 'Thanks for giving me this opportunity; is there anything else that you want to ask me please?'
- Thank the examiner.

Examples of photographs that could be presented:

- The Taj Mahal with a bench in front.
- High-rise buildings in London.
- A London bridge with vehicles and boats underneath.
- The New York Stock Exchange — an angry bull with a girl in front of it.
- A double-decker bus in London in front of the Houses of Parliament.
- A picture of a flower.
- A simple line drawing.

Question 63

Video-based communication station

Kaviarasan Karunanidhi

Question

Showing a video and asking the candidate to comment is often presented in an MMI. This might be a video clip for 1-3 minutes; it could be either a medical scenario or a non-clinical scenario.

If it is a medical scenario, the candidate is asked to communicate what went wrong in the video communication and what went well. If the communication station has not gone well, show your empathy: 'I am sorry that the consultation did not go well. I feel sorry for the patient'.

In non-medical scenarios, the candidate views the video and comments on what happened. Sometimes, it could be a simple day-to-day task and candidates can become worried that they are missing something; stay calm and just describe what you see.

How to manage this task

All the principles of effective communication apply in this scenario also:

- Stay calm and talk throughout the station.
- Introduce yourself and greet the role player.
- Once a question is asked, reflect it back to confirm the task: 'I am happy to describe the given video, thanks for asking me. I am happy to start the video'.
- Take it slowly and in a relaxed manner; enjoy the task rather than becoming stressed to finish it.
- Try to exhibit good body language; smile and be pleasant.
- Create a structure to describe the video: what is the scenario?; what happened?; how did the characters react and what was their purpose?; what went well or wrong?, etc.
- Expressing feelings based on the characters in the video might help.
- Conclude the answer.
- 'Thanks for giving me this opportunity; is there anything else that you want to ask me please?'
- Thank the examiner.

Question 64

Task-based communication station

Suresh Seetharaman

Question

Similar to the task in Question 61 on tying shoelaces, there can be different tasks that a candidate might be asked to do in an MMI station. These could include:

- The candidate is given a few LEGO® bricks and asked to build a structure and describe what they are doing.
- A magnetic screw set is given, and the candidate is asked to construct anything and describe it. The key is to talk while they do the task, and the examiner assesses how calm they are.
- The candidate is given a gift box which is wrapped and tied; the candidate has to advise on how it can be opened and the examiner will follow the instructions given by the candidate. This tests whether the candidate can give simple, clear instructions to follow.
- The examiner has guessed a thing in their mind; the candidate must ask questions to find this object. The examiner will only answer yes or no; questions need to be framed with this in mind. You can ask 20 questions in 5 minutes. The examiner will assess how you are

framing the questions and if there is a structure. The final task of finding the object is less important than the structure of the process.

- The candidate is asked to do two tasks at the same time, e.g. while building with LEGO bricks, they have to describe the way to their school; while drawing a picture, they have to describe the rules of how to play their favourite sport.

The principles of managing these stations are similar: keeping calm, communicating appropriately with verbal and non-verbal cues, being pleasant and engaging with the role player are important qualities that will be assessed.

It is difficult to predict what task could be given; candidates preparing for an MMI can practise a few similar tasks with their friends or relatives so that they are prepared for any unusual tasks in the real interview. Please note that the endpoint is not to finish the task, but it might help if you finish it; it is important to exhibit good communication skills throughout, both verbally and non-verbally.

Question 65

Map-based communication station

Kaviarasan Karunanidhi

Question

The candidate is given a map and asked to describe how to go from A to B. It looks very easy from the outset, but many candidates feel stressed to see an unfamiliar map and can become worried. Take a structured approach to manage this task:

- Introduce yourself to the examiner and thank them.
- Confirm what the examiner is asking: 'Thank you very much; you are asking me to describe how to go from A to B. Thanks, first let me have a look at this map'.
- Keep talking throughout in a slow and relaxed manner, engaging the examiner throughout.
- Start by describing what the map is: 'This is a map of the London underground with different tube rail paths'; 'this is a map of Leeds city centre'; 'this is a map of a shopping centre'.
- Explain from where you are starting: 'I am starting from A' and describe it first.
- Think in detail before you start which path you are going to take. Do not get confused in the middle.

- If you have made a mistake, apologise, say sorry, and ask if you can start again.
- Explain the route that you are taking; describe the landmarks: 'As I take the first turn, there will be a pub at the corner; when I walk a short distance, I should see a petrol station on the right, and I will take the immediate right there'.
- The aim is to reach B, but the examiner is assessing your communication skills in this station; stay calm and composed, talk in a friendly manner, and smile and keep talking.
- Use non-verbal cues for communication that might also be assessed.
- Once you have reached the destination, if there is time, summarise how you went from A to B.
- Conclude the station: 'I have now reached B'.
- Thank the examiner for giving you the opportunity to describe how to go from A to B.
- 'Is there anything else that you want to ask me?'

Question 66

Describing the way to your school

Gamma Manohara Prasad

Question

Assume that you are walking from your house to your school now. Describe the way that you will travel.

The examiner will assess your communication skills in this station.

Themes for discussion (■ Table 4.9)

Table 4.9.

Question themes	What is expected from the candidate?
1 The candidate greets the examiner and the actor, has good body language and speaks coherently.	'Hello, my name is [insert name].' The candidate maintains good eye contact and confident body language.

Table 4.9.

	Question themes	What is expected from the candidate?
2	The candidate clarifies the aim of the task at the start.	'My role is to describe the path of walking from my house to my school.'
		The candidate smiles at the examiner, receives the question properly and starts with an encouraging/positive statement.
3	The candidate explains what he is going to describe.	'Thank you for asking, I come from Leicester, and I study in X school.'
		'I am going to describe how I walk every day from my house to X school; it usually takes 20 minutes to walk.'
4	Describes the general details and then goes on to specifics in the path.	Having a structure helps in communication and the examiner will understand the candidate better.
		The process is more important than the exact directions in this scenario.
5	Able to communicate clearly; can describe the path to travel to school.	The candidate is relaxed and gives clear, easily understandable instructions. They ensure that the instructions include sufficient detail.
		Rather than becoming fixed with exact detail, the candidate should enjoy describing the path and stay positive.
6	Anyone listening to instructions can get from point A to point B easily.	The description is easy to understand and follow. The candidate should instil confidence in the examiner.

Table 4.9.

Question themes	What is expected from the candidate?
7 The candidate confirms that the examiner is listening to the description.	The candidate might reflect and talk to the examiner confirming that the message has been reached. 'I hope you can follow the path; we started at A and went through… and reached…' 'Are you OK and following me until now please?' 'Do you have any questions or doubts until now please?' 'Thank you, let me continue…'
8 Easy and simple instructions — focus on simplicity in directions, landmarks, and time taken.	It is important to include landmarks for easy identification and approximate time; however, please note that, rather than specifics, the communication should be clear and friendly. It is worth summarising the path once again so that the candidate is sure that the message has been conveyed to the examiner.
9 The candidate stays positive while describing the walk.	The candidate is smiling and feels happy to describe the path.
10 The candidate thanks the examiner and concludes the session.	The candidate makes sure that the path is described and engages with the examiner. 'Are you happy with the description? Is there anything else that you want to ask me?' 'Do you want me to describe the walk again?'

Discussion

In this communication station, rather than going to specifics, the candidate has to stay calm and use simple, easy-to-follow language. The examiner will observe both verbal and non-verbal cues in the communication.

It is prudent to summarise the path at the end and ask the examiner if they have followed it. Always conclude the session and thank the examiner.

Key Points

- Introduce yourself, reflect on the question and confirm the task.
- Start with the opening sentence, and explain what you are going to do.
- Be clear, have a structure, and explain this in simple language.
- Split the path into two or three parts if it is long, describe the structure, and then include a break in these sections to confirm that the examiner is following you.
- Conclude the station and thank the examiner at the end.

References

1.   British Medical Association. Good communication as a medical student. Available from: https://www.bma.org.uk/advice-and-support/ethics/medical-students/ethics-toolkit-for-medical-students/good-communication.

2.   General Medical Council. Achieving good medical practice: guidance for medical students. Communication, partnership and teamwork. Available from: https://www.gmc-uk.org/education/standards-guidance-and-curricula/guidance/student-professionalism-and-ftp/achieving-good-medical-practice/the-duties-of-a-doctor#communication-partnership-and-teamwork.

3.   General Medical Council. Good medical practice. Domain 3: Communication partnership and teamwork. Available from: https://www.gmc-uk.org/ethical-guidance/ethical-guidance-for-doctors/good-medical-practice/domain-3---communication-partnership-and-teamwork.

Section **5**

Medical framework/medical school

Section editor: Thanthullu Vasu

Introduction to medical framework/medical school

Medical framework

It is vital to know about the National Health Service (NHS) structure and the medical framework when you apply for medical school. Awareness of the General Medical Council (GMC) guidelines, including its code of conduct, will be tested in the Multiple Mini Interview (MMI) station. A medical career can be demanding, and the candidate needs to be aware of the challenges that they face before they take this career path. A good candidate will be aware of these challenges and will know how to balance their work-life conditions.

Teamwork is important in the healthcare sector; it is important to be aware of allied healthcare professionals that you might need to work together with in future and their roles.

The National Health Service (NHS) in the UK

In the UK, the NHS offers healthcare to most of the public; a candidate should be aware of the structure of the NHS, its constitution, and how funding is applied. The NHS was set up in 1948; it is the largest publicly funded health service. The NHS deals with over 1 million patients every 36 hours. Its core principle is to provide good healthcare to all, regardless of the ability to pay; it is a 'free for all' service. There is an exception with some charges, such as prescriptions, and optical and dental services.

The NHS constitution sets out rights to which patients, the public and staff are entitled and pledges its commitment to achieve these responsibilities. It states seven key principles:

1. The NHS provides a comprehensive service, available to all, without any discrimination.
2. The NHS is free of charge; access to the NHS is based on clinical need and not on the ability to pay.

3. The NHS aspires to the highest standards of excellence and professionalism.
4. The patient is at the heart of the NHS.
5. The NHS works across organisational boundaries.
6. The NHS provides the best value for taxpayers' money.
7. The NHS is accountable to the public, communities and patients.

NHS values

The six values in the NHS constitution include:

- Working together for patients.
- Respect and dignity.
- Commitment to quality of care.
- Compassion.
- Improving lives.
- Everyone counts.

The NHS structure in England

The Health and Care Act 2022 made major changes to the NHS structure; Integrated Care Systems (ICS) replaced the previous Clinical Commissioning Groups (CCG) that commissioned services for secondary care. There are approximately 220 NHS acute or foundation trusts in the country. Apart from these, there are ambulance trusts, mental health trusts, care trusts and other local primary care services. There are more than 112,000 doctors and 300,000 nurses in the NHS, with a total workforce of more than one million staff. Of these staff, one in eight originates from outside the UK. Despite these statistics, the demand for healthcare is rising, and the staffing need is causing challenges in the NHS.

Primary care is commissioned mostly by NHS England and is provided by GPs.

Integrated Care Systems (ICS) are partnerships that bring together providers and commissioners of NHS services across a geographical area with local authorities and other local partners to plan and meet the need for healthcare for the population.

Funding for the NHS

The NHS is funded by taxpayers' money. For the year 2022/2023, the commissioning budget is £153 billion. Out of this, £108 billion goes to integrated care boards, £30 billion goes to direct commissioning, and the rest is allocated to a service development fund, the NHS England central programme, an elective services recovery fund, and other system funds.

Training to be a doctor

In the UK, education in medical school is followed by foundation year training; this could be followed by core training and, depending on interest, lead to postgraduate training as a core trainee in a specialty or as a general practice trainee. The candidate should know the structure of the training and the pathway to becoming a consultant or GP.

Undergraduate medical training is a combination of university education with clinical placements in healthcare set-ups; this could last 4-6 years.

After this training, graduates must complete a 2-year programme of training called a foundation programme. This foundation year (FY) programme provides trainees with defined practical skills and competencies to proceed to specialist or GP training.

After completing this foundation training, doctors can proceed to either specialist training or general practice training. Specialist training can be in approximately 60 different specialties, and this can start as an initial 2 years of core training (CT) proceeding to higher specialist training (ST). This phase of training lasts for 3 years in general practice and 5-7 years in other specialties.

Foundation doctors, core trainees and specialist trainees are called junior doctors. On completion of the higher specialist training, doctors are awarded a Certificate of Completion of Training (CCT); this allows them to be registered by the General Medical Council, which allows them to practice in the UK.

Research the medical school

When you are selected for an interview in a particular medical school, you should have done some research on the structure, education pattern, and unique opportunities in that school. Some medical schools follow traditional teaching methods, whilst others follow problem-based learning; it is important to know about the structure used in that school. Some medical schools can offer intercalated degrees, and there could be some areas of interest that you can specify in interviews; speaking to students in the medical school, attending open days, and researching online can all help you to gather this information that could help you in a positive way in the interview. It is not only important to know about the medical school, but also it is vital to know about what the city has to offer; this awareness will provide an idea on how motivated the candidate is.

The Medical Schools Council is the representative body for all UK medical schools; their website provides collective details of different medical schools.

References

1. Department of Health & Social Care, United Kingdom Government. The NHS constitution for England. Available from: https://www.gov.uk/government/publications/the-nhs-constitution-for-england/the-nhs-constitution-for-england; January 2021.

2. British Medical Association. How the NHS works. Available from: https://www.bma.org.uk/advice-and-support/international-doctors/life-and-work-in-the-uk/toolkit-for-doctors-new-to-the-uk/how-the-nhs-works; June 2022.

3. NHS England. Our funding. Available from: https://www.england.nhs.uk/publications/business-plan/our-2022–23-business-plan/our-funding.

4. British Medical Association. Medical training pathway. Available from: https://www.bma.org.uk/advice-and-support/studying-medicine/becoming-a-doctor/medical-training-pathway.

5. Medical Schools Council. Studying medicine. Available from: https://www.medschools.ac.uk/studying-medicine.

Question 67

NHS framework and structure

Shivani Ganesh

Question

The NHS consists of many care providers in different sectors, working together in an integrated system. Patient services are organised and commissioned depending on the needs of the local area; the recent Health and Care Act 2022 aimed to aid further integration between NHS sectors.

In the next station, the examiner will question you on this NHS healthcare framework and structure and the recently proposed changes.

Themes for discussion (■ Table 5.1)

Table 5.1.	
Question themes	**What is expected from the candidate?**
1 Explain the sectors of service provision in the NHS and provide an example for each one.	Names and provides examples for primary, secondary, and tertiary care; candidates can also mention community health services for extra points.

Table 5.1.

Question themes	What is expected from the candidate?
	Primary care: GP, optometrist, dentist, community pharmacist.
	Secondary care: emergency, mental health, most hospital care.
	Tertiary care: specialist care, including transplant and neurosurgery.
	Community health: health visitors, district nurses, sexual health, etc.
2 Who commissions and organises patient services?	Understands the role of the Clinical Commissioning Groups (CCGs) in the allocation of patient services to the local population. Recently, Integrated Care Systems (ICSs) have been developed that bring NHS service commissioners and other local services together.
3 How is the quality of care in the NHS regulated?	CCGs (and ICSs) are accountable to NHS England and the Care Quality Commission (CQC).
4 The Health and Social Care Act 2022 was passed to allow more integration and collaboration within the NHS. Are you aware of any changes to the structure of the NHS as a result?	More authority will be given to Integrated Care Systems that will be legally established. The candidate is aware that Integrated Care Boards (ICBs) have replaced the Clinical Commissioning Groups (CCGs) in July 2022, and they work with Integrated Care Partnerships (ICPs) (made up of local authorities, people from the community, voluntary and social enterprises) that do not directly commission services.

Table 5.1.

	Question themes	What is expected from the candidate?
5	Judgement and clarity.	The candidate shows confidence and clarity in their understanding of the structure of the NHS or the local healthcare system.
		The candidate does not need to be an expert, but has a basic understanding of the pathway and the structure of the NHS.
6	Conclusion.	The candidate thanks the examiner and concludes the session.

Discussion

It is prudent that the candidate has a basic understanding of the structure of the NHS. The Department of Health, with the Health Secretary, leads the service with control of primary and secondary care at various levels. Knowledge of the ICS that replaces the CCG is advised.

Knowledge of the funding of the NHS and the need for an ethical and legal way of controlling it, as per the NHS code, is preferred. When there is an ethical dilemma about funding, it is wise to use the four pillars of medical ethics to detail the scenario (autonomy, non-maleficence, beneficence, and justice).

Key Points

- The Clinical Commissioning Groups (CCGs) are groups of primary healthcare providers who purchase services that benefit their local population using the money allocated to their area by the NHS; these include most of the secondary health services and GP care.
- NHS England commissions the rest of primary health services (e.g. dentistry, optometry).
- CCGs are now being replaced by ICSs (made up of ICBs and Integrated Care Providers [ICPs]).
- ICPs will not directly commission NHS services.
- ICBs will be made up of an independent chair, local NHS trust members, primary care clinicians and mental health professionals.

References

1. The healthcare ecosystem – NHS. Available from: https://digital.nhs.uk/developer/guides-and-documentation/introduction-to-healthcare-technology/the-healthcare-ecosystem#overview. Digital Press.

2. NHS England. Who commissions NHS services? Available from: https://www.england.nhs.uk/commissioning/who-commissions-nhs-services.

3. Kings Fund. Integrated Care Systems. Available from: http://www.kingsfund.org.uk/audio-video/integrated-care-systems-health-and-care-act.

4. Kings Fund. How the NHS works in England. Available from: http://www.kingsfund.org.uk/audio-video/how-does-nhs-in-england-work.

Question 68

The role of the MDT and allied healthcare professionals

Leena Naidu

Question

In the next station, the examiner will discuss the role of allied healthcare professionals and assess your awareness of the multidisciplinary team (MDT).

Themes for discussion (■ Table 5.2)

Table 5.2.		
	Question themes	**What is expected from the candidate?**
1	The candidate greets the examiner and has good body language.	The candidate is presentable and uses good communication skills; always recommended in any station.

Table 5.2.

	Question themes	What is expected from the candidate?
2	Are you aware of an MDT?	The candidate gives a good opening statement of the understanding of the situation.
3	Can you tell me what an MDT is?	A multidisciplinary team (MDT) is a scenario in which all the healthcare professionals in a team work together to ensure that all the needs of a patient are met. It could include doctors, nurses, allied healthcare professionals such as physiotherapists, pharmacists, radiologists, healthcare assistants, administrators, managers, etc.
4	Give me an example of an MDT that you are aware of.	This is an opportunity for the candidate to quote a work experience, if they have done any. It gives the candidate the ability to score more by explaining their motivation for attending the work experience and showing their passion and interest in medicine.
		They could quote any MDT either in primary care/GP service or in secondary care.
		For example, a cancer MDT could consist of a specialty consultant, surgeon, radiologist, oncologist, cancer nurse specialist, palliative care consultant and nurse, doctors responsible for managing this patient, ward nurses, pathologist, administrative staff and managers.
5	Are you aware of other allied healthcare professionals and their role in treating the patient?	The candidate should explain the role and importance of the whole team; this is again an opportunity to quote their workplace experience, if they have any.
		The candidate should be positive in their approach, appreciating the role of each healthcare professional in the NHS.
		They could give a few examples, such as: nurses help in administering drugs, monitoring vital parameters, and day-to-day care on the ward.

Table 5.2.

Question themes	What is expected from the candidate?
	Healthcare assistants help in the care of patients on the ward or in outpatient settings.
	A midwife helps in monitoring pregnant patients, taking care of and helping in the delivery of the baby.
	A physiotherapist helps in delivering gradual exercises, pacing and recovery/rehabilitation of patients.
	A pharmacist helps in the delivery of the right drug at the right doses.
	The candidate can give any number of examples, but having a structure and showing a positive approach are more important in this answer.
6 Give an example of how an MDT approach changed the care of the patient.	The examiner does not expect a huge amount of information from the candidate, but this question is an opportunity to express what the candidate has seen in their workplace experience.
	They could quote any MDT, even if it is a doctor/nurse meeting. Due to COVID restrictions and pressures on the healthcare system, most universities do not expect long work experiences, but having knowledge and awareness are vital.
7 Judgement and clarity.	The candidate has clarity in their answer and can clearly explain the benefits of an MDT. A clear presentation, smiling throughout and avoiding repetition — these steps can increase the scores in this station.
8 Conclusion.	The candidate concludes the session and thanks the examiner at the end. This gives extra bonus points.

Discussion

Use this station as an opportunity to express your workplace experience, observership or voluntary work experience. You can add positive marks to the whole interview by showing your motivation towards a medical career in this station.

A multidisciplinary approach draws appropriately multiple disciplines to explore problems outside normal boundaries and reaches solutions based on a new understanding of complex situations; it brings together all healthcare staff involved in patient care, with the sole aim of benefiting the patient.

Key Points

- You are expected to have a positive approach towards an MDT.
- It is prudent to know the role of all members of an MDT.
- An MDT works together for the benefit of the patient.
- An MDT helps to bring the different skills and expertise of all team members together.

References

1. NHS England. MDT development – working toward an effective multidisciplinary/multiagency team. Available from: https://www.england.nhs.uk/wp-content/uploads/2015/01/mdt-dev-guid-flat-fin.pdf.

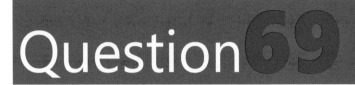

The GMC code of conduct for doctors

Shivani Ganesh

Question

Are you aware of the General Medical Council (GMC)? What do they do?

Can you detail the GMC's code of conduct for doctors?

Why is the GMC relevant to you when you are at medical school?

Do you know of any GMC guidance for medical students?

Themes for discussion (■ Table 5.3)

Table 5.3.	
Question themes	**What is expected from the candidate?**
1 What is the GMC? What does it do?	The candidate understands that the GMC is a statutory regulatory body that sets professional and ethical standards for doctors in the UK. They are aware that:

Table 5.3.

Question themes	What is expected from the candidate?
	• All doctors must be registered with the GMC to practice legally. • The GMC regulates medical education and investigates allegations of misconduct, and can assess fitness to practise. • The GMC produces documents to provide guidance for safe medical practice at a high standard (that are constantly updated).
2 Briefly describe the GMC's code of conduct for doctors	The student mentions 'Good medical practice' as a document and is aware of the four domains of 'duties of a doctor': • Knowledge, skills and performance. • Safety and quality. • Communication, partnership and teamwork. • Maintaining trust.
3 Why is the GMC relevant to you as a medical student?	The candidate is aware that, aside from being a future doctor registered with the GMC, the GMC is involved in medical schools in the following ways: • Outcomes for graduates, states the knowledge and competencies required for medical students to graduate as skilled doctors. • A student's fitness to practise hearings at medical school is based on GMC standards. • The GMC document 'Promoting excellence' sets required standards for students, such as promoting patient safety and raising concerns whilst in medical school.
4 Do you know of any guidance from the GMC for medical students?	The GMC has published 'Achieving good medical practice: guidance for medical students'.

Table 5.3.

Question themes	What is expected from the candidate?
	As a medical student, one is joining a trusted profession that will bring them into contact with patients and members of the public. The GMC expects that the medical student must demonstrate a high standard of behaviour at all times, which justifies the trust placed in them as a future member of the profession.
5 What sort of health concerns does the GMC regard as serious in cases of a medical student?	• Failure to seek appropriate treatment or advice from an independent healthcare professional. • Failure to tell the medical school or university if there is a serious medical condition. • Refusal to follow medical treatment or care plans. • Failure to comply with reasonable adjustments to ensure patient safety. • Failure to recognise the limits or lack of insight into health conditions. • Failure to be immunised against serious communicable diseases.
6 Judgement and clarity.	The candidate is aware of the GMC's guidance for medical students — 'Achieving good medical practice: guidance for medical students'; they have clarity and knowledge of the guidance.
7 Conclusion.	The candidate thanks the examiner at the end of the session.

Discussion

Before joining the medical school, it is expected that the candidate has some knowledge of the GMC's guidance for medical students. It is vital to understand the code of conduct that is expected of them by the GMC.

Key Points

- The GMC sets professional and ethical standards for doctors in the UK.
- The GMC's 'Good medical practice' guideline sets standards in four domains.
- The GMC has published guidance for medical students.

References

1. General Medical Council. Achieving good medical practice: guidance for medical students. Available from: https://www.gmc-uk.org/education/standards-guidance-and-curricula/guidance/student-professionalism-and-ftp/achieving-good-medical-practice.

2. General Medical Council. Promoting excellence. Available from: https://www.gmc-uk.org/education/standards-guidance-and-curricula/standards-and-outcomes/promoting-excellence.

3. General Medical Council. Ethical guidance for doctors. Available from: http://www.gmc-uk.org/ethical-guidance/ethical-guidance-for-doctors/good-medical-practice.

4. BMA guidance. Ethics toolkit for medical students. Available from: https://www.bma.org.uk/advice-and-support/ethics/medical-students/ethics-toolkit-for-medical-students.

Question 70

If you are the lead for the health service...

Leena Naidu

Question

If you are the lead for the health service in your area, tell me one change that you would make and detail the reasons for it.

Discussion

This question can come as part of testing the candidate's awareness of healthcare problems and present problems facing the health services.

The candidate can choose any problem, but should show an interest and motivation to keep updated with recent healthcare news.

As with any other answer, you need a framework for this answer; this could include the following:

- Start with a good introduction.
- Show motivation in your answer.
- Exhibit good body language.
- Introduce a problem; it could be an example.

- Detail the problem; explain how it is affecting healthcare and society.
- Explain why you chose this problem/example.
- Detail the solution that you propose.
- Show the problems that can happen with your solution, giving confidence to the examiner that you are aware of what can go wrong.
- Explain how you would bring about this change.
- Show awareness of how you will evaluate this change.
- Conclude with a summary.
- Thank the examiner.

Example scenario

Problem: you could take the problem of long-term workforce planning in the present NHS scenario.

Detail: workforce challenges are prevalent in all areas of the health service due to the ever-increasing demand and inability to match the capacity. Part of the mismatch may be due to leave, sickness and lack of cross-cover. There is little attention paid to 5-year strategic workforce planning and to predicting the increase in demand, population growth, influx, new advances in healthcare, and the introduction of new evidence-based pathways.

Why the problem needs attention: lack of planning leads to overworked staff and a stretched workforce, leading to absences. Currently, NHS hospitals have to outsource many services to private hospitals to keep the waiting lists down; this is not a cost-effective way of sustaining the services.

Solution: a team discussion to involve planning with all the team members, including clinicians, supporting staff, finance, and managers. Audit the reason why staff have left in the past. Discuss the reasons and how you could solve these problems. Evaluate what could lead to keep the staff retention rate higher. Work on a financial business plan to make these changes. Propose these plans to management and secure the funding. Evaluate the success of the plan and audit it regularly.

Key Points

- You could select any problem, but show an awareness of the problem.
- Have a structure to the answer with an introduction, detail of the problem, a solution and how you will evaluate the change.
- Show a positive approach and good body language.

References

1. General Medical Council. Leadership and management for all doctors. Available from: https://www.gmc-uk.org/ethical-guidance/ethical-guidance-for-doctors/leadership-and-management-for-all-doctors.

Question 71

Ethnic inequalities among patients

Shivani Ganesh

Question

Sir Michael Marmot's 2020 update to his 2010 Marmot Review stated that 'intersections between socioeconomic status, ethnicity and racism intensify inequalities in health for ethnic groups'.

In the next station, the examiner will question ethnic health inequalities among patients.

Themes for discussion (■ Table 5.4)

Table 5.4.	
Question themes	**What is expected from the candidate?**
1 Introduction.	The candidate introduces themselves and has good body language.

Table 5.4.

	Question themes	What is expected from the candidate?
2	Are you aware of health inequalities among different ethnicities?	The candidate starts with a good succinct introduction. The candidate can give an example of their work experience or volunteering, if they have seen different ethnicities and the problems faced in healthcare to gain additional extra points.
3	Are you aware of the Marmot review, as quoted in the question?	The candidate should be honest; if they are not aware of this review, they can apologise and say that they have read this statement in the question and have learnt a new fact. However, they are aware of the problem and understand the inequalities among ethnic groups.
4	What is your opinion on Sir Michael Marmot's statement?	Points to agree on: • Whilst a proportion of racial inequality in health outcomes is due to genetic variation, both direct and indirect racial bias plays a large role. • Racism directly affects health outcomes; physical and mental health/stress can be a big problem. • Factors such as low socioeconomic status and education also affect people of white ethnicity; however, certain ethnic groups are over-represented in measures of deprivation: e.g. 30% of overcrowded homes are of Bangladeshi ethnicity compared with 2% of the white population in the UK. • Any other relevant example of some ethnic groups facing adverse health outcomes from an intersectional perspective can be given to detail the answer. Points to disagree on: • Certain medical conditions that are more prevalent in some ethnic groups show a genetic link, e.g. there is evidence to state that type 2 diabetes is more likely in South Asians due to reduced lean muscle mass and impaired insulin secretion.

Table 5.4.

Question themes	What is expected from the candidate?
5 Can you provide some examples of ethnic health inequalities that people from minority ethnic groups face?	• Excess COVID-19 deaths, whilst people from some ethnic groups may have higher rates of comorbidities (e.g. diabetes), socioeconomic factors such as crowded housing, and the inability to work from home (taxi drivers, small store owners) could have affected the mortality rates. • Increased maternal mortality in women of African descent. • Increased sectioning of men from African ethnicity. • Reduced diagnosis of skin cancer in some ethnic groups. • Reduced health education awareness. • A disparity in pulse oximetry readings in darker skin.
6 What can be done to reduce ethnic health inequalities?	Any of the following (including reasons why it would help): • Active campaigning and awareness of ethnic health inequalities. • Community outreach, working with charities and grassroot organisations. • Health education in a wide range of languages. • Teaching health professionals the importance of cultural humility. • An appropriate representation of some ethnic groups in patient-facing roles. • Research into some ethnic groups and the use of focus groups to better suit patient needs.
7 Conclusion.	The candidate summarises the contents of the station and provides an appropriate conclusion.

Discussion

If there are any reports/reviews mentioned in the question that you are not aware of, please do not get worried. Read the question and you might be aware of the problem, but not the named review. Try to think about what is the problem behind the review and summarise your introduction statement.

Ethnic inequalities can affect healthcare and is an increasing problem in recent times. The candidate should respect this and look at ways of dealing with the problem in their practice.

Key Points

- Have a structure to your answer and show your awareness of the problem.
- The examiner does not expect the candidate to solve a major problem, but assesses the awareness and motivation to learn.

References

1. Pulse oximetry and racial bias rapid review. Available from: https://www.nhsrho.org/wp-content/uploads/2021/03/Pulse-oximetry-racial-bias-report.pdf.

2. BMA Response to the Race Report. Available from: https://www.bma.org.uk/media/4276/bma-analysis-of-the-race-report-from-the-commission-on-race-and-ethnic-disparities-june-2021.pdf.

3. Paradies Y, Ben J, Denson N, *et al.* Racism as a determinant of health: a systematic review and meta-analysis. *PLOS ONE* 2015; 10(9): e0138511.

4. Venkat Narayan K. Why are South Asians prone to type 2 diabetes? A hypothesis based on unexplored pathways. *Diabetologia*; 202(63): 1103-9.

5. Black Women's Maternity Experiences Report. Available from: http://www.fivexmore.com.

6. NHS Race and Health Observatory Annual Report. Available from: https://www.nhsrho.org/wp-content/uploads/2022/07/NHS-Race-and-Health-Observatory-Annual-Report-1.pdf; 2022.

Question 72

Equality and diversity inclusiveness

Shivani Ganesh

Question

A recent Workforce Race Equality Standard found that only 10% of NHS trust board executive posts are held by some minority ethnic individuals, whereas 22% of the NHS workforce identifies as being from a minority ethnic group.

The following questions are about race inequality in the NHS workforce.

Themes for discussion (■ Table 5.5)

Table 5.5.	
Question themes	**What is expected from the candidate?**
1 Introduction.	The candidate introduces themselves to the examiner. The candidate displays good body language and exhibits a positive approach.

Table 5.5.

	Question themes	What is expected from the candidate?
2	Are you aware of the problems faced by some minority ethnic groups resulting from inequalities in the healthcare workforce?	The candidate gives a good opening statement and explains the problem and their awareness. The candidate can show examples from their workplace experience or volunteering if they have any.
3	What could be the reasons for these inequalities?	The candidate is aware of barriers facing progression to leadership roles in the NHS from a minority ethnic group standpoint (colloquially referred to as the Snowy White Peaks). Some barriers include: • Lack of mentorship. • Not being involved in informal communications and networking. • Preconceptions about leadership ability in some ethnic groups are due to stereotyping. • Tokenism — just making a symbolic effort rather than real action.
4	Are you aware of the British Medical Association's (BMA) stance in this regard?	The BMA has stated that institutional racism is prevalent in the NHS, in response to the Government's Race Report. It works with the Government and the NHS to clear the obstacles to reduce these inequalities.
5	Can you explain why staff from some minority ethnic groups do not progress to leadership roles?	The candidate explains their understanding of institutional racism that can result in: • Unprofessional and unpleasant work environments; doctors from minority ethnic groups are two times more likely to report racial harassment. • Barriers to professional development, e.g. obstacles to GPs becoming partners, junior doctors becoming consultants, etc.

Table 5.5.

Question themes	What is expected from the candidate?
	• Ethnicity pay gap due to less progression. • Reduced confidence when raising concerns. The candidate can mention some timely examples, e.g. the impact of COVID-19 on minority ethnic groups, who were less likely to speak up when personal protective equipment (PPE) was inadequate.
6 How do you think the issues faced by NHS staff from minority ethnic groups can be alleviated?	The examiner does not expect the candidate to solve the problem, but this question assesses their awareness of the problems and dilemmas. Some examples that the candidate could offer include: • Continuing discussion about racism and equal opportunities, both informally and through equality, diversity and inclusion (EDI) panels or boards. • Improve mentorship opportunities. • Leadership development programmes. • Active bystander training for staff to support their colleagues from minority ethnic groups. • Involving minority support groups such as Black and Ethnic Minority (BAME) support groups.
7 Clarity.	The candidate has good clarity and can structure the answer.
8 Conclusion.	The candidate concludes and thanks the examiner.

Discussion

An awareness of equality and diversity issues is essential for the candidate. Institutional racism is defined by MacPherson as 'the collective failure of an organisation to provide an appropriate and professional service to people because of their colour, culture, or ethnic origin. It can be seen or detected in processes, attitudes and behaviour that amount to discrimination through unwitting prejudice, ignorance, thoughtlessness and racist stereotyping'.

Racial harassment can be perpetrated by individuals, but it is the workplace's duty to provide a safe work environment for its employees. Research has clearly shown that healthcare teams have increased innovation and better performance with increased diversity.

Key Points

- Awareness of equality and diversity issues is vital.
- Structure your answer and show a positive approach.
- It is a workplace's duty to provide a safe work environment for its employees.

References

1. Summary of key evidence on barriers to and initiatives to support career progression for ethnic minority doctors. Available from: http://www.bma.org.uk/media/5747/bma-summary-of-key-evidence-report-15-june-2022.pdf.

2. Mahase E. Covid-19: Ethnic minority staff felt "vulnerable" during pandemic, says senior leader. *BMJ* 2022; 378: o1715.

3. United Kingdom Parliament. The MacPherson Report: twenty-two years on. Available from: https://publications.parliament.uk/pa/cm5802/cmselect/cmhaff/139/13911.htm#:~:text=Sir%20William%20Macpherson's%20definition%20of,culture%2C%20or%20ethnic%20origin%E2%80%9D.

4. British Medical Association. A missed opportunity – BMA response to the race report. Available from: https://www.bma.org.uk/media/4276/bma-analysis-of-the-race-report-from-the-commission-on-race-and-ethnic-disparities-june-2021.pdf.

5.   The snowy white peaks of the NHS. Available from: https://www.mdx.ac.uk/__data/assets/
      pdf_file/0015/50190/The-snowy-white-peaks.

6.   Nagpaul C. The lived experience of many ethnic minority doctors is not an equality success story.
      Available from: https://blogs.bmj.com/bmj/2021/04/16/chaand-nagpaul-the-lived-experience-of-
      many-ethnic-minority-doctors-is-not-an-equality-success-story; April 2021.

Question 73

Problem-based versus traditional learning

Thanthullu Vasu

Question

Are you aware of the teaching style used in our university?

What is the difference between problem-based learning and traditional learning?

The examiner will ask you questions on these topics.

Themes for discussion (■ Table 5.6)

Table 5.6.	
Question themes	**What is expected from the candidate?**
1 The candidate greets the examiner, and has good body language.	The candidate is presentable and uses good communication skills; always recommended in any station.

Table 5.6.

	Question themes	What is expected from the candidate?
2	Are you aware of the teaching style used in our university?	When you go for an interview, it is prudent to research the university, its teaching style, and its modules in every year of medical school, as well as research about the city and living in that city.
		This will earn positive marks if you are aware of the practicalities in that particular medical school.
3	What are the teaching styles that you are aware of in medical schools?	• Traditional (conventional) teaching. • Problem-based learning (PBL). • Integrated style teaching.
4	What do you know about traditional type courses?	Usually, these courses have a preclinical and clinical separation; universities such as Cambridge, Oxford, Birmingham, and Nottingham use this type, but some have integrated approaches.
5	What is problem-based learning (PBL)?	PBL is taught in small groups, where a problem or scenario is given and key concepts are identified; the tutor or facilitator helps to guide students to research, brainstorm and discuss the objectives planned. Universities such as St Marys, Hull, Keele, and Manchester follow this pattern.
6	What is case-based learning (CBL)?	CBL is similar to PBL, but there is a clinical case over which objectives are framed, e.g. Liverpool and Cardiff.
7	What is integrated style (systems-based) teaching?	Both preclinical and clinical topics overlap, with many universities offering clinical contacts early in the medical school itself. Universities such as Kings, Bristol and Newcastle offer these types of courses.
8	What is enquiry-based learning (EBL)?	EBL poses questions, problems or scenarios rather than simply presenting established facts; this will be guided by a facilitator. Students are in charge of their own learning, e.g. Birmingham.

Table 5.6.

	Question themes	What is expected from the candidate?
9	Clarity and awareness.	The candidate has clarity in answering questions and has done some research about various teaching styles and medical schools before the interview.
10	Conclusion.	The candidate concludes the session and thanks the examiner at the end. This gives extra bonus points.

Discussion

The candidate should be aware of various teaching styles used in medical schools. More importantly, they should have researched the curriculum of the medical school for which they are giving the interview. The details mentioned in the above answer might have changed and we strongly recommend to check the curriculum and teaching details on the respective university website before the interview.

An awareness of educational style and an explanation of why they like that style can help in these interviews.

Key Points

- Traditional teaching has preclinical and clinical separation usually.
- PBL focuses on a problem and students work in a group with a facilitator.
- Integrated style teaching encompasses both, and clinical contacts happen early in medical school.

References

1. NHS Health careers. Choosing your medical school. Available from: https://www.healthcareers.nhs.uk/explore-roles/doctors/applying-medical-school/choosing-your-medical-school.

2. British Medical Association. Courses at medical school. Available from: https://www.bma.org.uk/advice-and-support/studying-medicine/becoming-a-doctor/courses-at-medical-school.

Question 74

Teacher-assessed grades

Thanthullu Vasu

Question

During the COVID-19 pandemic, students were graded by teachers rather than standard exams. What do you think about teacher-assessed grades?

In the next station, the examiner will discuss teacher-assessed grades.

Themes for discussion (■ Table 5.7)

Table 5.7.	
Question themes	**What is expected from the candidate?**
1 The candidate greets the examiner and has good body language.	The candidate is presentable and uses good communication skills; always recommended in any station.

Table 5.7.

Question themes	What is expected from the candidate?
2 Are you aware of the teacher assessments that happened during the COVID pandemic rather than exam-based assessments?	The candidate gives a good opening statement and is aware of the problems that happened during the pandemic.
3 What are the benefits of teacher assessment?	The candidate lists a few such as: • Face-to-face exams were not possible during the pandemic times. • Teacher assessment is a continuous process rather than the assessment on exam day. • Teachers know the student well, as they have followed and assessed them over the year or longer. • Some candidates might not do well with the pressures of exams; teacher-based assessment removes this bias. • To make the system fair, guidance is given by the exam boards for standardisation of the marking system and this reduces the bias. • Teacher-assessed grades have always been higher than exam grades in GCSE and A-level exams, as per the statistics until now.
4 What are the disadvantages of teacher assessment?	• There is an element of bias in this system. • Some candidates do well in exams rather than being expressive in class. • Some candidates are used to preparing hard at the last minute before the exam rather than constant preparation.
5 What do you prefer?	The candidate has a right to give any answer, but they should have listed both pros and cons, and then give reasons for their preference.

Table 5.7.

Question themes	What is expected from the candidate?
6 In medical school, tutors will assess your coursework. Are you prepared for this type of assessment?	At A-level stage, candidates would have already experienced a practical section in which the teacher gives an assessment. They are used to this system and the candidate shows a positive approach and is enthusiastic. Furthermore, if the candidate has gone on the medical school website and looked at how the assessment is done in a particular school, they can quote this and show their awareness about the medical school. This gives positive marks if the examiner is confident of the interest of the candidate in joining their medical school.
7 What happens if there is overprediction in A-level scores by teachers when they join medical school?	Overprediction leads to candidates with lower academic performance joining medical schools. This will lead to difficulty in coping and medical school should plan additional teaching for these entrants and offer extra support for the missed A-level teaching. The candidate explains that those selected for the medical schools will have confidence and they will work hard to reach the scores needed. The candidate stays optimistic throughout the answer.
8 Clarity and awareness.	The candidate has clarity in answering questions and has a fair knowledge of teacher assessment and the problems related to this.
9 Conclusion.	The candidate concludes the session and thanks the examiner at the end. This gives extra bonus points.

Discussion

The candidate should be aware of the benefits and problems related to teacher-marked grading systems. It is unavoidable that some of the marking systems in medical colleges will be tutor- or facilitator-based and the candidate should have a positive approach to this.

Research has shown that overpredicted grades in A-level can lead to the need for extra teaching and support when the candidates join medical school.

Key Points

- Teacher-based assessment has benefits and disadvantages.
- The candidate should show a positive approach, but can prefer any system giving reasons for their choice.

References

1.   McManus IC, Woolf K, Harrison D, *et al.* Predictive validity of A-level grades and teacher-predicted grades in UK medical school applicants: a retrospective analysis of administrative data in a time of COVID-19. *BMJ Open* 2021; 11(12): e047354.

Question 75

Compulsory working in rural areas for doctors

Arani Sridhar

Question

In some developing countries, there is a shortage of doctors; the governments in those countries have asked medical students to work compulsorily in rural areas for 1 year after their graduation.

What are the issues with this proposal? The examiner will discuss these in the next station.

Themes for discussion (■ Table 5.8)

Table 5.8.	
Question themes	**What is expected from the candidate?**
1 The candidate greets the examiner and has good body language.	The candidate is presentable and uses good communication skills; always recommended in any station.

Table 5.8.

	Question themes	What is expected from the candidate?
2	Introduction.	The candidate gives a good opening statement on compulsory working in rural areas after graduation from medical school. They understand the problems and benefits of this approach.
3	What are the reasons for the lack of interest in working in rural areas?	In some countries, there might be less interest in working in rural areas, which could be due to the following: • Lack of resources such as medical equipment or medications. • Lack of therapies for medical ailments. • Lack of staff and multidisciplinary team. • Living conditions can be demotivating in rural areas in these countries.
4	What are the motivating factors to work in rural areas?	• Desire to serve low-income and underprivileged people. • Better respect for medical staff in rural areas. • Better living conditions, less traffic, not a busy life, access to natural beauty, etc.
5	Do you see this problem in the UK?	The candidate could mention that some students prefer to work or study in university teaching hospitals in bigger cities rather than district general hospitals. District general hospitals in rural areas struggle to recruit staff in various disciplines.
6	What could be done to motivate young doctors to work in rural areas?	The candidate can give various reasons for these including: • Better pay to those working in rural areas. • Provide appropriate resources. • Educational and learning opportunities can be improved. • Facilitate links with bigger hospitals to support them. • Better living conditions can attract them to rural areas.

Table 5.8.

	Question themes	What is expected from the candidate?
7	Clarity and awareness.	The candidate has clarity in answering questions and has an understanding of how the medical system differs in developing countries.
8	Conclusion.	The candidate concludes the session and thanks the examiner at the end.

Discussion

This station tests the awareness of candidates of healthcare systems in different countries. The examiner is not expecting the candidate to solve the crisis/problem but is checking that the candidate is motivated/interested to know about various healthcare systems.

Key Points

- Lack of interest in working in rural areas could be due to various reasons.
- The candidate should be aware of factors that can motivate and change this scenario.

References

1. Barman P. Why are budding doctors hesitant to work in rural areas? *Res Matters*, Chandigarh. February 2019.

2. Budhathoki SS, Zwanikken PAC, Pokharel PK, Scherpbier AJ. Factors influencing medical students' motivation to practise in rural areas in low-income and middle-income countries: a systematic review. *BMJ Open* 2017; 7(2): e013501.

Question 76

Pharmaceutical industry sponsoring lunch

Kodaganallur Parthasarathi Krishnan

Question

You might have noticed that some pharmaceutical companies sponsor educational meetings and grand round meetings in hospitals. As part of this, they offer free samples and lunch, but also advertise their products.

The examiner will question the ethical dilemmas and problems with this scenario.

Themes for discussion (■ Table 5.9)

Table 5.9.	
Question themes	**What is expected from the candidate?**
1 The candidate greets the examiner, has good body language and speaks coherently.	The candidate introduces themselves clearly with good body language and maintains eye contact throughout the conversation.

Table 5.9.

	Question themes	What is expected from the candidate?
2	The examiner enquires whether the candidate has read the question.	The candidate is able to relay what they have read whilst waiting outside, such that their understanding of this station is clearly voiced; the opening statement could give a good idea of what the candidate has understood.
3	Why do companies sponsor events in general other than in medicine?	The candidate gives examples of areas where they come across sponsorship such as television programmes, sports such as football teams and major events, and large educational society events including charities. Sponsors help to finance conducting major events, thereby shouldering some financial burden. In turn, they expect that their products are well displayed, and given opportunities to interact with delegates to ensure good exposure of their products.
4	The examiner asks what to look for in choosing such sponsors.	Candidates are expected to say that sponsors are chosen such that their products are relevant to the topics being discussed on the day ideally. If not, it could be something that is new to the field that adds value to those involved in attending that particular educational meeting.
5	Are we obliged to allow our hospitals to then buy those products displayed?	There are two types of sponsorship; in the first type, the product(s) displayed and discussed are already in use. These events aid clinicians and help in their understanding. The other type of sponsor is to display new products or techniques that are on the market. The department will then be able to discuss within themselves and arrive at a conclusion if they would benefit from those. There is no obligation to buy these products for the trust or department, and this will be clearly agreed upon when the sponsorship is arranged.

Table 5.9.

Question themes	What is expected from the candidate?
6 Sponsors offer free lunch and samples during the meeting. Are doctors ethically correct in taking these offers? Is there a fear that they will inadvertently acknowledge the use of the product by that sponsor?	Historically, sponsors used to actively campaign for their products by offering lots of 'freebies' to doctors, including financial gains such as free travel. However, the newer legislation is very clear that such practices are not allowed. The offer of lunch is not to be considered, as this is ethically wrong. Samples offered usually are there to remind clinicians of these products and do not offer any other gain. The Association of the British Pharmaceutical Industry (ABPI) regulates these sponsorships.
7 Are clinicians allowed to work for such sponsors and if so what are they expected to do?	Occasionally, some doctors may undertake some form of research or talk in meetings that have relevance to some products. They are then expected to declare their involvement in the form of disclosure. If there are financial gains, this has to be declared in their tax return also.
8 Where should students or doctors declare if they receive gains?	Doctors/students do not need to declare if they receive lunch or free small-value items. If they are of considerable value, they have to declare it and be open and honest. Hospital trusts expect them to declare this openly and these declarations with their financial value are available in the public domain.
9 Pillars of medical ethics.	The candidate can use non-maleficence, beneficence and justice to discuss how this sponsorship dilemma could be argued. The GMC's 'Good medical practice' guidelines on probity and integrity could be quoted for extra points in this station.
10 Conclusion.	The candidate concludes the station and thanks the examiner.

Discussion

This is a very important question on the domain of probity/integrity of doctors; one such question will definitely be asked in the MMI, as this is taken seriously by the profession.

The UK General Medical Council (GMC) regulates the profession, and they have very important guidance, 'Good medical practice'; this guidance deals with the professionalism of doctors.

The GMC also has a similar guidance for medical students, and it is worth quoting this in the station to make sure that the candidate is aware of this — 'Achieving good medical practice: guidance for medical students'.

Key Points

- Always introduce yourself/thank the examiner and appropriately close the session.
- You should be able to reproduce the content of the station correctly.
- Be clear on your thoughts on sponsorship, and the types and nature of free material offered.
- When involved, such relationships are declared clearly to avoid probity issues.

References

1. General Medical Council. Good medical practice: Domain 4: maintaining trust. Available from: https://www.gmc-uk.org/ethical-guidance/ethical-guidance-for-doctors/good-medical-practice/domain-4---maintaining-trust#paragraph-65.

2. General Medical Council. Achieving good medical practice: guidance for medical students. Available from: https://www.gmc-uk.org/education/standards-guidance-and-curricula/guidance/student-professionalism-and-ftp/achieving-good-medical-practice.

Question 77

Ethics of charging patients

Thanthullu Vasu

Question

There was a proposal by politicians to charge patients who do not attend their NHS appointments; the proposal was to charge £10 for each non-attendance.

The Government withdrew this immediately due to controversies, but there is still a debate about whether it is feasible and whether it is a good idea.

What are your views on this dilemma? In the next station, the examiner will discuss these ethical dilemmas.

Themes for discussion (▓ Table 5.10)

Table 5.10.	
Question themes	**What is expected from the candidate?**
1 The candidate greets the examiner and has good body language.	The candidate introduces themselves and greets the examiner with good body language.
2 Explanation of the scenario.	The candidate has a clear knowledge of the problem and starts with a good introduction statement.
3 The candidate explains why it is a good idea to charge.	• NHS DNAs (did not attend) are costly (can cost £160 per non-attendance), and this is a waste of taxpayers' money. • This fine will encourage patients to attend. • The NHS is already consuming huge resources; this wastage should be avoided. • If the patient does not attend, they are taking slots away from people who need them and are wasting them; this is not ethically right.
4 The candidate explains why patients should not be charged.	• The NHS has a core principle of 'free for all at point of use'; this policy is against this NHS principle. • Unfair to those who cannot pay. • Will affect vulnerable people more than others (e.g. mental health conditions, people in poverty, etc.). • This will deter patients from coming to the NHS, especially the most underprivileged and most needed ones. • Ethically wrong. • The patient can have a valid reason for non-attendance, e.g. illness, family condition, caring for others, postal delays or errors in administrative work, etc. • To collect this fine requires more staff, resources, etc.; this can itself be difficult given the difficulty in recruiting staff in the NHS.

Table 5.10.

Question themes	What is expected from the candidate?
5 The candidate has a clear opinion on this issue and explains the reasons.	The candidate can choose any answer but should detail both pros and cons first, then give clear answers why they do or do not choose to support this policy.
6 The candidate uses three of the four pillars of medical ethics (non-maleficence, beneficence and justice).	• Non-maleficence — do no harm — this can deter patients from seeking help. • Beneficence: there are arguments about whether this can benefit or not, but it might not be beneficial for the patient. • Justice — an overall benefit to society — applying fines can save taxpayers' money.
7 Alternative ideas to reduce DNAs (motivate, remind, phone/text, advertise money lost)	• Spend money on advertising the need to attend, how much money is lost due to DNA, etc. • Send reminders to patients: phone SMS messages, text, phone calls, emails, etc. • Motivate patients to attend; GPs can do this when they send a referral to the hospital. • Place advertising boards in hospitals and GP surgeries on money lost due to DNAs. • Have a policy that the GP has to refer again if the patient does not attend after two DNAs. In this case, GPs will put more pressure on patients to not miss their appointment.
8 What are the views of doctors?	The British Medical Association (BMA) is strongly against this policy and does not want the Government to charge for non-attendance.
9 Judgement and clarity.	The candidate has good clarity on the issue and understands the problems.
10 Conclusion.	The candidate concludes and thanks the examiner.

Discussion

Approximately 1 in 10 outpatient appointments are missed every year in England; this can lead to wasted NHS resources. It is claimed that more than 15 million GP appointments are missed every year in the UK, wasting 1.2 million hours and costing the NHS £216 million. Reduced DNAs could lead to increased NHS productivity.

The British Medical Association (BMA) has strongly opposed charging patients for missed appointments. It opines that charging patients could undermine the essential trust between doctor and patient and threaten the fundamental principle that the NHS delivers free care at the point of need for all.

Many opine that rather than punishing patients who do not attend, the reasons should be investigated. Penalising patients affects the poorest and the most vulnerable in the community. This will discourage them from rebooking, which could worsen the already existing health inequalities; candidates can use one of the pillars of medical ethics — in particular, justice — to explain their view about this point.

A study showed that, rather than a standard reminder text for healthcare appointments, a message with information about the specific waste of not attending reduced the number of missed appointments by 23%.

Key Points

- Non-attendance of an NHS appointment is a waste of resources and taxpayers' money.
- Fining patients can lead to a worsening of healthcare inequalities; it will affect the poorest and most vulnerable to a greater extent.
- The candidate should use any of the pillars of medical ethics to detail their views.
- The BMA is strongly against charging patients for non-attendance.

References

1. United Kingdom Government. A zero cost way to reduce missed hospital appointments. Available from: https://www.gov.uk/government/publications/reducing-missed-hospital-appointments-using-text-messages/a-zero-cost-way-to-reduce-missed-hospital-appointments; January 2016.

2. British Medical Association. Charging patients for missed appointments is not the answer to tackling the NHS backlog, says BMA. Available from: https://www.bma.org.uk/bma-media-centre/charging-patients-for-missed-appointments-is-not-the-answer-to-tackling-the-nhs-backlog-says-bma; July 2022.

3. Wales online. Rishi Sunak wants to fine patients £10 if they miss NHS appointments. Available from: https://www.walesonline.co.uk/news/uk-news/rishi-sunak-wants-fine-patients-25375827; October 2022.

Section **6**

Personal qualities

Section editor: Shreya Shyam

Introduction to personal qualities

The three fundamentals of a good clinician are knowledge, skills and attitude. The three factors can be thought of as the legs of a stool, as without even one of them, the structure will topple. The MMI interview is designed to assess knowledge through fact-based questions, and skills will be assessed through communication stations and role-play stations. It is therefore the personal character station in which the candidate's attitudes and motivations are truly able to shine, and the candidate is able to present themselves as a future clinician.

One of the most likely lines of questioning in this station will be on the candidate's motivation behind studying medicine. A good candidate will be well versed in their personal statement and will be able to draw on aspects of this in their answer.

Studying medicine is rarely an overnight decision, and examiners will be keen to see a candidate who has a diverse range of reasons behind their goal as opposed to a single experience that encouraged them. In addition, medicine is a career that can be challenging both physically and emotionally. A candidate who addresses these challenges and their plan to manage them will show the examiner that they have deeply reflected on their career choice and are more prepared for any hurdles they will face.

Reflection is a key step in a doctor's continual professional development. One way in which reflection is assessed is through a candidate's ability to recall their use of personal skills in a variety of past situations, e.g. an instance in which they used teamwork/leadership skills. Questions such as this give a candidate the opportunity to put forward their own abilities, whilst also giving a chance to show how they can transfer this experience to their medical career. A good candidate will mention what went well in the situation, as well as what could have gone better, and how they will build on this reflection.

Finally, the personal qualities station will give a chance for the candidate to discuss their life outside education. For these questions, a candidate should be able to discuss any hobbies and interests and explain how these will give them a coping mechanism for tackling the demands of medical education. To exceed requirements, a candidate can also mention any transferable skills from their extracurricular activities that will aid their career. For example, a student who takes part in team sports can mention that they have developed physical stamina and good teamwork skills, both of which can aid them in a clinical setting.

In summary, the personal qualities station provides an opportunity for a candidate to truly sell themselves and give a personal touch to the interview setting. Make sure that you know your way around your personal statement and show a positive, enthusiastic attitude!

Question 78

Personal statement questions

Paul Sanjay Sundaram

Question

In the next station, the examiner will ask you about the points discussed in your personal statement, including your motivation to study medicine, your understanding of medicine as a career and your own personal qualities.

Themes for discussion (■ Table 6.1)

Table 6.1.	
Question themes	**What is expected from the candidate?**
1 The examiner asks the candidate why they want to be a doctor?	There is no right or wrong answer here; the examiner will instead assess the candidate's enthusiasm and delivery of their answer. The candidate gives reasons that are unique and meaningful to themselves. Some points that could be mentioned include the candidate's passion for science/biology, past people interactions, work experience and personal motivators. The candidate's passion will automatically shine throughout here and using specific examples will result in high marks.

Table 6.1.

	Question themes	What is expected from the candidate?
2	Which is more important, leadership or teamwork?	The candidate should give a balanced, thoughtful answer, which considers the merits of both leadership and teamwork. A top-level answer will include the personal experiences of the candidate involving leadership and teamwork, as well as the relevance of these qualities in a clinical setting. Examples of points the candidate could mention include: • Importance of teamwork for bettering patient care, e.g. in an MDT setting. • A good leader helps to put together the group's strengths and plan the goals of the team. • A good leader will enhance any teamwork, so the relationship is a two-way street. Candidates should consider both sides and then come to a conclusion.
3	The examiner asks the candidate to pick out any three qualities from their personal statement that they believe a doctor should have and why?	The candidate should have insight into qualities that are important in a medical profession. They may draw inspiration from the qualities outlined in the GMC's guideline, 'Good medical practice'. Examples of qualities the candidate could mention include effective communication, resilience/persistence and having a sense of compassion or empathy for others. Candidates should link these qualities to personal experiences of observing or demonstrating these qualities, e.g. in an academic setting, work experience or volunteering.
4	Where can you see yourself in 5, 10 and 15 years?	This question tests the candidate's understanding of the trainee doctor pathway. After 5 years, most candidates will be at the start of their FY1 career. After 10 years, candidates will be in their respective training (specialty training or core training) or finishing GP training. After 15 years, candidates can be senior registrars or attain consultant level.

Table 6.1.

Question themes	What is expected from the candidate?
5 Why do you want to do medicine and not nursing as a career?	The candidate shows appreciation for both doctors and nurses, demonstrating that they both play pivotal roles in providing the best patient care. The candidate is aware that advanced nurse practitioners can diagnose and treat but understands that doctors have more scope and opportunities to do this. The candidate expresses interest in lifelong learning and teaching that carries on throughout the career. They also understand the research opportunities that are available in medicine. The candidate may suggest they want a mix of science and caring in their career that is achieved in the role of a doctor.
6 The examiner asks the candidate to name a quality that is not desirable in a doctor.	The candidate thinks about antagonistic qualities here; for example, aggression, arrogance, and egoism. Many of these qualities are qualities that do not help a team dynamic and will make a doctor less approachable to their colleagues or patients. The candidate describes the repercussions of having a quality like this on patient care and inter-professional relationships. They may mention observations from work experience or volunteering to support their answer.
7 Conclusion.	The candidate concludes the session and thanks the examiner at the end.

Discussion

As you might have realised from the above, there are no fixed answers for any of the questions related to personal character. The examiners are experienced enough to assess the motivation and qualities of a candidate appearing for the MMI interview. The candidate needs to be positive and show motivation in their answers.

In any question, it is prudent to include, if possible, the nature of the workplace experience or volunteering that the candidate might have done; this will add more to the score achieved in this station.

Key Points

- Deliver your answer enthusiastically and let your passion come across.
- Give a balanced discussion and argument for evaluation questions.
- Use observations and experiences from work placements to support your answer.

References

1. General Medical Council. Good medical practice. Available from: https://www.gmc-uk.org/ethical-guidance/ethical-guidance-for-doctors/good-medical-practice/duties-of-a-doctor.

Question 79

Work experience-based questions

Paul Sanjay Sundaram

Question

Tell me about any work experience you have participated in.

How did it help you and what did you gain from the experience?

Themes for discussion (▇ Table 6.2)

Table 6.2.	
Question themes	**What is expected from the candidate?**
1 Introduction.	The candidate greets the examiner, has good body language and speaks coherently.

Table 6.2.

Question themes	What is expected from the candidate?
2 The examiner asks the candidate an opening question about work experience.	The candidate gives the details about their work experience, including: • Time frame. • Setting (primary, secondary or tertiary care). • The types of professionals shadowed (e.g. doctor, receptionist, nurse). • Roles the candidate undertook (observing, helping with minor tasks, talking to patients, etc.).
3 The examiner asks the candidate to describe a situation encountered in work experience that stood out to them.	The candidate explores a particular situation they encountered during their experience in detail. They ensure the information is descriptive, whilst maintaining patient confidentiality, e.g. 'I had an interaction with Mr X, a 74-year-old man in a care home'. STAR is a good mnemonic that can be used to ensure that the candidate discusses the relevant details of the experience; it includes Situation, Task, Action and Result.
4 The examiner asks the candidate to describe what they learnt from this situation.	The candidate should link what they learnt from the experience to skills they can practise and qualities they can embody as a medical student and a future doctor. For example 'When communicating with Mr X, I learnt the importance of active listening and open body language in building rapport. I can apply these skills to patient interactions as a medical student and as a doctor to form good patient-clinician relationships'. Other qualities or skills that the candidate may discuss include compassion, empathy, teamwork, resilience, etc.

Table 6.2.

Question themes	What is expected from the candidate?
5 The examiner asks what they found challenging during work experience.	This question is about reflection. Here, candidates can describe the realities and stresses of medicine. They may mention difficulties in communicating with patients or adjusting to the fast-paced environment. After describing the challenge, it is important for the candidate to show reflection on why they encountered this challenge and how they can work on overcoming it. For example, if the candidate struggled with communication, they may improve on this by volunteering in a local care home or partaking in a debate club.
6 Conclusion.	The candidate summarises the key points discussed in the station and thanks the examiner for their time.

Discussion

This station is an opportunity for the candidate to express their positive attitude towards medicine as a career; they should be enthusiastic but coherent in their description of the experience. Being positive and respecting all allied professions is prudent. Maintaining anonymity to the patient is essential, but describing where the candidate had the experience (e.g. primary care, secondary care hospital, which clinic, which situation, etc.) can add value to the answer.

Key Points

- Be descriptive, but avoid confidential details when describing work experience.
- Use the STAR mnemonic to describe experiences, as well as what you learnt (Situation, Task, Action and Result).
- Reflect and give examples of how you can develop your skills and attitude.

References

1. General Medical Council. Good medical practice. Available from: https://www.gmc-uk.org/ethical-guidance/ethical-guidance-for-doctors/good-medical-practice/duties-of-a-doctor.

Question 80

Teamwork and its importance

Arani Sridhar

Question

Why is teamwork important? What is an MDT and how does it work? How will you resolve conflict in a group? Conflict in a team setting: what are the problems with member participation?

Themes for discussion (■ Table 6.3)

Table 6.3.	
Question themes	**What is expected from the candidate?**
1 The candidate greets the examiner and has good body language.	The introduction and communication skills of the candidate will be assessed in all MMI stations.

Table 6.3.

Question themes	What is expected from the candidate?
2 What are your thoughts on teamwork?	The candidate gives a good opening statement about their understanding of the importance of teamwork, e.g. 'Communication and teamwork skills are essential for providing quality healthcare. When all clinical and non-clinical staff collaborate effectively, healthcare teams can improve patient outcomes, prevent medical errors, improve efficiency and increase patient satisfaction'. A possible team structure can include: patients, junior doctors/physician associates, nurses, consultants, allied health staff, ward clerks/admin, managers, and the hospital board. The exact team structure will vary from trust to trust, hospital to hospital and even ward to ward. Medical teams can be united through their shared principles, common goals and clear lines of accountability and responsibility.
3 Why do you think teamwork is important in the NHS/medical practice/patient care?	The candidate describes some benefits of effective teamwork (i.e. improved performance, productivity, patient satisfaction, clinical outcomes and staff morale). The candidate can give an example of a situation in which they personally witnessed the benefits of teamwork, e.g. during work experience or volunteering in a clinical setting. They can describe the situation, the types of clinicians involved in the team, and the features of the teamwork that were particularly effective.

Table 6.3.

	Question themes	What is expected from the candidate?
4	What makes a good team?	The broad principles are: effective leadership and governance, supportive team dynamics and clear roles/responsibilities of the team members.
		The candidate can discuss the characteristics of a good team, such as:
		<ul><li>A common sense of purpose.</li><li>A clear understanding of objectives.</li><li>Resources to meet targets.</li><li>Mutual respect among team members.</li><li>Understanding members' strengths and weaknesses.</li><li>Mutual trust.</li><li>Willingness to speak openly.</li><li>Range of skills to deal effectively with tasks.</li><li>Range of personal styles for team roles.</li></ul>
5	What are your thoughts on the MDT and how does it work in clinical practice?	Multidisciplinary team (MDT) working: how health and care professionals work together to support people with complex care needs who have been identified through risk stratification and case finding.
		An MDT is a group of healthcare staff who are members of different organisations and professions (e.g. hospital staff, GPs, social workers, nurses) who work together to make decisions about the treatment of individual patients and service users. MDTs are used in both health and care settings.
		Teamwork has become an important health intervention for several reasons. First, clinical care is becoming more complex and specialised. Therefore, when treating a patient, communication is required across a diverse range of specialties. An ageing population, and the increase in chronic diseases such as diabetes, cancer, and heart disease, have forced medical staff to take a multidisciplinary approach to healthcare:

Table 6.3.

Question themes	What is expected from the candidate?
	• Researchers have found that working together reduces the number of medical errors and increases patient safety. Teamwork also reduces issues that lead to burnout. • No longer is one person responsible for the patient's health; today, an entire team of health workers comes together to coordinate a patient's well-being. • Examples of MDT care: cancer care, elderly care, care of children with functional needs, stroke care, etc. • Advantages: gives patients access to an entire team of experts, improves service coordination, expedites the referral process, provides new avenues for service implementation, and allows patients to create goals for themselves. • Disadvantages: time pressure, can involve team members with varying experience/skills, requires frequent collaboration to be effective, needs resources and clear documentation of roles and responsibilities.
6 Do you think conflicts exist in teamwork and what are the possible reasons for conflict within teams?	Conflict can range from minor misunderstandings to highly destructive behaviours. Generally, conflicts have two aspects: • The relationship between the people involved: relationship conflict. • The issue that is the basis of the disagreement: task and process conflict. Reasons for conflict in the NHS are: • Poor communication. • Personality clash and unwillingness to assist. • Power difference: hierarchy. • Organisational problems. • Heavy workloads, stress and fatigue.

Table 6.3.

Question themes	What is expected from the candidate?
7 How would you resolve conflict within a team?	The candidate gives a comprehensive answer and may draw on their own experiences in the answer.
	Examples are shown below.
	DOs:
	• Ensure the issues are fully outlined. • Acknowledge emotions and different styles. • Make sure you have a comfortable environment for any meeting. • Set a time frame for the discussion. • Establish good rapport. • Use names throughout the process to personalise the approach. • Seek advice from a manager or mediator if necessary.
	DO NOTs:
	• Conduct your conversation in a public place. • Leave the discussion open; instead create an action plan. • Use jargon. • Interrupt or talk over others. • Distort the truth. • Use inappropriate humour.
8 You are in a group project with three other people. One member is very talkative and frequently interrupts others, whilst another member is very quiet and rarely contributes. How will you manage this situation?	The candidate should first acknowledge the challenges that low or excessive member contribution can pose to the team dynamic and productivity. The emphasis should be on effective communication and empathy towards their team members. For example, a candidate could mention the importance of understanding the reasons behind the overenthusiasm/lack of enthusiasm of their team members and use this background to frame their approach.

Table 6.3.	
Question themes	**What is expected from the candidate?**
	The candidate can mention past experiences in which they may have used similar skills to overcome a difficult team dynamic. They may also mention the principles of NHS core values and the GMC's 'Good medical practice' guideline that they could apply in their approach. The NHS strategy for conflict resolution is: • Prevention is better than cure. • Mediation. • Team healing. • Constructive conversation.

Discussion

One of the most common questions asked in an MMI station is about teamwork. The NHS cannot work efficiently without this key characteristic. The candidate should be very motivated and positive towards teamwork.

In an MMI interview, it will secure bonus points if the candidate uses their experience from the past to explain efficient teamwork; even if it is not from their work experience or volunteering experience, it could come from some other aspect of their life, including that from school/college or from community experience.

Key Points

- Being a good team leader is equally important as being a good team player.
- Give an example of past experiences to exemplify your abilities in a team setting.
- Learn about the professionals and team dynamics within an MDT.

References

1. Royal College of Physicians. Improving teams in healthcare: Resource 1: building effective teams. Available from: https://www.rcplondon.ac.uk/projects/outputs/improving-teams-healthcare-resource-1-building-effective-teams; 2017.

2. Rosen MA, DiazGranados D, Dietz AS, *et al.* Teamwork in healthcare: key discoveries enabling safer, high-quality care. *Am Psychol* 2018; 73(4): 433-50.

3. NHS England. MDT development. Available from: https://www.england.nhs.uk/wp-content/uploads/2015/01/mdt-dev-guid-flat-fin.pdf; 2014.

4. Taberna M, Gil Moncayo FG, Jané-Salas E, *et al.* The multidisciplinary team (MDT) approach and quality of care. *Front Oncol* 2020; 10: 85.

5. NHS England, NHS improvement. Quality, service improvement and redesign tools: managing conflict. Available from: https://www.england.nhs.uk/wp-content/uploads/2022/01/qsir-managing-conflict.pdf.

Question81

Improving teamwork

Thanthullu Vasu

Question

The next station will discuss teamwork and its role in healthcare. You will be asked about a situation in which you worked in a team and how well it went.

The dynamics of the team, things that can go wrong and how to make it effective will all be discussed in this station.

Themes for discussion (■ Table 6.4)

Table 6.4.	
Question themes	**What is expected from the candidate?**
1 Introduction.	The candidate greets the examiner, has good body language and speaks coherently and clearly.

Table 6.4.

	Question themes	What is expected from the candidate?
2	Have you worked in a team?	The candidate gives an example of when they worked in a team. Examples could include: • Academic setting. • Sports team. • Job/volunteering. STAR is a good mnemonic that can be used to ensure that the candidate discusses the relevant details of the example; it includes Situation, Task, Action and Result.
3	What was your role in the team?	The candidate explains the various components of the team, the team working style, and the candidate's own contributions that they brought to the task.
4	What made the team successful?	Examples of qualities the candidate could discuss are: • Effective communication. • Good leadership. • Good understanding of individual strengths and weaknesses. It is important that the candidate shows reflection on the more effective and less effective parts of the team; they may also link this to anything they observed during work experiences or other teamwork experiences.
5	Are you a leader or a follower?	The candidate explains the importance of being both a good leader and a good follower and can give personal examples of both roles. The use of the STAR mnemonic can aid the description of past experiences.

Table 6.4.

	Question themes	What is expected from the candidate?
6	Who is a good leader?	The candidate outlines qualities for good leadership: communication, reaching out and listening to all, organisation and delegation.
7	Have you been in a situation in which teamwork failed?	The candidate gives an example and may make effective use of the STAR mnemonic. It is important that they describe the situation in a reflective tone instead of pointing out blame. A good candidate will explain the key lessons they learnt from this situation and how they adapted in future team settings to avoid the same mistakes.
8	Concludes the session.	The candidate thanks the examiner for their time and concludes the session.

Discussion

One of the most common questions asked in an MMI station is about teamwork. The NHS cannot work efficiently without this key characteristic. The candidate should be very motivated and positive towards teamwork.

In an MMI interview, it will secure bonus points if the candidate uses their experience from the past to explain about efficient teamwork; even if it is not from their work experience or volunteering experience, it could come from some other aspect of their life, including that from school/college or from community experience.

Key Points

- Use the STAR mnemonic to describe past situations; the acronym helps to ensure that the relevant points are shared without excess detail.
- Ensure that you show reflection and explain how you have learnt from your past experiences and adapted for future events.
- Relate the teamwork skills you have learnt from past experiences to work within multidisciplinary teams in a clinical setting.

References

1. Royal College of Physicians. Improving teams in healthcare: Resource 1: building effective teams. Available from: https://www.rcplondon.ac.uk/projects/outputs/improving-teams-healthcare-resource-1-building-effective-teams; 2017.

2. Rosen MA, DiazGranados D, Dietz AS, *et al.* Teamwork in healthcare: key discoveries enabling safer, high-quality care. *Am Psychol 2*018; 73(4): 433-50.

3. NHS England. MDT development. Available from: https://www.england.nhs.uk/wp-content/uploads/2015/01/mdt-dev-guid-flat-fin.pdf; 2014.

4. Taberna M, Gil Moncayo FG, Jané-Salas E, *et al.* The multidisciplinary team (MDT) approach and quality of care. *Front Oncol* 2020; 10: 85.

5. NHS England, NHS improvement. Quality, service improvement and redesign tools: managing conflict. Available from: https://www.england.nhs.uk/wp-content/uploads/2022/01/qsir-managing-conflict.pdf.

Question 82

Leader versus follower

Kodaganallur Parthasarathi Krishnan

Question

In a team setting, you will find both leaders and followers. What type of personality do you think you have?

Themes for discussion (■ Table 6.5)

Table 6.5.	
Question themes	**What is expected from the candidate?**
1 Introduction.	The candidate greets the examiner and has good body language.

Table 6.5.

	Question themes	What is expected from the candidate?
2	What are the personality types that you can find in a team?	The candidate gives a good opening statement about what a team involves. They explain, possibly with an example, how a team consists of individual members of varying personalities, e.g. leaders, followers, managers, observers, etc.
3	Can you explain who a leader is?	Leaders are those who have a vision about what the team needs to achieve and help guide the path for the team to reach the goal. Good qualities in a leader include enthusiasm, excellent communication skills, being good listeners, adaptability and an understanding of the strengths and weaknesses of the team.
4	What are the attributes of a follower?	Followers are key and valuable components of any team. Good followers need to be good communicators to ensure that their ideas are voiced, as well as good listeners, so that they are open to discussion. In addition, followers in a team should be ready to work together and support the guidance of the leader, to ensure that the whole team functions as one cohesive unit.
5	Who do you think a manager is?	Managers are those who build a work culture, focus on team members' strengths, are assertive, handle pressure and are good at people management.
6	Based on the descriptions you have given, which personality suits you best?	There is no one correct answer to this, as this is not a test of one's personality. The candidates can choose to pick any one of the above or even state that they are still developing different characteristics in themselves and adapting based on different settings.

Table 6.5.

	Question themes	What is expected from the candidate?
7	Are you aware of any methods to identify what personality one belongs to?	Whilst a variety of tools and questionnaires exist for assessing personality, one popular example is the Myers-Briggs Type Indicator (MBTI). It is a well established questionnaire that, after extensive probing, identifies up to 16 different personalities.
8	Why do you think this question was asked in the MMI interview?	Working as a doctor, both in primary and secondary care, involves dealing with many different types of people, including leaders, followers and managers. It is vital for the candidate to understand and explain the importance and existence of different personalities to avoid conflicts and ensure smooth working environments.
9	Should the selection of candidates be a mixture of these personalities based on personality tests such as the MBTI?	The candidate explains that these tests carry uncertainty. They are more useful as supporting tools to identify personality attributes and individual strengths, which in turn can fuel more tailored working and learning styles. However, the tests alone are not accurate or definite enough to make important decisions.
10	Conclusion.	The candidate summarises the points covered in the station and thanks the examiner for their time.

Discussion

A team consists of different personalities and the candidate should be aware of these. The candidate should be able to distinguish the characteristics of a leader and a follower and be able to identify key personalities that can aid the team in working efficiently.

Key Points

- Have an understanding of the different personality types and the key characteristics of each type.
- Understand the importance of teamwork in both clinical and non-clinical settings.
- Personality tests are useful tools but carry a degree of uncertainty and inaccuracy.

References

1. General Medical Council. Leadership and management for all doctors. Available from: https://www.gmc-uk.org/ethical-guidance/ethical-guidance-for-doctors/leadership-and-management-for-all-doctors.

Question83

Probity: a medical student stealing equipment

Siva Thanthullu

Question

You have just started medical school and have been posted to attend a GP surgery for learning.

On the way back to your accommodation on your first day, your friend/flatmate tells you that she has taken the stethoscope from the clinic room; she tells you that she has taken it so that she can train herself to listen to the heart sounds that was taught in the teaching that day. You ask her 'Have you stolen the stethoscope?' She says that she has only taken it temporarily and will return it in a few weeks after improving her auscultation clinical skills.

What would you do now? The next station will discuss this complex scenario and how you would approach the problem.

Themes for discussion (■ Table 6.6)

Table 6.6.		
	Question themes	**What is expected from the candidate?**
1	Introduction.	The candidate greets the examiner, has good body language and speaks coherently.
2	Can you explain the scenario?	The candidate summarises the scenario into four or five key points, as opposed to repeating it word for word.
		It is important that the opening summary is succinct and clear, as it gives a good impression of the candidate to the examiner.
3	What ethical principles play a role in this scenario?	A good candidate will reference the importance of the GMC's 'Good medical practice' guideline, especially the principles of integrity and maintaining trust, which are discussed in Domain 4.
		Whilst integrity and honesty go hand in hand, they are not one and the same. Honesty is the act of being truthful; in this scenario her friend should show honesty by telling the truth about her actions. By contrast, integrity involves consistently showing moral behaviour, including honesty. A medical student should consistently show honesty that will, in turn, develop into integrity. Integrity inspires trust within the patient-clinician relationship and can increase the quality of patient care.
		Furthermore, patient care and safety can be compromised due to the non-availability of this vital equipment in the clinical area. Patient safety is of prime concern in the clinical context here.
4	What will you do?	A good candidate is one who balances empathy with moral principles. On the one hand, it is important that they encourage their friend to be honest about her mistake and return the stethoscope, as this is in line with the GMC ethical principles. On the other hand, the candidate should also be understanding of the reasons behind their friend's actions and approach her with empathy.

Table 6.6.

Question themes	What is expected from the candidate?
	An example of an appropriate course of action would be to encourage the friend to talk to her supervising clinician, explain her actions, apologise and ask the clinician if they can suggest a different way she can practise auscultation.
5 What will you do if your friend does not listen and does not take your advice seriously?	The candidate remains empathetic but firm in their moral principles. The candidate should once again suggest that the friend herself owns up; if not, they themselves will tell the tutor or supervisor. This is due to the fact that integrity and patient safety are compromised by missing equipment.
6 Conclusion.	The candidate summarises the key points of the situation and thanks the examiner for their time.

Discussion

Probity is vital for any healthcare professional. The GMC takes probity seriously and any medical student should be aware of these principles. The GMC's document, 'Achieving good medical practice: guidance for medical students', clearly mentions that they should be honest, open and act with integrity (see the section on maintaining trust). The GMC clearly mentions that, as medical students, they are studying to join a trusted profession that will bring them into contact with patients and members of the public. It expects medical students to demonstrate a high standard of behaviour at all times, which justifies the trust placed in them as future members of the profession.

Key Points

- Have a good understanding of the GMC's 'Good medical practice' guideline.
- Understand how the principles of honesty and integrity translate to patient safety and quality of patient care.
- Balance empathy and moral principles to create a more persuasive approach.

References

1. General Medical Council. Achieving good medical practice: guidance for medical students. Available from: https://www.gmc-uk.org/education/standards-guidance-and-curricula/guidance/student-professionalism-and-ftp/achieving-good-medical-practice.

2. General Medical Council. Good medical practice. Available from: https://www.gmc-uk.org/ethical-guidance/ethical-guidance-for-doctors/good-medical-practice/duties-of-a-doctor.

Question 84

Clinical error: a probity issue

Kodaganallur Parthasarathi Krishnan

Question

You are a junior doctor. Yesterday, you discharged a patient without senior input or consultation as the patient was stable. Unfortunately, the patient became unwell and is readmitted to the ward the next day. Currently, you are the only clinician who is free on the ward and you meet the patient.

In the next role-play station, you will talk to the patient and explain the events.

Themes for discussion (■ Table 6.7)

Table 6.7.	
Question themes	**What is expected from the candidate?**
1 Introduction.	The candidate introduces themselves to the examiner.

Table 6.7.

	Question themes	What is expected from the candidate?
2	The examiner introduces the patient (actor) to the candidate.	The candidate introduces themselves to the patient and confirms their name and date of birth.
3	The candidate makes enquiries about the reason for admission.	The candidate undertakes a reasonable history-taking to ascertain why this patient had been readmitted to the hospital. Questions they can ask include: 'What brings you to the hospital today?' 'When did the feelings of being unwell begin yesterday? Did anything occur just before you started feeling poorly?' 'Can you describe where the pain is? Does it come and go?' 'Does anything make the pain better or worse?'
4	The candidate identifies that symptoms were similar to his previous admission. The patient shows signs of unhappiness and some element of discontent.	The candidate apologises to the patient and is empathetic to his views. They are open and honest about their mistake in discharging the patient without discussion with a supervisor or senior consultant. A good candidate will assure the patient that they will address their mistake with their supervisors, reflect on it, and change their actions appropriately next time. The candidate may try to regain the patient's confidence by reassuring them that the team will look after him well, and identify and treat the reasons for his readmission.
5	The actor is still unhappy and wants to know why he was discharged so early yesterday.	The candidate continues to be calm and composed. They show empathy and understanding through their words (saying sorry, I understand your frustration, etc.) and their body language (non-verbal cues are important also).

Table 6.7.

	Question themes	What is expected from the candidate?
		Keeping eye contact, staying on the same level and listening to the angry patient are all important active actions here.
6	The actor insists on speaking to any senior on the ward; they say they are not satisfied with the explanation.	The candidate remains calm and explains to the patient that currently they are the only clinician on the ward, but they will seek out a senior clinician as soon as one is available. The candidate can offer to address the patient's concerns to the best of their abilities in the meantime.
7	The patient asks how sure he is that he will be safely discharged this time.	The candidate should reassure the patient that they will reflect on their previous actions and will take steps in consultation with seniors to ensure that safe discharge will happen only when all symptoms are resolved.
8	The examiner asks the candidate what they will do next.	The candidate explains that they will go and speak to their senior, either a registrar or consultant. They will have an open and clear conversation as to what happened, explain the reasons for their action and seek guidance. They should show evidence of being receptive to learning if any potential mistakes may have happened.
9	Conclusion.	The candidate thanks the patient and conveys their apologies again. The candidate concludes the session by asking, 'Is there anything else that I can do please?'

Role play for the actor

The actor was told to be unhappy and upset about their readmission. They will not reveal their symptoms unless the candidate tries to take their history with simple, easy-to-understand language. They will initially be stubborn about not engaging with the candidate and insist on speaking to a senior. Towards the end of the role-play station, they will ask how the past mistake will be avoided this time and will calm down following reassurance from the candidate.

Discussion

Many MMI interviews will include questions on dissatisfied patients. This is done to assess that the candidate can listen, communicate and show empathy. Apologising is an important step in any situation in which a mistake has been made or something untoward has happened (to express empathy for how the patient feels). The candidate's main task is to de-escalate the situation and reassure the patient's trust in the healthcare system.

The UK General Medical Council's (GMC) 'Good medical practice' guideline (Domain 2: Safety and quality) clarifies the need to respond to concerns openly and safely. Domain 3 (Communication partnership and teamwork) stresses that doctors must listen to patients, take account of their views, and respond honestly to their questions. The GMC's guidance for medical students also promotes the same messages but advises informing supervisors involved in the care.

One of the key traits that a candidate should demonstrate in this station is to stay calm but show empathy at the same time. Listening is an active skill and needs to be developed; at the same time, most stations are 5-7 minutes long, and the candidate must apologise and explain what happened, and reassure that corrective steps will be taken. Practising with mock actors can give confidence to the candidate for facing the real MMI scenario.

Remember the mnemonic ICE (Ideas, Concerns, Expectations) when talking to an unsatisfied patient: ideas, concerns and expectations of the patient.

Perhaps most importantly, the candidate should be able to demonstrate the skill of reflection; this should be expressed in this station. As a medical student, the General Medical Council expects that they not only learn the scientific and clinical aspects but have the professional skills and identity that will help them to provide a high standard of care for their patients; the practice of reflection will assist in this process.

Key Points

- Take note of ICE: the Ideas, Concerns and Expectations of the patient.
- An empathetic approach and saying 'sorry' are vital in these situations.
- Reflect and explain how your actions will change to prevent the mistake from reoccurring.

References

1. General Medical Council. The reflective practitioner – a guide for medical students. Available at: https://www.gmc-uk.org/education/standards-guidance-and-curricula/guidance/reflective-practice/the-reflective-practitioner---a-guide-for-medical-students.

2. General Medical Council. Good medical practice: Domain 2: safety and quality. Available from: https://www.gmc-uk.org/ethical-guidance/ethical-guidance-for-doctors/good-medical-practice/domain-2----safety-and-quality#paragraph-22.

3. General Medical Council. Good medical practice: Domain 3: communication partnership and teamwork. Available from: https://www.gmc-uk.org/ethical-guidance/ethical-guidance-for-doctors/good-medical-practice/domain-3---communication-partnership-and-teamwork#paragraph-31.

4. General Medical Council. Achieving good medical practice: guidance for medical students. Domain 4: maintaining trust. Available from: https://www.gmc-uk.org/education/standards-guidance-and-curricula/guidance/student-professionalism-and-ftp/achieving-good-medical-practice/domain-4-maintaining-trust#act-with-honesty-and-integrity.

5. American Medical Association. Ethics – patient rights. Available from: https://www.ama-assn.org/delivering-care/ethics/patient-rights.

Question85

A patient complains that she does not like you

Prabhu Gandhimani

Question

You are a junior doctor. A patient who you visited yesterday on the ward has complained to the manager that she does not like your bedside manner and has requested a different clinician to see her in the future. How will you respond?

This is not a role-play station; it will involve discussion with the examiner.

Themes for discussion (■ Table 6.8)

Table 6.8.	
Question themes	**What is expected from the candidate?**
1 Introduction.	The candidate introduces themselves to the examiner and summarises the key points of the scenario.

Table 6.8.

	Question themes	What is expected from the candidate?
2	The examiner asks the candidate about the key themes in this situation.	The candidate starts with an apology to the patient feeling dissatisfied with the consultation/appointment and says 'sorry' for how the patient felt. The candidate understands that a doctor's visit can be a stressful experience for a patient as it demonstrates their vulnerability. A situation such as this is a good test of a doctor's communication skills, active listening skills and empathy.
		The candidate defines empathy as the art of putting oneself in another's shoes and the ability to share and understand the feelings and emotions of the other person. The candidate explains that a doctor can display empathy by listening to the patient's concerns, avoiding medical jargon and involving patients in decision making. There is evidence that a good empathetic doctor has a positive influence on patients' health.
3	The examiner asks the candidate how they, as a doctor, would respond to this situation.	The candidate understands the importance of empathy and acknowledging the feelings of the patient. This can include understanding the Ideas, Concerns and Expectations of the patient to understand why the care that was provided was not deemed satisfactory.
		The candidate puts an emphasis on openness and honesty. This includes apologising to the patient for any distress that was caused. An apology opens the path for conversation, allowing the candidate to find out more about how their actions affected the patient and how they can change this behaviour next time.
		Finally, a good doctor is not afraid to ask for help. The candidate should mention the availability of support from supervisors, colleagues and other support networks within the workplace.

Table 6.8.

Question themes	What is expected from the candidate?
4 The examiner asks the candidate whether they should assign the patient to a different doctor.	The candidate understands that sometimes, despite one's best efforts, patients may not be satisfied with the care and may want to see a different clinician. The candidate understands that this lies within the patient's rights and is a key concept in patient-centred care, a shift from the paternalistic care of the past.

The patient-clinician relationship and the trust it inspires is the backbone of providing high-quality and satisfactory care to a patient. If this relationship has been compromised and cannot be restored by the doctor's reflection and change in actions, the moral choice would be to assign the patient to a different doctor whom they trust and are comfortable with. It is important to ensure continuity of care and ensure that the patient is not put to harm or suffering due to this incident. |
| 5 Conclusion. | The candidate thanks the patient and conveys apologies again. The candidate concludes the session by asking if there is anything else that they can do for this patient. |

Discussion

Reflection is a key skill of any clinician. Feedback forms a crucial part of personal and professional development. NHS hospitals regularly collect feedback through patient surveys and 'Friends and family tests'. Doctors collect feedback from patients, supervisors and colleagues as part of their appraisal (once a year) and revalidation (once every 5 years). Positive feedback reassures doctors and makes them aware of their strengths, whilst negative feedback provides an opportunity for reflection and improvement. Reflection forms the backbone of continuous professional development (CPD).

Key Points

- An apology opens the pathway for communication; saying sorry does not mean a mistake always, but it is an empathetic expression for what the patient experienced.
- Reflect on why a mistake has occurred, to reduce the chance of recurrence.
- A strong patient-clinician relationship is the backbone of high-quality care and patient satisfaction.

References

1. General Medical Council. The duties of a doctor registered with the General Medical Council. Available from: https://www.gmc-uk.org/ethical-guidance/ethical-guidance-for-doctors/good-medical-practice/duties-of-a-doctor.

2. General Medical Council. Good medical practice. Available from: https://www.gmc-uk.org/ethical-guidance/ethical-guidance-for-doctors/good-medical-practice.

3. Kelm Z, Womer J, Walter JK, Feudtner C. Interventions to cultivate physician empathy: a systematic review. *BMC Med Educ* 2014; 14(1): 219.

Question 86

Motivation to do medicine

Siva Thanthullu

Question

In the next station, the examiner will ask you reasons for selecting medicine as a career.

Themes for discussion (■ Table 6.9)

Table 6.9.	
Question themes	**What is expected from the candidate?**
1 Introduction.	The candidate greets the examiner, has good body language and speaks coherently and clearly.

Table 6.9.

	Question themes	What is expected from the candidate?
2	Can you summarise your personal statement?	The candidate should be able to give a succinct summary of their personal statement in this session in a minute or two. They should have adequately practised this before, as this can often be asked in an MMI station. Try practising all positive points, but categorise them within a minute into academic achievements, workplace/volunteering achievements, sports/hobbies, and other achievements. Having a systematic approach, classifying/categorising and concluding appropriately will fetch good marks in this section.
3	What motivated you to choose medicine as a career?	This is an opportunity to show positive enthusiasm by the candidate. Please do not use boring, previously used reasons! It should be simple and practical and show your enthusiasm in the correct manner.
4	What work experience have you had with medicine?	The candidate can use this opportunity to explain their workplace experience, volunteering or even online experience. It is prudent to categorise them so that the examiner knows what you are going to explain. Then, it is easier to explain where you did, what you did and what you learnt from that experience. Reflection is a key skill for doctors and medical students, and it is good to reflect on the experience and explain how it helped you to choose medicine as a career.
5	Why do you want to come to our medical school?	The candidate should have researched the medical school, its curriculum, what positive advantages the school offers, etc., clearly before the interview. They can also explain about the city, what it offers and what attracts the candidate.

Table 6.9.

Question themes	What is expected from the candidate?
	In some universities, this question is taken seriously; for example, if the school offers problem-based learning and if the candidate erroneously says that it is integrated teaching, it can be marked down significantly. It shows that the candidate has not made an effort to even look at the teaching style or curriculum of the university before applying for the interview.
6 Having witnessed a doctor's career, what aspect attracts you to it?	The candidate should show positive emotions towards this question. They can give a list of reasons, but showing positive emotion is the key. The reasons could include the following: • Satisfaction helping patients. • Rewarding career. • Multifaceted, teamwork. • Real change to others in the way we work. • Patient care. • Financially rewarding. The candidate can use their work experience or volunteering experience to explain what attracted them to this career.
7 What aspect of a doctor's work do you not like?	Despite the negative question, the candidate has to show a positive outlook and say that the career is rewarding, but they are aware of the problems. A doctor's career can be demanding and stressful, and the examiner is assessing whether the candidate is well prepared for this. The candidate can use workplace experience here to explain that they are aware of these problems. Examples could include a busy life, demanding patients, work-life balance, etc.

Table 6.9

	Question themes	What is expected from the candidate?
8	All the positive aspects you mentioned are present in a nursing career; why did you not select nursing instead of medicine?	The candidate has to show respect to all allied professions and understand their role and importance in healthcare delivery. Although nursing is rewarding, the candidate can give a few reasons why it differs from a medical career: a more scientific approach, more hands-on approach including interventions, leading a team, better decision-making skills, more financially rewarding, etc. Few nurses become leaders and do all the above, but the majority of doctors have to take on this role. The candidate can quote their workplace experience here to maximise the scores.
9	If you are not successful in getting into medical school, what will you do?	This tests the passion and commitment of the candidate. The candidate can show optimism, but they should have a back-up plan if not successful. Persevering and looking at options to come back is good; the candidate should not express arrogance or lack of commitment in this question.
10	Concludes the session.	The candidate thanks the examiner for their time and concludes the session. The candidate should have given confidence to the examiner that they are motivated and committed to the demands of a medical career and understand the difficulties in such a career.

Discussion

The candidate should exhibit passion, positive emotions and motivation in this station. Researching the medical school, its curriculum and the city is vital before attending any interview. This is one of the most common questions in an MMI station and is an opportunity for the candidate to prepare themselves to show their optimistic, positive approach.

Key Points

- Show your motivation and positive attitude for a medical career.
- Research the university, its curriculum and practicalities before going to the interview.
- Respect all professions allied to medicine and know their importance in the teamwork.

References

1. General Medical Council. Good medical practice. Available from: https://www.gmc-uk.org/ethical-guidance/ethical-guidance-for-doctors/good-medical-practice.

Question 87

A positive attitude

Roshni Francis

Question

This station will include questions about a positive attitude and its importance in a clinical setting; the examiner will ask questions based on these topics.

Themes for discussion (■ Table 6.10)

Table 6.10.	
Question themes	**What is expected from the candidate?**
1 Introduction.	The candidate greets the examiner, has good body language and speaks coherently.

Table 6.10.

Question themes	What is expected from the candidate?
2 Give an example of a situation in which a 'positive attitude' has benefited you.	When describing a past experience, the candidate could use the mnemonic STAR, to ensure that they include relevant information without going into excessive detail. STAR stands for Situation, Task, Action and Result. An example is: Situation: 'Duke of Edinburgh award, gold expedition. My group was very tired and we were reaching the end of our day. We had been incorrectly led by one of my peers and we were now lost in the dark'. Task: 'To help everyone calm down and to work on finding the way back to camp'. Action: 'I first reassured my peer that everyone makes mistakes and not to worry. I then got everyone to sit down and assess the situation, reassuring them that if, all else failed, we could seek advice from our supervisors'. Result: 'Everyone began to calm down and think more practically. It allowed us to come together and work as a team'. This is only an example; using the same standard examples can mark you down. Please think and select a simple example from your real-life experience.
3 How can having a positive attitude be applied in medicine?	Medicine can be an emotionally challenging career, and a positive attitude can be the make or break of the mental health of clinicians and the quality of care they provide.

Table 6.10.

Question themes	What is expected from the candidate?
	A candidate can give an example of a situation in which they saw a clinician with a positive attitude (e.g. during work experience or volunteering), and the effect that their attitude had on the patient-clinician relationship and the quality of care that was provided.
4 Conclusion.	The candidate concludes the session, giving good assurance to the examiner that they understand the importance and role of a good attitude in a medical career.

Discussion

The candidate shows enthusiasm and positive energy throughout the MMI station. The candidate gives assurance to the examiner that they are motivated towards a medical career.

Key Points

- Use the STAR mnemonic when describing past experiences.
- Reflection is a key tool in learning from experience.
- A positive attitude can make a big impact on your own experience of clinical care, as well as on the type of clinician you become.
- Do not just tell; show! Enthusiasm and an optimistic tone during the interview will further demonstrate your positive attitude to the examiner.

References

1. General Medical Council. Professionalism in action. Available from: https://www.gmc-uk.org/ethical-guidance/ethical-guidance-for-doctors/good-medical-practice/professionalism-in-action.

2. General Medical Council. Achieving good medical practice: guidance for medical students. Available from: https://www.gmc-uk.org/education/standards-guidance-and-curricula/guidance/student-professionalism-and-ftp/achieving-good-medical-practice.

Question88

A patient that inspired you

Roshni Francis

Question

Tell me about a patient that you saw during your volunteering or work experience who motivated you to find out more about their condition.

Themes for discussion (■ Table 6.11)

Table 6.11.	
Question themes	**What is expected from the candidate?**
1 Introduction.	The candidate greets the examiner, has good body language and speaks coherently.

Table 6.11.

	Question themes	What is expected from the candidate?
2	The examiner asks to describe the setting.	The candidate introduces the setting, for example, volunteering at an old people's home.
		When describing the setting, the key points the candidate should mention are:
		• The type of location. • Time frame (how long ago was this experience). • What type of role did the candidate play in this setting (employee, volunteer, etc.).
		However, the candidate should not breach confidentiality by giving any patient identifiable details (e.g. full name of the patient, date of birth and exact details of location).
		'During my weekly volunteering this past year in a care home for older residents with dementia, I was involved in mainly feeding and keeping them company. I became involved in the care of one particular resident, Mary, who I began to spend time with regularly.'
3	What were the different challenges encountered by this patient?	The candidate can describe the different biopsychosocial challenges encountered by the patient due to their condition:
		Medical challenges: difficulty eating, frailty, prone to injuries, etc.
		Psychological challenges: poor mental health, anxiety, depression.
		Social challenges: lack of contact with family, minimal interactions with friends and other care residents.

Table 6.11.

	Question themes	What is expected from the candidate?
		'I was in charge of giving food to Mary; however, she would often have difficulty eating and would often forget whether or not she had eaten. Towards the evening, Mary would become very distressed and agitated; she would repeatedly ask when Bill (her late husband who passed away a couple of years ago) would be coming to take her home. I found this very distressing to watch and I was initially unsure how to react or respond to the patient in this situation.'
4	How did this motivate you to learn more about the problem?	The candidate explains how they were motivated to learn more about the situation, for example:
		'I spoke to the matron and staff about the problems and situations they encountered as part of their daily routines and work in general.'
		'Witnessing the difficulties surrounding dementia that residents mainly and also the staff go through motivated me to find out more about the condition: who it affects, the aetiology behind it and currently available treatments.'
		(The candidate should give an example of an article or research, i.e. evidence that they found out more. For example 'I read a book about dementia or read *BMJ* articles'.)
5	How do you think this experience/exposure will help you in your career?	'The knowledge I gained subsequently allowed me to remain calmer and more at ease around Mary, particularly when she was getting agitated. It allowed me to develop more empathy and this enabled me to handle the situation appropriately.'

Table 6.11.

Question themes	What is expected from the candidate?
	'It gave me insight into the hardships that accompany committing to a career in healthcare provision. I came to appreciate the importance of patience and empathy for healthy and fruitful interactions in such distressing circumstances.'
6 Conclusion.	The candidate thanks the examiner and concludes the station.

Discussion

Reflection is a key skill expected from a medical student and this station will assess this characteristic. Whenever a candidate mentions a work experience or volunteering, they should reflect on their experience and explain what they learnt from this experience.

Key Points

- Describe how the experience helped you and what you learnt: REFLECTION.
- Make a link between the importance of learning more about conditions to having a better approach to communicating with the patient and managing difficult situations.
- The candidate should mention that they are keen to continue to learn and find out more (maybe the candidate can evidence this, i.e. volunteering for a dementia charity/support group).

References

1. General Medical Council. The reflective practitioner – guidance for doctors and medical students. Available from: https://www.gmc-uk.org/education/standards-guidance-and-curricula/guidance/reflective-practice/the-reflective-practitioner---guidance-for-doctors-and-medical-students.

Question89

Enhancing learning when the clinical supervisor is late

Roshni Francis

Question

You are a first-year medical student who is doing a placement in a GP surgery. The GP has phoned the secretary to let you know that he will be late by one hour.

How will you enhance your learning experience during this hour?

Themes for discussion (■ Table 6.12)

Table 6.12.	
Question themes	**What is expected from the candidate?**
1 Introduction.	The candidate greets the examiner, has good body language and speaks coherently.

Table 6.12.

Question themes	What is expected from the candidate?
2 What would you do in this situation?	The candidate should first acknowledge their position as a medical student, meaning that there are limitations on some of the activities they could carry out, such as talking to a patient.
	They can suggest talking to a supervisor and asking for advice as to what tasks they could participate in.
3 How can you enhance your learning experience?	The candidate makes several suggestions as follows:
	• Talking to the receptionist(s) about their day-to-day roles and duties and learning more about their administrative role including any challenges they face.
	• Talking to patients in the waiting area and making them aware that the doctor is running late, reassuring them and thereby improving communication skills.
	• The candidate makes sure to specify that they will correctly introduce themselves to ensure that they do not mislead the patient or affect the patient's care.
	• Talking to the practice nurse about their roles and duties to learn about some of the other professionals in a multidisciplinary team.
	• Reading the information leaflets and adverts for self-management groups available in the surgery can be very informative and can direct the candidate towards further learning about specific diseases and conditions.
	• Talking to the administrative personnel about referral pathways (to get a better understanding of the interface between primary and secondary care).

Table 6.12.

	Question themes	What is expected from the candidate?
4	Conclusion.	The candidate shows motivation to learn and uses the opportunity to talk to the multidisciplinary team members including the administrative staff and realises the importance of teamwork. The candidate concludes the session and thanks the examiner at the end.

Discussion

One way in which the transition from school to university has been described is 'moving from a pond to an ocean'. Whilst students receive tailored care and a fixed curriculum in school, in a university there is a large focus on self-directed learning. It becomes the responsibility of the student to organise their learning, find appropriate resources and seek any necessary support.

The examiner will assess the candidate's ability to take ownership of their learning, within the limitations of their role as a medical student.

A good candidate will also need to have some understanding of the workings of primary care, the types of professionals involved and the different needs of the patients. A good resource for any aspiring medic is the Observe GP interactive video platform created by the Royal College of General Practitioners (RCGP). This is a free alternative to work experience and provides valuable insights into the workings of general practice and the type of setting a medical student would face.

Key Points

- Show confidence and the ability to take the initiative in your learning.
- Be aware of the limitations of a medical student's role; refrain from advising patients.
- There are many learning opportunities in a GP practice other than observing a GP; awareness of multidisciplinary teamwork is essential.
- Use platforms such as 'Observe GP' and any work experience to give better informed answers.

References

1. Royal College of General Practitioners, Observe GP. Available from: https://www.rcgp.org.uk/observegp.

Question 90

A mistake that you did and what you learnt

Paul Sanjay Sundaram

Question

This station will be about mistakes you have made in the past and how you learnt from them. You will also be asked about mistakes taking place in a clinical setting.

Themes for discussion (■ Table 6.13)

Table 6.13.	
Question themes	**What is expected from the candidate?**
1 Introduction.	The candidate greets the examiner, has good body language and speaks coherently.

Table 6.13.

	Question themes	What is expected from the candidate?
2	The examiner asks the candidate to describe a mistake they committed in the past.	The candidate selects a relevant example of a mistake they committed, ideally in a recent time frame.
		STAR is a good mnemonic that can be used to ensure that the candidate discusses the relevant details of the example; it includes Situation, Task, Action and Result. For example:
		Situation: a friend lent their laptop.
		Task: the candidate was using the laptop to submit a project.
		Action: the candidate accidentally mishandled the laptop and broke it.
		Result: the friend became angry at the candidate.
3	What did you learn from this mistake?	The key skill required in this answer is reflection. The candidate is honest and admits to their mistake. They may pick out specific actions that led to the mistake, e.g. 'I am sorry that I was careless with the equipment'. Honesty will show that the candidate embodies the GMC's 'Good medical practice' values of probity and integrity.
		The candidate can mention any actions they took at the time of the mistake to make remedies. They can also show that they acted on their reflections to improve future behaviour, e.g. 'I understood that I was clumsy and now I take care of other people's possessions more carefully'.

Table 6.13.

	Question themes	What is expected from the candidate?
4	What happens if a mistake happens in clinical practice?	The candidate should mention the stages of the duty of candour. These include: telling the person about the mistake you made, apologising, offering an appropriate remedy and fully explaining any short-term and long-term effects of the mistake that you made. To attain top marks, candidates should ensure that they show an understanding of the reporting system in hospitals or general practice.
5	How will you stop mistakes happening such as this in the future?	The candidate shows a good understanding that when a mistake happens, it can be the result of individual and/or systemic factors. For the individual, they can reduce the risk of the mistake recurring through reflection and appropriate training. On a systemic level, there may be a need to carry out root cause analysis and change policies.
6	Relevant topics in the news.	The candidate may mention a recent and relevant case of medical error in the news, describing the mistake, the consequences and the actions that were taken to remedy it.
7	Conclusion.	The candidate shows awareness that as a student and doctor it is possible to make mistakes. They understand the importance of honesty, reflection and seeking appropriate support.

Discussion

Openness and honesty are vital for a medical student and a doctor; the candidate should be aware that mistakes can happen and learning from mistakes to avoid them happening in the future is important. A culture of openness can reduce these errors. It is important to apologise openly to patients and do the needful clinically and make sure that clinical governance systems are put in place to avoid these errors in future.

Key Points

- For any mistake, honesty is the best policy; this links to the GMC's principles of probity and integrity.
- If a clinician makes a mistake, they must follow the principal actions outlined in GMC guidance on the duty of candour.
- Ensure that you are aware of the relevant systems to prevent another error from occurring in clinical practice.

References

1.   General Medical Council. Openness and honesty when things go wrong: the professional duty of candour. Available from: https://www.gmc-uk.org/ethical-guidance/ethical-guidance-for-doctors/candour---openness-and-honesty-when-things-go-wrong/the-professional-duty-of-candour.

Question 91

What are your weaknesses?

Prabhu Gandhimani

Question

This station will be about your weaknesses, how you manage them and how they could affect a future clinical career.

Themes for discussion (▦ Table 6.14)

Table 6.14.	
Question themes	**What is expected from the candidate?**
1 Introduction.	The candidate greets the examiner, has good body language and speaks coherently.

Table 6.14.

	Question themes	What is expected from the candidate?
2	The examiner asks the candidate to give an example of one of their weaknesses.	The candidate gives a well developed description of one of their weaknesses. Examples can include: • Taking on too many tasks at a time. • Taking criticism too personally. • Finding difficulty in saying no to people. The candidate can flesh out their answer by giving an example of when their weakness was a hurdle, and how they overcame it. A good mnemonic to use when giving descriptions is STAR, which stands for Situation, Task, Action and Result.
3	The examiner asks the candidate if their weakness will affect their ability to be a good clinician.	The key skill required in this answer is reflection. The candidate is honest and admits that their weakness can pose a hurdle to a healthy work-life balance and a good clinical career. Then, the candidate should explain the ways in which they currently overcome those challenges and action plans that they have taken to move past the weakness in the future. For example, 'My weakness is that I am afraid of public speaking. I know that this can pose a challenge for clinicians who must interact with patients and other clinicians in a team setting. I am working on building my confidence by attending the debating club at my school'.
4	Conclusion.	The candidate shows awareness that doctors are human and that everyone has weaknesses. However, they are focused on working to overcome this weakness and have an action plan for tackling this in the future.

Discussion

This is an important question and candidates might struggle if they do not consider it before an interview setting:

- This question tests the candidate's personal insight and how comfortable the candidates are to acknowledge their weaknesses and speak about them.
- The interviewer can test the candidate's skills of reflection and resilience.
- The question also gives an opportunity to test how a candidate might perform under pressure.

A good answer is one in which the candidate describes the weakness and gives an example of how they became aware of it, how it limited them and what they have done to overcome it. A quick answer may come across as being arrogant, lacking insight and showing someone who is not keen to reflect. Reflection and learning are key qualities expected of a doctor. The interviewers are not looking for perfect candidates, but rather someone who is aware of their limitations and is keen to learn and improve.

When candidates mention weakness, it is better to avoid giving examples that relate to the key qualities required to be a doctor.

These are:

- Being knowledgeable and keen to learn.
- Having effective communication skills.
- Being an active listener.
- Being a good team player.
- Honesty and probity.
- Having empathy and a caring attitude.

In addition, avoid cliché answers such as 'I am a perfectionist' and 'I can't say no'. These answers are given frequently by candidates and interviewers will quickly lose interest in the answer. A unique and personal answer will draw more attention and are likely to be better received.

Some of the general themes one can consider include procrastination, too much attention to detail, taking on too many tasks, taking criticism too personally, lacking organisation, trying to please everyone, getting embarrassed to ask questions in class, etc.

Although the question is about weaknesses, you can use this as an opportunity to highlight some of your strengths. The examiner is assessing your attitude and positive attitudes like empathy and care in this section. Reviewing the GMC's guidance, 'The reflective practitioner — guidance for doctors and medical students' and 'Professionalism in action' can help the candidate to answer this section in a better way.

Key Points

- Weaknesses are simply areas where there is room for further improvement.
- Use this question as an opportunity to also highlight some of your strengths.
- Show the interviewer your self-awareness as well as your keenness to reflect and improve.

References

1. Stone D, Heen S. *Thanks for the feedback: the science and art of receiving feedback well*. Penguin; 2015.
2. General Medical Council. The duties of a doctor registered with the General Medical Council. Available from: https://www.gmc-uk.org/ethical-guidance/ethical-guidance-for-doctors/good-medical-practice/duties-of-a-doctor.
3. General Medical Council. The reflective practitioner – guidance for doctors and medical students. Available from: https://www.gmc-uk.org/education/standards-guidance-and-curricula/guidance/reflective-practice/the-reflective-practitioner---guidance-for-doctors-and-medical-students.

4.   General Medical Council. Professionalism in action. Available from: https://www.gmc-uk.org/ethical-guidance/ethical-guidance-for-doctors/good-medical-practice/professionalism-in-action.

Question 92

Book or movie

Paul Sanjay Sundaram

Question

What type of media is better? Books or films? Give reasons for your decision.

Themes for discussion (■ Table 6.15)

Table 6.15.	
Question themes	**What is expected from the candidate?**
1 Introduction.	The candidate greets the examiner, has good body language and speaks coherently.

Table 6.15.

	Question themes	What is expected from the candidate?
2	The examiner asks the candidate what media they prefer: books or films.	The candidate gives points in the argument for both books and for films: Example points for books: • More accessible to everyone as less technology is required. • Often cheaper and sometimes free to access, e.g. through libraries. • Books can go into more detail than films. • Everyone's imagination and interpretation of a book are unique. • Books can increase brain cognition, reasoning and thinking. Example points for films: • It can be quicker to watch than books, and this can be useful in a time-pressured life. • Films can be more relaxing and easier to engage in. • Films often include music and have aided the rise of many notable composers. • Everyone watching the movie has the same version with little difference in imagination. • More social activity going to a movie. • More visual and audio stimulation in a movie. • The film industry supports the careers of a vast number of people.
3	Conclusion.	The candidate evaluates points both in favour of books and movies. They show a balanced and logical decision making but come to a clear choice.

Discussion

A question such as this may initially throw off an unprepared candidate, as it stands out among other medically themed questions. When faced with a question such as this, the candidate should first try to understand the purpose behind the question. On the one hand, the examiner is testing the candidate's ability to react quickly when facing an unexpected, unprepared for question. Clinicians need to be able to quickly adapt to new scenarios, particularly in emergency settings; therefore, this is an important skill for prospective candidates to display.

On the other hand, clinicians must also be skilled at logical reasoning and balanced decision making. This question also tests the candidate's ability to show balanced reasoning and the ability to consider arguments for both sides before coming to any decision.

Another question that can come up in an MMI is to describe your favourite book or movie; it is easier for the candidate to think about this before and describe in simple language what the book is about, a few words about the author, why you liked the book and why you would recommend it to others.

Key Points

- When facing an unexpected question, first try and understand the reasoning behind it.
- Give points for both sides and show logical reasoning in your evaluation.
- Come to a clear choice and summarise your reasons for choosing it.

References

1. CNBC news. Bill Gates' advice to his younger self is simple: "Read a lot". Available from: https://www.cnbc.com/2022/05/21/bill-gates-advice-read-a-lot-and-find-a-skill-you-enjoy.html#:~:text=Gates%20reads%2050%20books%20each,during%20a%202021%20Reddit%20AMA.

Question 93

Empathy versus sympathy

Paul Sanjay Sundaram

Question

What is the difference between sympathy and empathy? Which one is more important?

Themes for discussion (■ Table 6.16)

Table 6.16.

	Question themes	What is expected from the candidate?
1	The examiner asks the candidate about sympathy and empathy.	The candidate first defines these two terms and explains the differences:
		'Sympathy involves understanding from your own perspective.'
		'Empathy involves putting yourself in the other person's shoes and understanding why they may have these particular feelings.'

Table 6.16.

	Question themes	What is expected from the candidate?
2	Why is sympathy important?	The candidate gives a definition of sympathy:
		Sympathy is an acknowledgement of the thoughts and feelings of a person but in a superficial context. It is not as deep as empathy and generally does not require the person to feel the same feelings the other person has. Often it involves 'feeling sorry for another person'. In clinical practice, this is useful, but often this is not deep enough to fully appreciate the patient's situation.
3	Why is empathy important?	The candidate gives a definition of empathy, making clear how it differs from sympathy:
		Empathy is understanding someone's feelings and putting oneself in another's shoes. In clinical practice, empathy can help a clinician understand how a patient feels and why they feel that way. This can improve a patient-clinician relationship, as the doctor will better understand the motivation behind a patient's actions. A doctor can use this understanding to try and better tailor their patient interactions to improve patient compliance and the quality of care provided. An example of an empathic statement would be 'I'm sorry this has happened; I understand this must be hard for you'.
4	How will you develop these qualities?	These qualities can be developed through people interaction and the skills of active listening when communicating with people during everyday life. The candidate can mention undertaking experience themselves in care homes or other volunteering settings and may give an example of how they themselves showed sympathy or empathy in the past.

Table 6.16.

	Question themes	What is expected from the candidate?
5	Conclusion.	The candidate summarises the points, and thanks the examiner for their time.

Discussion

This topic of the difference between sympathy and empathy can often come up in an MMI station. Showing empathy is a key quality of any communication or role-play station in an MMI.

Key Points

- Sympathy often involves 'feeling sorry' for another person.
- Empathy involves understanding how someone feels and why they feel that way.
- Empathy is generally more useful in clinical practice.
- One can develop these qualities through practising active listening during everyday life.

References

1. Psychiatric medical care. The difference between empathy and sympathy. Available from: https://www.psychmc.com/blogs/empathy-vs-sympathy.

Question 94

Making a positive difference

Sheena Abraham

Question

Give an example in which you made a positive difference in someone's life. What did you learn from this experience?

Themes for discussion (■ Table 6.17)

Table 6.17.	
Question themes	**What is expected from the candidate?**
1 Introduction.	The candidate greets the examiner, has good body language and speaks coherently.

Table 6.17.

	Question themes	What is expected from the candidate?
2	The candidate introduces the scenario.	The candidate gives a good opening statement, setting the scene and giving background information: • Who did you impact? • When did this happen? • Where did it take place?
3	Describe the instance.	The candidate gives a description of the experience. STAR is a good mnemonic that can be used to ensure that the candidate discusses the relevant details of the example; it includes Situation, Task, Action and Result. The candidate could also follow the general framework below: • Choose an example: e.g. assisting a team member in a group project, tutoring someone, helping a sibling, a unique/unconventional experience, etc. • Explain their actions: e.g. listening to an individual's personal goals, setting attainable targets, encouraging them, implementing an idea, etc. • Ensure details of any people are non-identifiable. • Remain humble when delivering the answer.
4	The outcome of your actions.	The candidate describes the outcome of their actions: • What positive impact did the candidate make? • How did the person change? • How did the person benefit?
5	Relate the skills learnt to their relevance in a clinical career.	The candidate understands the ways in which their actions may be transferable to medicine: • Demonstrating empathy, communication skills, teamwork, etc.; try to use a work placement example and explain the skills learnt in that scenario. • Relate why this skill is essential in medicine.

Table 6.17.

Question themes	What is expected from the candidate?
	For example: 'When I helped the old lady share her grief, I learnt the importance of active listening, and the ability to give people a comfortable space in which they can share their feelings. I believe I can apply these skills to patient interaction in a clinical setting, as better communication can improve the patient-clinician relationship and the quality of care that I provide'.
6 Conclusion.	The candidate concludes the session, summarising the key points if possible, and thanks the examiner at the end.

Discussion

The candidate should use this question as an opportunity to demonstrate their qualities such as empathy, communication skills, teamwork, etc. Always reflect on the situation and relate it to clinical medicine if possible.

Key Points

- Use the STAR structure to describe the situation: Situation, Task, Action and Result.
- Clarify the skills you practised and learnt in this experience, as well as any reflection that you made.
- Explain how these skills are transferable to a clinical career.

References

1. Interview questions answered: tell me about a time when you influenced someone else. Available from: https://interviewpenguin.com/tell-me-about-a-time-when-you-influenced-someone-else.

Question 95

Maintaining a work-life balance

Sheena Abraham

Question

What is your understanding of a work-life balance, and do you believe it is important? How will you maintain a good work-life balance in your medical career?

Themes for discussion (■ Table 6.18)

Table 6.18.		
	Question themes	**What is expected from the candidate?**
1	Introduction.	The candidate greets the examiner, has good body language and speaks coherently.

Table 6.18.

Question themes	What is expected from the candidate?
2 What is a work-life balance?	The candidate gives a good opening statement about the meaning of a work-life balance. For example 'My understanding of a work-life balance is prioritising what is important to you alongside maintaining your career. You should not forsake one for the other'.
3 Why is a work-life balance important?	The candidate explains the importance of a work-life balance. They explain its benefits to an individual as well as its benefits in a clinical setting to patients and to wider society: • Improves mental and physical health and subsequently reduces the risk of burnout (a state of physical and emotional exhaustion caused by prolonged stress). • Burnout may hinder patient care; e.g. may lead to a lapse in judgement, poor decision making, sharps injuries, etc. It is of utmost importance to do no harm to patients. • Improves quality of work and productivity: working long hours may feel like you are doing more; however, it is likely that the quality of your work decreases. • Fewer problems with physical health: chronic stress due to a poor work-life balance can lead to various health issues. • Having balance improves relationships: nurturing relationships can also contribute to good mental health and social well-being.
4 How can a work-life balance be affected by a medical career?	The candidate understands that a medical career can be physically and emotionally challenging; therefore, clinicians may need to take extra steps to ensure a good work-life balance. The candidate may draw on their own observations and conversations with clinicians during work experience.

Table 6.18.

Question themes	What is expected from the candidate?
	'During my work experience, I talked to a young junior doctor. She told me that occasionally she compromises her physical and mental well-being to prioritise working long hours. She also needs to take care to ensure she spends enough time with her family and friends, as otherwise she feels lonely. From this, I learnt that when a work-life balance is not managed, there is a risk of biopsychosocial impacts on a clinician's life.'
5 How would you create a work-life balance?	The candidate gives a variety of examples and may mention their own hobbies or extracurricular activities: • Organise your day: allocate time towards rest and other activities you enjoy. Try to avoid working during this time. • Do not sacrifice your hobbies. Having an interest or hobby outside of medicine to nurture will help you to wind down after a long day and relax. It is important to continue to do things that bring you joy. • Set boundaries: do not take on more than you can handle and prioritise your well-being. It is important to learn how to say no. Remember that a work-life balance is ultimately created through your choices. • Spend time with loved ones: it is important to have people around you whose company you enjoy, and make time to do so.
6 Conclusion	The candidate concludes the session, summarising the key points if possible, and thanks the examiner at the end.

Discussion

Medicine can be a demanding and stressful career; it is natural that the universities check that the candidate is well rounded about understanding the need for a work-life balance.

Every candidate should have done lots of extracurricular or non-academic work and it is important to explain this systematically if there is an opportunity. Rather than just explaining what you did (for example, the Duke of Edinburgh award gold expedition), reflect on what you learnt in this expedition and what skills were acquired in the process; you could split these skills into physical, first aid, mental skills, teamwork skills, communication skills, perseverance, resilience, etc. and explain each in detail. Reflection is key in this process.

An explanation of how your hobbies (e.g. music) help you to unwind and remove stress can be a better explanation than just saying that you have passed the grade 4 music exam.

Key Points

- A work-life balance is a key aspect of a healthy life and safe clinical practice.
- Draw on your own work experience to give your understanding of a clinician's work-life balance.
- Mention your current hobbies and extracurricular activities to add a personal touch to the answer.

References

1. Moulder H. 10 Reasons why work life balance is important. Available from: https://www.coursecorrectioncoaching.com/reasons-why-work-life-balance-is-important.
2. American Society of Clinical Oncology. Balancing your life at work and home. *J Oncol Pract* 2009; 5(5): 253-5.

Question 96

Supporting a friend who has an eating disorder

Sheena Abraham

Question

You are a first-year medical student. You have a friend who is concerned about their body image. They have been overweight since this academic year started, and recently you saw them vomiting in the bathroom during lunchtime. How will you approach this situation?

This is a discussion station and no actor is involved.

Themes for discussion (■ Table 6.19)

Table 6.19.	
Question themes	**What is expected from the candidate?**
1 Introduction.	The candidate greets the examiner, has good body language and speaks coherently. The candidate shows a supportive, empathetic approach.

Table 6.19.

	Question themes	What is expected from the candidate?
2	How will you approach this situation?	The candidate outlines a series of logical steps, with an emphasis on confidentiality, compassion and providing appropriate support. Here are a few examples of some of the steps the candidate could outline:

- Finding an appropriate setting for the conversation, e.g. quiet and private room.
- Gently broaching the topic, without pressuring the friend into saying anything if she is reluctant to talk. You may open with phrases such as, 'Is it OK if I talk to you about something important? I just want to talk as your friend because I care about you'.
- Showing patience and being a good listener. If and when the friend opens up, it is important not to advise or criticise them.
- Ask the friend why they were vomiting. This will ensure that the candidate does not make any false assumptions.
- If the friend's vomiting is related to body image issues, it is imperative to ask whether she has a support system to confide in and receive help from.
- If not, then recommend appropriate forms of support such as student support services, eating disorder support groups, or GP guidance. The candidate may offer to accompany the friend to seek support, but should not overstep any boundaries.
- Thank the friend for opening up to them and offer to be a listening ear if the friend wants to talk again.

3	Conclusion.	The candidate should summarise the key points from their answer, e.g. the importance of active listening, being open-minded and maintaining confidentiality.

Table 6.19.	
Question themes	**What is expected from the candidate?**
	The candidate may relate the question to any experiences or similar situations they have faced in the past.
	Finally, the candidate thanks the examiner for their time and concludes the session.

Discussion

This is a complex, sensitive problem; the candidate should show confidence in taking a step-wise approach whilst maintaining confidentiality (asking to talk in a private or quiet area). It is vital that the candidate is empathetic in their approach and knows where to signpost the friend to get help. It is important not to advise or criticise as this can make the friend angry rather than receptive.

In some MMI stations, this can be given as a role play in which an actor will act as the friend with the eating disorder and an examiner will observe the communication skills.

Key Points

- Approach the situation with an open mind without making any assumptions.
- Be clear that you will find a quiet and private setting before beginning the conversation.
- Give importance to active listening and patience.
- Give specific examples of support that you could refer the friend to or signpost them.

References

1. Reachout. How to help a friend with an eating disorder. Available from: https://au.reachout.com/articles/how-to-help-a-friend-with-an-eating-disorder.

2. National Health Service. How to help someone with an eating disorder. Available from: https://www.nhs.uk/mental-health/advice-for-life-situations-and-events/how-to-help-someone-with-eating-disorder.

Question 97

Coping with sleep difficulties in your career

Sheena Abraham

Question

You are a junior doctor. Recently, you have been given a much larger workload and you find that you do not have enough time to sleep. How will you approach this situation? The examiner will ask you questions on this topic in the next station.

Themes for discussion (■ Table 6.20)

Table 6.20.	
Question themes	**What is expected from the candidate?**
1 Introduction.	The candidate greets the examiner, has good body language and speaks coherently. The candidate gives a good succinct introduction statement of the problem read in the question.

Table 6.20.

Question themes	What is expected from the candidate?
2 Why is sleep important?	The candidate understands clearly the importance of appropriate sleep, considering both themselves and the risk to patients during clinical practice.
	Examples of points the candidate could mention include:
	• Long-term effects on health: 'Sleep deprivation increases the risk of cardiovascular disease, primary sleep disorders, overweight/obesity, type 2 diabetes, depression and anxiety, and is likely to contribute to an increased risk of some cancers, and dementia'. • Risk to mental health. • The danger of harming patients: you may make poor decisions, may not remember correct patient history, sharps injuries, clinical errors, etc. • Risk of an accident in the workplace or travelling to and from the workplace.
3 How can you reduce the risk of sleep deprivation?	There are various possible answers:
	• Maintain a good night-time routine and sleep hygiene. • Plan ahead for night shifts. • Take rest whenever possible and appropriately during night shifts. • Set boundaries: do not accept extra tasks if exhausted, and tell your supervisor when you are unable to cope. • Try to separate home life from work life. • Seek professional help for any concerns about lack of sleep and fatigue.
4 Conclusion.	The candidate concludes the session, summarises the key points and thanks the examiner at the end.

Discussion

Sleep is important and this could be deprived significantly in a junior doctor's career. It is vital for doctors to take care of themselves in order to take good care of patients.

Key Points

- Sleep deprivation is not compatible with a healthy life and safe practice.
- Mention the importance of seeking support if you are overwhelmed with tasks.
- Explain the importance of a good work-life balance for both individual health and good clinical practice.

References

1. British Medical Association. Anticipating and managing fatigue associated with doctors' working patterns. Available from: https://www.bma.org.uk/media/1073/bma_fatiguesl-sleep_deprivation _guidance_oct_2019.pdf.

2. General Medical Council. Good medical practice. Domain 2: safety and quality. Available from: https://www.gmc-uk.org/ethical-guidance/ethical-guidance-for-doctors/good-medical-practice/domain-2----safety-and-quality.

Question 98

Coping with a high intellectual environment

Sheena Abraham

Question

When medical students first begin university, they often need to adjust from an environment in which they were at the top of the class to one in which they are surrounded by similarly well achieving academics. How would you adapt to this new environment?

Themes for discussion (■ Table 6.21)

Table 6.21.	
Question themes	**What is expected from the candidate?**
1 Introduction.	The candidate greets the examiner, has good body language and speaks coherently.

Table 6.21.

Question themes	What is expected from the candidate?
2 How would you adapt to a medical school environment filled with high academic achievers?	The candidate gives a logical series of points, potentially relating their answer to their own past experiences. Here are some examples of points they could include:

- Accept that this is the reality of medical school, as entry is highly competitive, and therefore everyone is of a similar academic mindset and level.
- The initial transition into medical school and university may be difficult and may take some time to adjust, which is normal and nothing to worry about.
- Finding that academic performance is different from before is a common experience amongst most medical students, as the content is harder and the workload is substantial.
- Medical students should be kind to themselves and ensure that they do not compromise hobbies and activities that make them feel happy.
- If a medical student feels overwhelmed, there are a variety of support sources, including friends, family, university student support and, in some circumstances, a GP.
- A medical student can learn from the strengths of others to adapt their own working technique to one with which they are comfortable.
- Students can befriend like-minded people and form new connections and relationships.
- Relate to the future as a doctor: medicine is constantly evolving, and there may be times in the future when a practising professional feels similarly overwhelmed due to a new generation of discoveries and methods of treating patients.
- End on a positive note: medical school is a challenging, but nevertheless enjoyable experience, and competition encourages students to set new goals for themselves.

Table 6.21.

Question themes	What is expected from the candidate?
	• Add a word about the university's medical societies that can help give support and distract with new extracurricular hobbies; it is prudent to do some research or go to their open days to find what the societies offer and mention them in the interview, which can give bonus marks in this station.
3 Conclusion.	The candidate concludes the session, summarises the key points and thanks the examiner at the end.

Discussion

Medicine can be a demanding career and it is natural for the university to check that the candidate has the resilience to carry on successfully with medical school. It is vital that the candidate has done some research about the university and shows confidence in how to deal with stress and a high-achieving academic environment.

Key Points

- Adjusting for the first time at university can be a universally challenging experience.
- Support services for students include family and friends, university student support, and if health is compromised, it is vital to let the GP know and get appropriate help.
- Medical school is an exciting and enjoyable experience; challenges pave the way for self-improvement.

References

1. General Medical Council. Our guidance for medical students. Available from: https://www.gmc-uk.org/education/welcome-to-medicine/our-guidance-for-medical-students.

Question99

A patient is unwell whilst the doctor is away on holiday

James Francis

Question

You are a doctor. Your patient with arthritis, who sees only you regularly, declined a clinic appointment as you were on holiday, insisting that she would only see you. On your return from holiday, you are informed that she collapsed and was admitted to intensive care. She believes that this is your fault and that the event could have been avoided if you were not on holiday. How would you approach this situation?

This is a role-play station, an actor is present who is acting as a patient, but the examiner will assess the communication skills and ask a few questions at the end.

Themes for discussion (■ Table 6.22)

Table 6.22.	
Question themes	**What is expected from the candidate?**
1 Introduction.	The candidate greets the examiner and the actor, has good body language and speaks coherently.
2 The candidate begins to talk to the patient.	The candidate introduces themself and their position; the candidate confirms the patient's identity by asking for their name and date of birth. As the scenario mentions that it is your regular patient, you can call them by their name but still check the details.
3 The candidate apologises to the patient.	The candidate apologises to the patient and shows regret that their patient has been seriously ill, requiring admission to intensive care whilst they were on holiday. The candidate establishes and summarises the facts and circumstances that led to the patient's non-attendance at the clinic and subsequent deterioration leading to hospitalisation.
4 Is it wrong for the doctor to go on holiday?	The candidate should be clear that it is not wrong for the doctor to go on holiday. Health professionals, like other people, also have families with social and personal needs. In fact, it is important for health professionals to take regular breaks from work to reduce work-related stress and avoid burnout.
5 What are the precautions/steps that need to be put in place when the doctor is away?	It is very important to ensure there is appropriate cross-cover for the doctor/health professional(s) when they are away and that the patients under their care know who to contact in their absence. In case of any emergency, they should be directed to attend the appropriate emergency services.

Table 6.22.

	Question themes	What is expected from the candidate?
6	The patient only wanted to be seen by a particular doctor/specialist (you)! What are your thoughts about this?	The candidate explains that it is ideal for patients to be willingly seen and treated by any appropriately trained and suitable doctor/clinician, and not only by a particular individual, whoever that may be.
		It is important that patients do not delay seeking medical help as this can lead to very serious consequences.
		One important step is for the candidate to understand why the patient was not willing to talk to other clinicians. Understanding the motivation for the patient's actions could help the clinician to ensure a similar incident does not reoccur in the future.
7	How can such incidents be avoided in the future?	The candidate says that they will take steps to prevent this from happening again in future (reflecting on themselves and the process).
		It is very important that patients are appropriately informed and educated about their medical condition(s), in this case 'arthritis', and its treatment, and be made aware of any complications and consequences of delaying medical intervention.
		They should also be informed that the doctor/specialist is part of the multidisciplinary team (MDT) and that patients will not always be seen by the same doctor/specialist all the time.
		At the very outset, appropriate contact details, including emergency contact numbers, have to be provided to all patients.

Table 6.22.

	Question themes	What is expected from the candidate?
8	Conclusion.	The candidate summarises the points that have been discussed and asks the patient if there is anything else they can do for them. They thank the patient and examiner for their time.

Discussion

This station combines both communication skills through role play and the questioning by the examiner; this can be complex in the given time. The examiner will guide you and it is key to apologise/regret what has happened and be empathetic whilst talking to the patient. At the same time, the candidate should realise that healthcare cannot rely on a single person and it is important to hand over care to the right person or the MDT. It is important that the doctor takes care of themselves also.

Key Points

- Always apologise when the patient has had a bad experience; this can help to improve the patient-clinician relationship.
- The clinician is not at fault for being on holiday, but they should reflect on how to reduce the risk of this incident reoccurring.
- Patients should be provided with important information about their medical condition(s) and relevant emergency contact details.

References

1. British Medical Association. Chapter 1. The doctor-patient relationship. Available from: https://www.bma.org.uk/media/1987/bma-met-chapter-1-update-aug-2016.pdf. In: Medical Ethics Today. 3rd edn update (August 2016).

2. General Medical Council. Maintaining a professional boundary between you and your patient. Available from: https://www.gmc-uk.org/-/media/documents/Maintaining_a_professional_boundary_between_you_and_your_patient.pdf_58833579.pdf.

Section **7**

Health and clinical topics

Section editor: Shyam Balasubramanian

Introduction to health and clinical topics

It is common that a candidate will face a health and clinical topic in the MMI station. Awareness of the recent clinical topics in the news will help to answer the questions in this station. It might be prudent to look in the news column (e.g. BBC Health) for recent health topics.

Given the recent COVID pandemic problems, there is a chance that the candidate might get asked about COVID, the vaccine and its effects.

Chronic health problems such as obesity, smoking, high blood pressure, etc., can come up as topics, with questions on what interventions and priorities should be given; this will test the candidate's knowledge and how they would tackle these chronic conditions.

Triage scenarios (such as whom to give a liver or kidney transplant) will test the ethical knowledge and judgement of the candidate; in these scenarios, there is no right or wrong answer, but the examiner will test the decision-making capability of the candidate and the ethical/clinical basis behind this decision.

Question 100

COVID disease and the pandemic

Selvakumar Panchatsharam

Question

In the next station, the examiner will assess your knowledge and awareness of COVID disease and the pandemic.

Themes for discussion (■ Table 7.1)

Table 7.1.

	Question themes	What is expected from the candidate?
1	What do you understand by the term COVID?	COVID-19 stands for coronavirus disease 2019. It is caused by a novel coronavirus called SARS-CoV-2, which stands for severe acute respiratory syndrome coronavirus 2 (SARS-CoV-1 caused the 2003 outbreak). The World Health Organization (WHO) coined these terms on 11 February 2020 after confirming the origin of the virus from Wuhan, China, in late 2019.

Table 7.1.

	Question themes	What is expected from the candidate?
2	What is a coronavirus?	Coronaviruses are a large group of respiratory viruses that cause viral illnesses among humans and several mammals, including pigs, cats and dogs. Bats are considered to be the natural host of coronaviruses; however, when other mammals come into close contact, the virus can jump from its natural host to an intermediate host that acts as an animal reservoir, and subsequently is transmitted to humans. It is worth noting that approximately one-third of common colds is caused by coronaviruses. Therefore, not all coronaviruses cause COVID-19 disease. However, SARS-COV-2 was a novel coronavirus, meaning that the human immune system was naïve to this new virus.
3	What is the theory of the origin of the coronavirus?	According to the WHO, the SARS-CoV-2 virus originated from the wet markets of Wuhan, China. Although the virus is naturally harboured in bats, it is possible that the virus may have been transmitted to an intermediate host such as civet cats or racoon dogs from which it may have been transmitted to humans.
4	How does COVID spread?	SARS-CoV-2 spreads predominantly by the inhalational route, i.e. transmitted by respiratory secretions, although the virus has been isolated in most bodily fluids during an active infection. Droplets carrying the virus are transmitted from infected people when they cough, sneeze, sing or breathe in close proximity. These microdroplets, when inhaled by another person, are deposited in their respiratory tract and the virus enters the host cell to initiate a new infection.

Table 7.1.

Question themes	What is expected from the candidate?
	Occasionally the virus can be contracted by touching contaminated surfaces and subsequently touching one's nose or eyes. Therefore, simple barrier precautions such as wearing a face mask, and hand sanitisation can reduce the risk of transmission by up to 90%. Importantly, infected people can transmit the virus for up to 48 hours before developing symptoms (asymptomatic carriers), which made it difficult to contain the virus; therefore, lockdown measures were used to reduce virus spread.
5 What is the difference between COVID and flu illnesses?	Common flu, seasonal flu and previous flu pandemics in 1918, 1957, 1968 and 2009 (swine flu) were caused by a different group of viruses called influenza viruses, although flu and SARS-CoV-2 are both respiratory viruses.
6 What are the effects of COVID disease in humans?	Because viruses cannot self-replicate, they require a host cell to multiply. After viruses enter human cells in the upper respiratory tract by attaching to special receptors on the cell membrane, they integrate their genetic material with the host DNA. Therefore, when the host cell multiplies, the viruses also multiply and, thereby, increase the host viral load. The human immune system that detects the viruses releases several chemical mediators that are primarily aimed at killing the virus. These can damage host cells, which results in severe harm to alveolar cells in the lungs, causing severe acute respiratory syndrome (SARS). Furthermore, SARS-CoV-2 can affect many other organs, including the heart, circulatory system and kidneys, causing a multi-system disease with a high risk of death.
7 What are the common symptoms of COVID illness?	The common symptoms of COVID include cough, fever, fatigue, muscle aches and headache. Although the loss of smell and taste was commonly reported in the initial variants, it has been less commonly seen with the Omicron variants.

Table 7.1.

	Question themes	What is expected from the candidate?
8	What are the different variants of the COVID virus?	As the genetic material of the virus has changed constantly during the pandemic, there have been several variants and subvariants that were given common names following the Greek alphabet. The most common variants were Alpha, Beta, Delta and Omicron.
9	What is a pandemic and how does it differ from an outbreak and epidemic?	When a disease spreads rapidly, depending on its prevalence and the size of the outbreak, it is classified accordingly:
		Epidemic: refers to an increase, often sudden, in the number of cases of a disease above what is expected in the population in that area.
		Outbreak: this is the same definition as an epidemic but confined to a limited geographic area.
		Pandemic: refers to an epidemic that has spread over several countries or continents, usually affecting many people.
		The WHO issues pandemic alerts based on risk levels from Phase 1 (low risk) to Phase 6 (full pandemic).
10	Do you know of any other pandemics?	The biggest pandemic of all time was the Black Death caused by the plague in the 14th century that killed an estimated 70-200 million people worldwide.
		Other recent pandemics include the flu pandemic (Spanish flu) in 1918, which killed 20-50 million people and the Asian flu pandemic of 1956-1958 that killed 2 million people worldwide; also the smallpox pandemic and polio pandemic that have caused millions of deaths.

Table 7.1.

	Question themes	What is expected from the candidate?
11	What is the burden of COVID disease in the UK and the world?	As of December 2022, the WHO has reported that more than 642 million people have been affected by COVID-19 infection and 6.6 million people have died in the world.
		In the UK alone, more than 24 million people were infected and more than 197,000 people have died due to COVID-19.
		(More than 13 billion vaccine doses have been administered in the world until November 2022.)
12	What are the treatment options for COVID illness?	In the initial waves, it was estimated that approximately 80% of people who had COVID would have a mild illness; 20% of infected people would require hospitalisation and 5% would require intensive care treatment. Some specific patient population groups were deemed high risk, particularly people with coexisting illnesses such as chronic respiratory conditions, diabetes, heart disease, immunosuppression and older people. For hospitalised patients, the main treatment options were oxygen, supportive treatment and artificial breathing support by ventilators. Specific medications, including steroids, blood thinners and drugs that modulate the immune function (such as tocilizumab) were proven to be effective at reducing deaths.
13	What modalities were adopted to contain this virus?	The main preventative strategies used to contain this virus were community lockdowns, minimising socialisation, face coverings, social distancing and hand washing (hands, face, space). After the advent of vaccines in 2021, they remained the main defence against COVID.

Table 7.1.

	Question themes	What is expected from the candidate?
14	What types of COVID vaccines are used?	Although there were several vaccines produced across the world, in the UK, the main vaccines that were approved by the Medicines and Healthcare products Regulatory Agency (MHRA) were Pfizer-BioNTech, AstraZeneca, Moderna and Janssen (Johnson & Johnson) vaccines.
		When these vaccines are injected into the body, it initiates an immune response to the specific protein molecules (spike protein) on the virus. When a human catches the virus, the preformed antibody attaches to these specific protein molecules on the virus to either prevent infection or dampen down the infection to a milder form.
15	What is long COVID syndrome?	In some patients, the symptoms of COVID illness can last longer, up to weeks and months after the initial infection has subsided. This is called post-COVID syndrome or long COVID.
		Although it is not directly related to the severity of the initial infection, people with milder infections can also develop long COVID, but it is more commonly associated with hospitalised patients, underlying health conditions and being unvaccinated.
		Patients can report a wide range of symptoms of varying severity, including extreme tiredness (fatigue), shortness of breath, fever, chest pain, digestive symptoms, joint pains, sleeping difficulty (insomnia), memory and concentration problems (brain fog), anxiety and depression. The cause of long COVID syndrome is not clearly understood. There is no specific treatment that can immediately reverse the symptoms. Therefore, symptom management, supportive treatment and rehabilitation remain the mainstay in managing this condition.

Discussion

As COVID illness-related questions can be asked in an MMI station, we have given more options for this particular question than could be asked in the specific timeframe. An awareness of COVID illness, vaccines and the pandemic is expected from the candidate.

Key Points

- COVID-19 is caused by a coronavirus, a respiratory virus.
- Coronavirus spreads by the inhalational route by droplets.
- Vaccines are effective in controlling the pandemic.

References

1. World Health Organization. Coronavirus disease (COVID-19) pandemic. Available from: https://www.who.int/emergencies/diseases/novel-coronavirus-2019.

2. European Centre for Disease Prevention and Control. Clinical characteristics of COVID-19. Available from: https://www.ecdc.europa.eu/en/covid-19/latest-evidence/clinical.

3. World Health Organization. Coronavirus (COVID-19) Dashboard – Overview. Accessed 6 December 2022. Available from: https://covid19.who.int.

4. WHO Health Emergency Dashboard – WHO (COVID-19) homepage. Accessed December 6 2022. Available from: https://covid19.who.int/region/euro/country/gb. The United Kingdom.

5. Centers for Disease Control and Prevention, Long C. Available from: https://www.cdc.gov/coronavirus/2019-ncov/long-term-effects/index.html.

6. Vasu T. What is long COVID syndrome? In: Vasu T. *Managing Long COVID Syndrome*, 1st ed. Shrewsbury, UK: tfm publishing Limited; 2022: pp9-13.

Question 101

The UK Government's response to the COVID pandemic

Selvakumar Panchatsharam

Question

In the next station, the examiner will discuss the UK Government's response to the COVID pandemic.

Themes for discussion (■ Table 7.2)

Table 7.2.	
Question themes	**What is expected from the candidate?**
1 The candidate greets the examiner and has good body language.	The candidate is presentable and uses good communication skills; always recommended in any station.

Table 7.2.

Question themes	What is expected from the candidate?
2 What do you think about the COVID pandemic compared with other pandemics?	The candidate gives a good opening statement of the understanding of the situation. The COVID-19 pandemic was a pandemic that was unprecedented, at least in modern times. Although there have been other recent outbreaks, such as SARS 2003, swine flu 2009, Ebola 2013 and MERS 2015, the scale of the COVID-19 pandemic was much larger. As the pandemic spread very quickly, healthcare resources across the world were scarce and most countries struggled to find the resources to tackle the disease.
3 What healthcare demand did the COVID-19 pandemic create in the UK and why?	The UK's annual healthcare budget is more than 130 billion for the NHS. But the UK has fewer critical care beds per 100,000 population compared with other high-income countries (8 beds per 100,000 population in the UK, compared with 34 in the USA, 29 in Germany and 11.6 in France). This caused an enormous burden on the health service in the UK as it was at risk of being overwhelmed due to the high demand.
4 Did the UK Government manage the COVID pandemic well?	The candidate gives a good introductory statement; this will be followed by what went well and what could have gone better. In the end, the candidate gives his own personal opinion based on the balance of the facts discussed above. The candidate has a good flow of thought and a systematic approach; they have good judgement based on the facts given.

Table 7.2.

Question themes	What is expected from the candidate?
5 The candidate voluntarily lists the good aspects of COVID management by the UK Government.	The candidate can mention a few good things done during the pandemic by the UK Government: • Scientific approach: setting up the Scientific Advisory Group for Emergencies (SAGE) committee, a coronavirus taskforce. As the data were fast emerging and constantly evolving during the pandemic, it was important to ensure any decisions that were made, which had a significant impact on people's lives, were taken on a scientific basis by a panel of experts who worked closely to guide the policymakers. • Vaccination: this is perhaps regarded as the biggest success of the UK Government's policies. The UK established a Government-led vaccine task force. After the vaccine trials, in December 2020, the UK was the first country in the world to approve a COVID-19 vaccine, which was a watershed moment in the pandemic's history. The UK Government ordered 340 million doses of the vaccine early on, and rapidly rolled out the vaccination to the population to boost herd immunity. It is now very clear that vaccines played an important role in reducing the severity of the infection and, thereby, COVID-related mortality. • Research: the National Institute for Health and Care Research (NIHR), an independent body, was provided additional funding by the UK Government to carry out high-quality research, including the RECOVERY and REMAP-CAP trials that provided life-saving drugs for treating COVID, including dexamethasone in June 2020 and tocilizumab in February 2021. These studies proved the lack of benefit or harm of several other drugs that were in wider use during the pandemic and helped to streamline the treatment pathways based on evidence.

Table 7.2.

Question themes	What is expected from the candidate?
	<ul><li>Test and Trace: this started well when all new infections were actively screened, and contacts were traced. However, once the community numbers rose significantly, the system was unable to meet the demand due to the high numbers, as it relied heavily on volunteers.</li><li>Furlough scheme: this was also called the Coronavirus Job Retention Scheme. The UK Chancellor pledged £330 billion on 20 March 2020 to offer employers a grant from HM Revenue & Customs (HMRC) to cover up to 80% of employees' wages. This ensured that employees were still kept on the payroll and did not lose their jobs when businesses were struggling.</li><li>Nightingale hospitals: there were seven Nightingale hospitals at the cost of £530 million; the largest of them was the 4000 bedded hospital in the London ExCel centre with 500 ventilator beds and was the headline news built by the consortia (joint effort by the NHS, military and private sector) in a very short span of time, which was highly praised. However, the Nightingale hospitals did not admit any critically ill patients and the London ExCel centre admitted fewer than 100 patients. As they were deemed to be inefficient, they were decommissioned soon afterwards. However, it provided a safety net at the peak of the pandemic when hospital beds were at the critical point of being overwhelmed.</li><li>Critical Care Networks: although Critical Care Networks existed before the pandemic, they worked more coherently during the pandemic. Daily critical care situation reports (SitReps) identified hospitals that did not have intensive care unit (ICU) capacity and patients were transferred by a dedicated critical care transfer service to another hospital. This ensured that patients received vital critical care, even when their local hospital ran out of critical care beds.</li></ul>

Table 7.2.

Question themes	What is expected from the candidate?
6 The candidate mentions facts in which the UK Government could have done better.	The candidate also mentions a few examples in which the UK Government could have done better: • At the beginning of the pandemic, although community testing was started well, due to a shortage of testing kits, tests were prioritised mainly for hospitalised patients. This resulted in the loss of surveillance in the community that may have led to the exponential rise in cases. • Delays in lockdown: the WHO declared a world health emergency on 30 January 2020. The UK Government implemented a strict lockdown on 23 March 2020, which was weeks later than Spain, Italy and France. This, along with the open border, led to a rapid rise in cases, despite a clear signal from other countries, especially in Italy, where hospitals became overwhelmed. The *British Medical Journal* (*BMJ*) was critical of the delay in implementing the lockdown, which resulted in London hospitals being overwhelmed. A further delay in lockdown during the second wave and mixed messages before the lockdown resulted in much higher mortality during the second wave. • Pandemic preparedness and personal protective equipment (PPE) shortage: a BBC Panorama programme showed that the UK Government failed to stockpile enough PPE and there were several failures in the UK Government's pandemic plan, including expired PPE stock. This meant that there was rationing of PPE in hospital and social care settings, which resulted in many healthcare staff contracting COVID and becoming ill and, sadly, some died due to the illness. However, this was rectified in subsequent waves by better stockpiles and by establishing good international and national supply chains.

Table 7.2.

Question themes	What is expected from the candidate?
	• Care home resident handling: it was evident that there were not enough hospital beds to care for COVID patients based on mathematical modelling, to create more bed capacity. Older and vulnerable patients were rapidly discharged to care homes without any testing. This resulted in outbreaks in care homes, and sadly very many lives were lost. • Disproportionate allocation of resources: as the UK had fewer hospital beds per 100,000 population to meet the surge demands, the NHS had to cut back on other activities to prioritise the COVID pandemic. This included the cancellation of all non-emergency work, including cancer screening and treatment, which meant unfortunate delays in diagnosis and treatment. Although this work was resumed after the first wave, with subsequent waves due to hospital beds being filled with COVID patients coupled with high staff sickness, hospitals were not able to fully restart treatment to pre-pandemic levels for non-emergency work. • Mixed messages and Downing street parties: after the first wave, COVID outbreaks continued, which were managed by local lockdowns. This was proven subsequently to be ineffective at reducing case rates, and instead caused financial losses to local businesses. Before Christmas 2021, the UK Government was criticised for sending mixed messages about wearing masks and initially made a statement that people would be able to mix during Christmas, but quickly reverted to not allowing mixing between families.

Table 7.2.		
	Question themes	**What is expected from the candidate?**
		These confusing messages meant that the public was unclear about the COVID rules and, therefore, some rules were broken knowingly and, unknowingly, which resulted in a spike in cases of the Alpha variant (Kent variant) and in the Government losing public confidence. The recent penalties for Downing Street COVID parties in which policymakers had broken the COVID rules have significantly dented the credibility of the UK Government, and particularly in Downing Street.
7	Balanced view.	The candidate gives their personal opinion based on the facts listed above and concludes the debate.
8	Conclusion.	The candidate concludes the session and thanks the examiner at the end. This gives extra bonus points.

Discussion

This is a health-related political topic. Many discussions have happened regarding the strengths and weaknesses of the UK Government's handling during the pandemic. It is also important to note that the Government has ordered an independent inquiry: the UK COVID-19 Public Inquiry, which is ongoing, to look at the UK's preparedness and handling of the COVID-19 pandemic and the lessons to be learnt.

It is important that the candidate gives a balanced answer, however strongly they may feel about the way the pandemic was handled.

Key Points

- The COVID pandemic was met with unprecedented demand for healthcare resources.
- Some good aspects of the UK Government's management of the pandemic include the scientific approach, early vaccination, research, the test and trace scheme, the furlough scheme, and Nightingale hospitals.
- Some aspects in which the management could have been better include the problems in the supply of testing kits at the beginning of the pandemic, delays in lockdown, the shortage of PPE kits, care home resident handling, cancer and other specialties being affected, mixed messages from politicians, etc.

References

1. Coronavirus: lessons learned to date. Sixth Report of the Health and Social Care Committee and Third Report of the Science and Technology Committee of Session; 2021–22. Available online: https://committees.parliament.uk/publications/7496/documents/78687/default.

Question 102

Clinical examination of non-accidental injuries in a child

Subramanian Ganesan

Question

You are a junior doctor working in a GP surgery. You are seeing Jamie, who is a 6-month-old baby who has presented with vomiting, along with his mother. During your examination of Jamie, you find multiple bruises on his body that are not explainable: what are the issues here and how would you manage them?

The examiner will ask questions based on this scenario in the next station.

Themes for discussion (■ Table 7.3)

Table 7.3.		
	Question themes	**What is expected from the candidate?**
1	The candidate greets the examiner and has good body language.	The candidate is presentable and uses good communication skills; always recommended in any station.

Table 7.3.

	Question themes	What is expected from the candidate?
2	Explain the situation and examination findings.	The candidate gives a good description of the findings.
		The candidate should give the impression that there is no explanation given by the mother for the bruises.
3	What is the main issue here?	Bruises/injuries are not common in immobile babies. If there is no explanation for the injuries, it is a safeguarding issue.
4	How would you manage this issue?	The candidate should mention the following:
		• To discuss this with his senior doctor/supervisor for further advice.
		• To contact the social worker/social care for further investigation and medical examination/assessment by a trained paediatrician/children's doctor.
		• To explain to his mother about the referral to social care.
		• Clear documentation of the injuries noted on the body with measurements using a tape measure and use of a body map if available.
5	The mother refuses to be referred to a social worker. What would you do?	The candidate listens to the mother calmly to find out the reason for refusal; they will be empathetic throughout, but will keep the safety of the baby as the prime objective.
		They should mention that it is the legal duty of every doctor to make sure that a child is safe and that an appropriate referral to expert doctors/other agencies, such as social workers, is made when needed. This is to ensure the safety and welfare of the child.

Table 7.3.

	Question themes	What is expected from the candidate?
6	The mother asks what will happen now.	Ask the mother to continue with the routine baby care at home. The social worker will contact the parents by phone.
		The candidate can check the telephone numbers to be used to contact the mother.
		The baby and parents will be seen in the hospital for examination by an expert doctor/paediatrician, and they will explain what happens next.
7	The mother starts crying in the clinic. What would you do?	The candidate should explain the support available and show empathy for the mother and baby. They can enquire about and offer to contact any family member/partner to accompany her back home.
8	Conclusion.	The candidate can explain the importance of safeguarding children, especially babies, as they are very vulnerable to physical abuse; the candidate is aware of the need to protect them by involving various agencies. The candidate concludes by thanking the examiner at the end.

Discussion

Safeguarding children is everyone's responsibility: whether you are the child's parent, relative, family friend, neighbour or professional. Child protection means protecting children from physical, emotional and sexual abuse or neglect, thereby providing a safer environment to grow up into confident, healthy and happy adults.

Most children acquire bruises, broken bones and other injuries accidentally during their childhood whilst they are playing or in sports activities. Very rarely, broken bones or bruising can be caused by a medical condition that may require further tests. But if the bruises or injuries in children are caused by the deliberate acts of adults (parents/carers/strangers), this is known as physical abuse.

Physical abuse should be suspected if injuries are noticed in babies who are not mobile, or in children when:

- No explanation was given by the parents or carers.
- An explanation that does not fit the pattern of the injury is seen during the examination.
- Multiple explanations were given by the parents for the same injury.

All workplaces, educational institutions, leisure and sports centres have a safeguarding policy and a designated safeguarding officer who knows the procedure/policy well. In the UK, there is a designated line for safeguarding contactable through the police.

Referrals should be made through social workers who will arrange for medical examinations to be done by expert doctors/paediatricians. Doctors will be asked to provide parent details, home addresses, and details of any key agencies involved in the care, e.g. health visitors, school nurses, etc. The referrer will need to fill in a Multi-Agency Referral Form (MARF).

More detailed information about safeguarding children is available from the National Society for the Prevention of Cruelty to Children (NSPCC), the UK children's charity (https://www.nspcc.org.uk/).

The General Medical Council has published a guidance in 2012 called 'Protecting children and young people: the responsibilities of all doctors' to guide medical professionals in the safeguarding aspects.

Key Points

- Safeguarding concerns should be raised if there is an injury in a baby or child that cannot be explained.
- It is the legal duty of every doctor to make sure that the child is safe; appropriate, timely referral to social workers and experts is vital.

References

1. The Royal College of General Practitioners (RCGP). The child safeguarding toolkit. Available from: https://elearning.rcgp.org.uk/mod/book/view.php?id=12531.

2. National Institute for Health and Care Excellence. Child abuse and neglect: recognising, assessing and responding to abuse and neglect of children and young people. Available from: https://www.nice.org.uk/guidance/ng76; October 2017.

Question 103

Timing of introduction of COVID vaccination

Pritika Kandamaran

Question

In the next station, the examiner will question you on your knowledge of the COVID-19 vaccine and the timing of applying the COVID-19 vaccine in the UK. Was it right to introduce it early? A few critics have argued that it was brought out too early. What are your thoughts?

Themes for discussion (■ Table 7.4)

Table 7.4.	
Question themes	**What is expected from the candidate?**
1 The candidate greets the examiner and has good body language.	The candidate is presentable and uses good communication skills; always recommended in any station. This is a complex scenario; the candidate understands this complexity but stays calm and has a good approach.

Table 7.4.

	Question themes	What is expected from the candidate?
2	The candidate showcases their understanding of COVID vaccines.	The candidate gives a good opening statement with a clear understanding of the COVID-19 pandemic and the role of vaccines: • The COVID-19 pandemic was an unprecedented crisis faced by the world that killed millions of people over several years. • During this period, vaccines were encouraged throughout the world as a form of protection to reduce the risks of contracting the virus. • The vaccines were also said to reduce the severity of the virus if contracted. • According to the NHS, vaccines are the most effective way of preventing the spread of infectious diseases.

3	The candidate showcases their knowledge of the different COVID vaccines.	The candidate showcases their knowledge of the different COVID vaccines:
		
		• Various COVID vaccines were used, including:
		  - mRNA vaccines: Pfizer-BioNTech, Moderna;
		  - vector vaccine: AstraZeneca, Johnson & Johnson (Janssen);
		  - protein subunit vaccine: Novavax.
		• In both the UK and USA, the Pfizer-BioNTech, Moderna and Novavax vaccines are the currently approved and available vaccines.

4	The candidate highlights the ethics and procedure for releasing a vaccine.	The candidate gives some insight into how a vaccine is developed for release: • Vaccines undergo preclinical and clinical phases before they are approved and licensed. • In the UK, the Medicines and Healthcare products Regulatory Agency approves vaccines only if the standards of quality, safety, and effectiveness are met. The United States Food and Drug Administration approves vaccines in the USA.

Table 7.4.

Question themes	What is expected from the candidate?
	• The vaccines appeared to have been developed quickly, but the technologies used to develop some of the COVID-19 vaccines had been a 'work in progress' for many years, as a preparation to combat infectious diseases. • As a provider, you must promise beneficence and non-maleficence towards patients (do benefit, do no harm). Quoting pillars of medical ethics can fetch extra marks in any MMI ethics station. • According to the GMC, the benefits of the research should outweigh the risks. Moreover, participants should be protected from harm.
5 The candidate highlights the ethics and controversial issues surrounding taking vaccines.	The candidate understands clearly the controversial topic of taking vaccines: • The initial introduction of vaccines caused mixed reactions among people. Some people were pro-vaccine, some were confused, and others were against the vaccine. • Whilst there was increased encouragement to take the vaccine by healthcare systems and governments, the choice to take the vaccine was ultimately the individual's decision. • One cannot be forced to take the vaccine without consent (UK General Medical Council's 'Good medical practice' guideline and the American Medical Association's Code of Medical Ethics). • In England, the Public Health (Control of Disease) Act 1984 specifically prevents ministers from creating new rules that would make vaccines mandatory (it would have to pass approval through Parliament).

Table 7.4.

	Question themes	What is expected from the candidate?
6	The candidate volunteers the pros for administering the vaccine.	The candidate clearly understands the pros of introducing the vaccines at an early stage of the pandemic: <ul><li>Masks, social distancing and contact tracing were proven to be insufficient in preventing the spread of the virus. Immediate action was required.</li><li>There was a reduction in expected mortality rates and transmission rates for countries after administering the vaccine.</li><li>It increased herd immunity.</li><li>It allowed many institutions and workforces to return to a face-to-face setting (this reduced economic losses for a country).</li><li>The vaccines had passed clinical trials, so there was no need to delay their introduction.</li><li>Moreover, most side effects of the vaccine were tolerable.</li><li>Vaccines were only given to those who met the requirements to ensure their safety (people over 60 and young children were not allowed to take the vaccines initially).</li></ul>
7	The candidate volunteers the cons for administering the vaccine.	The candidate clearly understands the cons of administering the vaccines at that early stage: <ul><li>The early rollout of the vaccine was not effective enough in counteracting misinformation surrounding the COVID-19 vaccine.</li><li>Some side effects of certain vaccines were only seen later on. For example, a few cases of Guillain–Barré syndrome were reported following use of the Johnson & Johnson vaccine.</li><li>The duration of protection was unknown for the vaccines.</li><li>Some people thought they were fully immune to the virus and started taking the social distancing measures lightly.</li><li>After its introduction, vaccines were made mandatory in many workforces, especially in the private sector. As a result, those who refused to be vaccinated lost their jobs.</li></ul>

Table 7.4.

Question themes	What is expected from the candidate?
8	The candidate has a clear opinion and explains the reasons behind this opinion.	The candidate can choose any path, but their judgement and its reasons should be clear. For example, if the candidate chooses to agree that the vaccines were indeed brought out too early, the points on cons should be stressed and explained precisely.
9	Conclusion.	A clear presentation, smiling throughout and avoiding repetition — these steps can increase the scores in this station. The candidate concludes the session by saying 'thank you' to the examiner. This gives extra bonus points.

Discussion

Do not worry about finding the right answer; most candidates become distracted with choosing one side and lose their clarity. Please make sure that you can explain both the pros and cons of the early release of the vaccines. Showcase that you are confident in choosing one side and explaining the reasons for this stance. Explaining ethical dilemmas is the key to this station.

Vaccine development is a long procedure that requires many trials and regulations in order for a vaccine to be released to the public. According to the UK General Medical Council's 'Good medical practice' guideline and the American Medical Association's Code of Medical Ethics, an individual must always be protected from harm from research products. Additionally, it is stated that an individual has the right to make decisions about any medical test or treatment they receive, as long as they have the mental capacity to do so.

Key Points

- Always introduce yourself/thank the examiner and appropriately conclude the session.
- There are pros and cons to any ethical dilemma; the candidate must express an understanding of both sides.
- The candidate should be able to clearly conclude their discussion and explain their reasoning.
- The candidate should quote the General Medical Council's 'Good medical practice' document or the American Medical Council's or a similar body's code of ethics to show that they are aware of the ethics behind the scenario.

References

1. World Health Organization. COVID-19 vaccines. Available from: https://www.who.int/westernpacific/emergencies/covid-19/covid-19-vaccines.

2. National Health Service. Coronavirus (COVID-19) vaccine. Available from: https://www.nhs.uk/conditions/coronavirus-covid-19/coronavirus-vaccination/coronavirus-vaccine.

3. Centers for Disease Control and Prevention. COVID-19. Stay up to date with vaccines. Available from: https://www.cdc.gov/coronavirus/2019-ncov/vaccines/stay-up-to-date.html; December 2022.

4. Rahman MA, Islam MS. Early approval of COVID-19 vaccines: pros and cons. *Hum Vaccin Immunother* 2021; 17(10): 3288-96.

5. General Medical Council. Good practice in research. Available from: https://www.gmc-uk.org/ethical-guidance/ethical-guidance-for-doctors/good-practice-in-research/good-practice-in-research#paragraph-5.

6. General Medical Council. Ethical hub: COVID-19 questions and answers. Available from: https://www.gmc-uk.org/ethical-guidance/ethical-hub/covid-19-questions-and-answers#[Vaccines].

Question 104

A sportsperson missing a tournament due to the vaccine

Pritika Kandamaran

Question

A prominent sportsperson is not allowed to play in an international tournament as he refused to have the COVID-19 vaccine. There are ethical challenges in this scenario and the examiner will discuss your thoughts on this in the next station.

Themes for discussion (■ Table 7.5)

Table 7.5.	
Question themes	**What is expected from the candidate?**
1 The candidate greets the examiner and has good body language.	The candidate is presentable and uses good communication skills; always recommended in any station. This is a complex scenario. The candidate understands this complexity, but stays calm and has a good approach.

Table 7.5.

Question themes	What is expected from the candidate?
2 Is it right for the sportsperson to refuse the COVID vaccine?	The candidate gives a good opening statement of the understanding of the situation. The summary should be attractive and bring the main ethical problems into discussion.
3 The candidate volunteers the pros for the sportsperson using his right to refuse the vaccine.	The candidate understands clearly the pros of not taking the vaccine: • Any sportsperson or human being has the right to refuse a vaccine or any medical intervention. • Anyone cannot be forced to take a vaccine without their consent (UK General Medical Council's 'Good medical practice' guideline and the American Medical Association's Code of Medical Ethics). • In England, the Public Health (Control of Disease) Act 1984 specifically prevents ministers from creating new rules that would make vaccines mandatory (it would have to pass the approval of Parliament); in the case of COVID-19, this was applied very early. • As influential public figures, they can represent the beliefs of certain groups in not taking the vaccine.
4 The candidate volunteers the cons for the sportsperson not taking the vaccine to participate in the event; why it should not be the preferred path.	The candidate understands clearly the cons for not taking the vaccine: • As a public figure, their life will be majorly impacted. • As a prominent sportsperson, they will not be able to participate in many tournaments and further progress their career. • They are losing out on tournament earnings as well as sponsorships and endorsement earnings from brands due to their vaccination status. • Their fans may be disappointed in them not being able to play in the tournaments. • They may even cause a stir among some of their fans who may be pro-vaccination, whilst others support their decision. They may lose the support of some of their fans.

Table 7.5.

	Question themes	What is expected from the candidate?
5	Is it right for the tournament/country to stop this sportsperson from playing?	• The sportsperson may not be able to participate in tournaments due to the travel restrictions of overseas countries. Ultimately, the country's governing body has control over its borders. • Maybe, at that time, the COVID-19 virus had just reached its peak in some countries, and it was the cause of many deaths worldwide. • Therefore, governments were trying to protect their people by enforcing travel restrictions. • However, whilst they can encourage travellers to take vaccines, they cannot force them. • The current situation has changed; we have reached a stage of the pandemic in which countries are reducing travel restrictions. • For example, the UK currently does not require COVID tests or quarantine if you have been administered the vaccine, but some other countries might still have restrictions on entering their country.
6	How could the situation be handled better?	• Notify all the tournament players beforehand of both the tournament's COVID-19 requirements as well as the hosting country's requirements. • Organise international events in countries with fewer travel restrictions to accommodate all players. • The players should be prepared beforehand and be able to make a well thought-out decision. There would be no last-minute withdrawals, such as in this particular case that would be a disappointment for both the sportsperson and their fans, who would have been expecting their participation in the tournament.
7	The candidate has a clear opinion/conclusion and explains the reasons.	The candidate can choose any path, but their judgement should be clear. For example, if the candidate chooses to support the sportsperson's refusal of the COVID-19 vaccine, their pro arguments should be stressed and explained precisely.

Table 7.5.

	Question themes	What is expected from the candidate?
8	Judgement and clarity.	The candidate has clarity in their answer, can explain the pros and cons, concluding clearly. A clear presentation, smiling throughout and avoiding repetition — these steps can increase the scores in this station.
9	Conclusion.	The candidate concludes the session by saying 'thank you' to the examiner. This gives extra bonus points.

Discussion

Do not worry about finding the right answer; most candidates become distracted with choosing one side and lose their clarity. Please make sure that you can explain both the pros and cons and are confident in choosing one side and explaining the reasons for this stance. Explaining ethical dilemmas is the key in this station.

According to the UK General Medical Council's 'Good medical practice' guideline and the American Medical Association's Code of Medical Ethics, an individual has the right to make decisions about any medical test or treatment they receive as long as they have the mental capacity to do so. The Public Health (Control of Disease) Act in England prevents making vaccines mandatory. Therefore, whilst the Government may encourage those who are eligible to take the vaccine, it will always be the choice of the individual. This also means that an individual cannot be punished for refusing the vaccine.

Key Points

- There are pros and cons to any ethical dilemma; the candidate must be aware of both.
- The candidate should be able to clearly conclude their discussion and explain their reasoning.
- The candidate should quote the General Medical Council's 'Good medical practice' document or the American Medical Council's or a similar body's code of ethics to show that they are aware of the ethics behind the scenario.
- Express an understanding of the situation (and be prepared to give a recent example from the news/press, e.g. the case of Djokovic in Australia).

References

1. Liberty. Coronavirus vaccinations: Can I be forced to get the vaccine? Available from: https://www.libertyhumanrights.org.uk/advice_information/coronavirus-vaccinations-can-i-be-forced-to-get-the-vaccine.

2. Age UK. What standards you should expect from NHS services. Available from: https://www.ageuk.org.uk/information-advice/health-wellbeing/health-services/healthcare-rights.

3. American Medical Association. Code of medical ethics – patient rights. Available from: https://www.ama-assn.org/delivering-care/ethics/patient-rights.

4. United Kingdom Government. Guidance: travel to England from another country during coronavirus (COVID-19). Available from: https://www.gov.uk/guidance/travel-to-england-from-another-country-during-coronavirus-covid-19#:~:text=You%20do%20not%20need%20to%20take%20any%20COVID%2D19%20travel,you%20qualify%20as%20fully%20vaccinated.&text=The%20testing%20and%20quarantine%20rules,will%20change%2011%20February%202022.

5. Centers for Disease Control and Prevention. International travel to and from the United States. Available from: https://www.cdc.gov/coronavirus/2019-ncov/travelers/international-travel-during-covid19.html.

Question 105

Monkeypox disease and prevention

Pritika Kandamaran

Question

Monkeypox disease: what do you understand by this? If you are in charge and have the power to make plans to prevent this, what would you do?

In the next station, the examiner will question you on these topics.

Themes for discussion (■ Table 7.6)

Table 7.6.	
Question themes	**What is expected from the candidate?**
1 The candidate greets the examiner and has good body language.	The candidate is presentable and uses good communication skills; always recommended in any station.

Table 7.6.

	Question themes	What is expected from the candidate?
2	The candidate showcases their understanding of monkeypox disease.	The candidate has an understanding of monkeypox disease: • Monkeypox is caused by the monkeypox virus. • There is an increasing amount of cases in Europe and North America. • Clinical presentation is similar to that of smallpox. • It spreads through skin-to-skin contact with a person who has the monkeypox virus. • Symptoms may last for 2-4 weeks.
3	The candidate highlights how they would identify a patient with monkeypox disease.	The candidate has an understanding of the symptoms related to monkeypox disease: • Flu-like symptoms (fever, intense headache, muscle aches, etc.) followed by rashes (starting from the face and spreading throughout the body). • Confirmed by a polymerase chain reaction (PCR) test.
4	The candidate highlights the treatment for a patient with monkeypox disease.	The candidate briefly explains the treatment for a patient with monkeypox disease: • Treatment is similar to that of smallpox. • In most cases, treatment is not required. • However, if a person is severely ill, they may be admitted to hospital.
5	The candidate gives an overview of plans they would make to prevent monkeypox disease from spreading.	The candidate states clearly the plans they would enforce: • Reaching out to organisations and sending healthcare teams to spread awareness about monkeypox diseases (precautions, symptoms, vaccines, testing centres, additional facilities). • Making changes to the healthcare system and facilities to accommodate for virus-related morbidities. • Reaching out to the Government to take action at a country level.

Table 7.6.

	Question themes	What is expected from the candidate?
6	The candidate explains self-measures one can take to minimise their chances of being exposed to the disease.	The candidate emphasises the importance of measures one can take to protect themselves from the virus: • Avoiding close contact with people who have a rash that looks like monkeypox or those who have been confirmed to have the virus. • Washing your hands often and following good hygiene. • Wearing a well fitting mask in public. • Staying up-to-date with the news on monkeypox. • Choose to take the vaccine if you are at high risk.
7	The candidate explains measures that can be taken in the clinical setting.	The candidate explains what can be carried out at the clinical level: • Preparing teams of trained staff specifically for the management of monkeypox cases. • Having isolated areas in hospitals and facilities to treat monkeypox cases. • Having patients' and staff's temperatures checked before entry to hospital. • Frequent cleaning and disinfection of common areas. • Ensuring that there are multiple centres for testing and vaccines, making them accessible to all communities.
8	The candidate explains measures that can be taken at the community level.	The candidate explains actions the community and community-based organisations can take: • Educating the public, including children, about monkeypox disease. • Advocating for personal hygiene and safety measures on the radio and news. • Initiating vaccine drives to encourage uptake. • Encouraging the wearing of masks. • Refraining from mass gatherings. • Distributing posters with safety measures.

Table 7.6.		
	Question themes	**What is expected from the candidate?**
9	The candidate explains what the Government can do to prevent the spread of monkeypox disease.	The candidate explains how they would reach out to the Government and the actions they can take to prevent the spread of this virus: • Controlling borders (limiting visitors from high-risk countries). • Implementing social distancing measures in workplaces, hospitals and schools. • Ensuring the country has sufficient vaccines, masks and other medical equipment. • Keeping track of the number of cases and relevant data related to the virus. • Keep reassuring the public, but letting them know the truth about the current situation of their country.
10	Conclusion.	The candidate summarises their points clearly. The candidate concludes the session by saying 'thank you' to the examiner.

Discussion

The candidate should showcase their knowledge about monkeypox disease. There is no single management plan, so candidates can create plans and provide explanations why they chose to incorporate each measure. The candidate should highlight the precautions that can be taken at home, in a clinical setting and in a community. Additionally, the candidate can explain some measures the Government can put in place to ensure the safety of the country.

The WHO and NHS websites can give the candidate a basic understanding of monkeypox disease, including precautionary measures that can be taken to reduce exposure to the disease, and up-to-date information pertaining to treatment and vaccines.

Monkeypox is a rare infection usually reported in Africa, but recently there has been an increase in cases in the UK. The risk of catching monkeypox virus is low. It is caused by the monkeypox virus, an orthopoxvirus belonging to the *Poxviridae* family. It is usually a self-limiting disease lasting 2-4 weeks, but severe cases can occur and mortality has been 3-6% in recent times.

It is recommended that the candidate keeps up-to-date with recent healthcare-related topics in the news; visiting the BBC Health news page and other health-related news pages will be useful before the MMI interviews.

Key Points

- Always introduce yourself/thank the examiner and appropriately close the session.
- Showcase your understanding of monkeypox disease, including what it is, its current relevance, symptoms and treatment.
- Clearly state your plans to prevent monkeypox disease from spreading.
- Highlight precautionary measures that can be taken at home, in a clinical setting, and as a community, as well as measures that the Government can put in place.

References

1. World Health Organization. Monkeypox. Available from: https://www.who.int/news-room/fact-sheets/detail/monkeypox.

2. National Health Service. Monkeypox. Available from: https://www.nhs.uk/conditions/monkeypox.

Question 106

Managing obesity in young children

Pritika Kandamaran

Question

Obesity is a big problem in healthcare and it affects children also. What steps can you suggest for managing obesity in young children? The examiner will ask for your views on this problem in the next station.

Themes for discussion (■ Table 7.7)

Table 7.7.	
Question themes	**What is expected from the candidate?**
1 The candidate greets the examiner and has good body language.	The candidate is presentable and uses good communication skills; always recommended in any station.

Table 7.7.

	Question themes	What is expected from the candidate?
2	The candidate gives a brief overview of obesity in children.	The candidate gives a good opening statement showcasing their knowledge and understanding of obesity and its prevalence in young children.
3	The candidate provides a brief framework of how they would manage obesity in young children.	The candidate gives a brief overview of their approach to managing childhood obesity: • Confirm the diagnosis of childhood obesity and classify it (overweight, obese, severely obese). This can be confirmed by checking their body mass index (BMI); BMI is calculated by dividing weight in kilogrammes by the square of the height in metres. • Chat with the child and their parent/guardian(s) to learn about the daily routine and lifestyle of the child. • Listen to the parents'/guardians' knowledge about obesity, further educating them and making them aware of the risks associated with obesity. • Work as a team with the child and parent/guardians to create a personalised, multidisciplinary approach to manage obesity in the child. • Follow-up appointments are key to seeing the child's progress and ensuring adherence to the plan.
4	The candidate involves the parents/guardians of the children.	The candidate understands that the patient is a young child who lacks the ability to make informed decisions and therefore depends on their parents for consent to treatment and adherence to the treatment plan. Helping the parents to understand their child's situation will help them to communicate with the child. Additionally, teachers, the child's siblings and friends can help to motivate the child.

Table 7.7.

Question themes	What is expected from the candidate?
5 The candidate provides the causes of obesity in young children.	The candidate highlights factors that can lead to childhood obesity (and can classify the causes into diet-related, genetic, endocrine, environmental, family, mental health, etc.): • More calories consumed than calories burnt. • Little to no physical activity/sedentary lifestyle (common now with the increased use of electronics and online classes). • Consuming energy-dense foods: high in fats and sugars, but low in healthy micronutrients (fast food). • Underlying health conditions: hypothyroidism and genetic diseases. • Stress, anxiety and depression. • Having a parent who is obese increases the risk.
6 The candidate explains why obesity is a health risk and why it should be treated.	The candidate understands the health risks associated with childhood obesity: • Cardiovascular diseases. • High blood pressure and high cholesterol. • Type 2 diabetes. • Liver and kidney disease. • Sleep apnoea. • Joint pain. Severe cases of obesity may lower the life expectancy of the child due to the high risks of various diseases.
7 The candidate volunteers lifestyle and other approaches to treat obesity.	The candidate explains the lifestyle changes that can be made, including healthy eating (e.g. snacking on fruits instead of chips and avoiding fast food, etc.), limiting screen time and encouraging the physical activities in which the child shows interest. Ensure that the child is not stressed or showing signs of insecurities.

Table 7.7.

	Question themes	What is expected from the candidate?
8	The candidate explains the medical approaches to treating obesity.	The candidate explains the involvement of the clinical setting as a part of the treatment plan. The plan may involve a combination of expertise, including physicians, nurses, registered dieticians, psychologists and exercise specialists, to name but a few. The clinical setting is mostly to counsel the family, create goals, motivate them, and provide them with the tools and knowledge they can apply to the child's daily life and routine. In some cases, medication may be prescribed by physicians as a part of their weight-loss plan.
9	The candidate explains the preventative measures.	The candidate highlights some ways to prevent obesity in young children: • Groups in the community and community-based organisations can educate the public, making them aware of this prevalent issue and lower the social stigma associated with it. • Schools can encourage healthy eating habits and physical activity. • Schools can encourage social interaction between students and provide health-related sessions to educate children from a young age.
10	Judgement and clarity.	The candidate provides a clear management plan for a young child with obesity. A clear presentation, smiling throughout and avoiding repetition — these steps can increase the scores in this station.
11	Conclusion.	The candidate concludes the session and thanks the examiner at the end. This gives extra bonus points.

Discussion

Please make sure to provide clear steps in the management plan for childhood obesity. There is no single management plan, so candidates can create a plan and provide explanations why they chose to incorporate each step. The candidate should highlight the teamwork required between the family, clinicians and community to help with the progress of the child.

The GMC's guide to medical students can give the candidate an understanding of how to approach the treatment of a child based on age and maturity. These are young children and not adults who are fully responsible for themselves and so parents are usually involved, and their involvement is also encouraged.

Key Points

- Always introduce yourself/thank the examiner and appropriately close the session.
- Showcase your understanding of obesity and clearly highlight a management plan to treat the young child with obesity.
- Highlight the involvement of the child and their parents/guardians when creating the management plan.
- Highlight the various approaches required to treat obesity; mention the clinical, familial and community efforts required.
- Ensure that the child is adhering to the treatment plan.

References

1. British Medical Association. Ethical toolkit for medical students: treating children and young people as a medical student. Available from: https://www.bma.org.uk/advice-and-support/ethics/medical-students/ethics-toolkit-for-medical-students/ethics-of-treating-children-and-young-people.

2.   General Medical Council. 0-18 years: guidance for all doctors. Making decisions. Available from: https://www.gmc-uk.org/ethical-guidance/ethical-guidance-for-doctors/0-18-years/making-decisions.

3.   General Medical Council. Treatment and care towards the end of life: good medical practice in decision making. Neonates, children and young people. Available from: https://www.gmc-uk.org/ethical-guidance/ethical-guidance-for-doctors/treatment-and-care-towards-the-end-of-life/neonates-children-and-young-people.

4.   World Health Organization. Noncommunicable diseases: childhood overweight and obesity. Available from: https://www.who.int/news-room/questions-and-answers/item/noncommunicable-diseases-childhood-overweight-and-obesity.

Question 107

Smoking cessation

Pritika Kandamaran

Question

You are the lead in a healthcare team for smoking cessation in the community. What can you suggest to help people stop smoking in the population? The examiner will discuss this in the next station.

Themes for discussion (■ Table 7.8)

Table 7.8.	
Question themes	**What is expected from the candidate?**
1 The candidate greets the examiner and has good body language.	The candidate is presentable and uses good communication skills; always recommended in any station.

Table 7.8.

	Question themes	What is expected from the candidate?
2	The candidate briefly introduces the topic of smoking.	The candidate gives a good opening statement and a brief overview of smoking: • Smoking is one of the biggest public health threats that the world is facing, killing millions of people each year. • Tobacco in the form of cigarettes is the most common product used for smoking. • Smoking affects not only the smoker, but also those who are around the smoker through second-hand smoke (passive smoking). • Smoking is addictive, so it is difficult to stop.
3	The candidate provides reasons why people may smoke.	The candidate highlights reasons why people start smoking: • To cope with stress and negative moods. • Peer pressure. • Simply to relax. • The appealing marketing of tobacco products.
4	The candidate highlights the negative effects of smoking.	The candidate highlights the increased health risks and overall negative impact associated with smoking: • Smoking causes cancer (lung, mouth, throat and more). • The greater risk of cardiovascular and respiratory disease (coronary artery disease, stroke, emphysema, chronic bronchitis). • Reduced fertility. • Pregnant women are at an increased risk of preterm delivery, stillbirth and ectopic pregnancy. • Passive smokers are at increased risk of obtaining the same illnesses as that of a smoker.

Table 7.8.

	Question themes	What is expected from the candidate?
5	The candidate emphasises the benefits of smoking cessation.	The candidate understands clearly the benefits of smoking cessation: • Overall improved health status and quality of life. • Immediately reduced risks of the previously mentioned diseases associated with smoking. • After 20 minutes of smoking cessation, blood pressure returns to normal; after 8 hours, the chances of having a heart attack start to reduce; and after 48 hours, taste and smell start to improve. • Reduces the financial burden for the smoker, as well as healthcare facilities in the long term.
6	The candidate understands how smoking affects our society.	The candidate highlights the negative impact of smoking on society: • Workplace absenteeism and productivity are decreased. • Emotional instability causes a strain in relationships. • Increased accidents.
7	The candidate highlights ways to minimise smoking in the population.	The candidate provides some ways to minimise smoking in the population. The WHO response involves MPOWER: • **M**onitoring tobacco use and prevention policies. • **P**rotecting people from tobacco use. • **O**ffering help in quitting tobacco use. • **W**arning about the dangers of tobacco. • **E**nforcing bans on tobacco advertising, promotion and sponsorship. • **R**aising taxes on tobacco.

Table 7.8.

	Question themes	What is expected from the candidate?
8	The candidate highlights some difficulties the healthcare team may face.	The candidate understands why it may be difficult for individuals to stop smoking: • Nicotine addiction: nicotine stimulates the brain to release chemicals that make your body feel 'good'. An individual's brain has to become used to the absence of nicotine and to a daily routine without smoking. • Withdrawal symptoms: irritability, anxiety, urge to smoke, inability to concentrate, weight gain, difficulty in falling asleep. • Emotional issues as a result of their environment may encourage them to continue smoking to relieve stress and anxiety. • Some individuals may not be able to afford healthcare options.
9	The candidate explains how they would lead their healthcare team in accomplishing this.	The candidate explains how to accomplish this: • Healthcare teams can be split into groups. • Some members can be a part of the advocacy team, for a 'Quit Smoking' campaign. The community can be educated about the health risks associated with smoking and to whom smokers can reach out to start their smoking cessation. • The healthcare team can also provide counselling services to create a personalised smoking cessation plan and also identify and treat any underlying cause that may stimulate the urge to smoke. • Instead of compelling everyone to stop smoking immediately, provide alternatives for them and introduce 'quit smoking' medications, setting more realistic goals for individual compliance in their path to quitting.

Table 7.8.	
Question themes	**What is expected from the candidate?**
	• Support programmes can be organised for those ex-smokers and people who have begun their smoking cessation, so they can share their experiences and progress, as an encouragement to move forwards. • The healthcare team can work with the Government to implement tobacco control regulations, more smoke-free zones, and prohibit advertisements related to smoking. • Ensure that patients comply with their plans by having follow-up appointments with healthcare officials.
10 Conclusion.	The candidate summarises their points clearly. The candidate concludes the session by saying 'thank you' to the examiner.

Discussion

The candidate should showcase their knowledge about smoking and smoking cessation. The candidate should explain clearly the plans and measures that can be taken to help people to quit smoking. The candidate should portray their leadership skills by explaining how they would work with their team to promote smoking cessation. The candidate should showcase their understanding of the challenges they may face in helping people to quit smoking.

The WHO and NHS websites can give the candidate a basic understanding of the prevalence of smoking and the health risks associated with it. Additionally, the WHO has highlighted six measures as a part of their plan to promote smoking cessation in a practical, cost-effective way.

Key Points

- Always introduce yourself/thank the examiner and appropriately close the session.
- Showcase your understanding of smoking as a public health threat.
- Highlight why people should quit smoking and understand why it is a difficult process.
- Explain in detail how you would lead your healthcare team to help people in your community stop smoking.

References

1. National Health Service. What are the health risks of smoking? Available from: https://www.nhs.uk/common-health-questions/lifestyle/what-are-the-health-risks-of-smoking.

2. World Health Organization. Available from: https://www.who.int/news-room/fact-sheets/detail/tobacco.

3. Centers for Disease Control and Prevention. Health effects of cigarette smoking. Available from: https://www.cdc.gov/tobacco/data_statistics/fact_sheets/health_effects/effects_cig_smoking/index.htm.

4. Centers for Disease Control and Prevention. Smoking and tobacco use. Cessation. Available from: https://www.cdc.gov/tobacco/data_statistics/fact_sheets/cessation/smoking-cessation-fast-facts/index.html.

Question 108

Triaging: the scene of a bomb blast

Thanthullu Vasu

Question

You are a year 13 student attending a concert with your mother and your brother. There is a bomb blast; fortunately, you are unharmed.

However, others are injured. Sort out the most important and least important scenario when triaging those injured or close by (six scenarios given below):

- Brother crying for help with pain in his leg.
- A mother who has chest pains.
- Unconscious older person.
- Run away immediately from the scene.
- People are stealing things from those injured.
- Pick up your own laptop.

Themes for discussion (■ Table 7.9)

Table 7.9.	
Question themes	**What is expected from the candidate?**
1 The candidate greets the examiner and has good body language.	The candidate is presentable and uses good communication skills; always recommended in any station.
2 What is triaging? Why is it needed?	Triaging helps to decide the order of treatment; triage is the preliminary assessment of patients or casualties so that we can decide the urgency of treatment.
	Triage is needed to balance the available resources versus needs. It helps to assess who is most in need of intervention and who will benefit the most from our treatment or actions.
3 In what order will you triage the six scenarios from most needed to least needed?	The candidate can choose any order; there is no right or wrong answer, but they should give a clear description of why they chose that order. The candidate should have a scientific, medical or ethical reason for choosing this order. They will not be scored for the order, but for the reasoning behind the order.
	The candidate is able to think and make a judgement; they know who is a priority, but at the same time, what is practicable for a year 13 student.
4 Run away immediately from the scene, as the first option.	Safety is a priority; in any blast, there is always a chance of an after blast that can happen. The candidate should run away from the scene, and check that it is safe to approach before coming back.
5 A mother who has chest pains versus a brother with leg pain.	There is no right or wrong answer but, as said before, the candidate should give clear reasoning. A brother with leg pain might just need immobilisation if there is a fracture, whereas the mother with chest pain can have a serious problem.

Table 7.9.

	Question themes	What is expected from the candidate?
		This is an opportunity for the candidate to describe their first aid skills, resuscitation skills or their workplace experience. For example, the candidate may say that they would choose to go to the mother first as they are trained in Airway, Breathing, Circulation (ABC) resuscitation and as they have done a resuscitation or defibrillator course (if any was done in the past).
6	Unconscious older person.	The candidate realises that there is a serious airway problem here; there could be a head injury, or even the patient might have died. The understanding of priorities, limitations and restrictions in the concert arena, limitations due to the skills available, calling an ambulance or 999, putting in the recovery position; there are many such options, but these should be reasonably balanced with the candidate's ability to give a reason.
7	People stealing things from those injured and picking up your own laptop.	The candidate understands the limitations of material value in this scenario and gives priority to what is needed. This is an opportunity to test the professionalism of the candidate.
8	Would you oppose doing anything about people stealing things from those injured?	The candidate has to stay safe; it might not be prudent to confront those doing unprofessional things at this time, whilst saving lives is a priority.
9	If you had training in first aid, would your order of priorities change?	The candidate has knowledge of the importance of first aid, resuscitation and defibrillator training. If they had this training, they might try to resuscitate the unconscious older person or the mother with chest pain instead presenting a different order. The candidate should clarify how they would do this with their training.
		This is an opportunity for the candidate to express their resuscitation training or workplace experience in a prudent manner.

Table 7.9.

	Question themes	What is expected from the candidate?
10	Conclusion.	The candidate concludes the session and thanks the examiner at the end.

Discussion

Triaging can come up as a station in an MMI; the main aim is to assess whether the candidate has the ability to give reasoning behind the order of the triage. It is wise to practice a few such scenarios with your friends or parents, as this can be stressful for many candidates. Most of the time the candidates fail, because they think that there is a correct order to give, rather than realising that they should just give the right reasoning for their choice of order.

Key Points

- There is no right or wrong answer in triaging; the key is to give the right reasoning behind the chosen order in a scientific and ethical manner.
- Triaging helps to decide the order of the treatment.
- Triage is the preliminary assessment of patients or casualties so that we can decide the urgency of the treatment.
- Triage is needed to balance the available resources versus need.

References

1. National Health Service (England). Guidance for emergency departments: initial assessment. Available from: https://www.england.nhs.uk/guidance-for-emergency-departments-initial-assessment/#:~: text=Triage%20is%20part%20of%20the,unwell%20patients%20are%20seen%20first.

Question 109

Triaging: a liver transplant recipient

Selvakumar Panchatsharam

Question

You are asked to triage who should receive a liver transplant among these five patients; unfortunately, there is only one liver available. You should give valid reasons for your order of triage:

- A 47-year-old man with alcoholism who is a father of two children.
- A 73-year-old fit healthy gentleman.
- A 32-year-old lady with well-controlled AIDS.
- A 6-year-old boy with genetic liver disease.
- A 34-year-old pregnant lady.

The examiner will question the order of the triage, its ethical dilemmas and the problems with this scenario.

Themes for discussion (■ Table 7.10)

Table 7.10.

	Question themes	What is expected from the candidate?
1	The candidate greets the examiner, has good body language and speaks coherently.	The candidate is presentable and uses good communication skills; always recommended in any station.
2	The candidate gives an introduction to this problem.	There is no right or wrong answer in this type of triage; even experienced doctors can differ in their order of triage. This is a complex question and the examiner will assess the reasoning and judgement of the candidate. Whatever order is chosen, the score is given only for the correct reasoning explained by the candidate.
3	Usually, this is a team or MDT decision.	The candidate is aware that, usually, this is not one person's decision and the final decision will be made based on a consensus from the multidisciplinary team (MDT).
4	What will be your key factor in considering who will be the right recipient?	The key factor in deciding who will be the right recipient will be to assess which recipient would 'most benefit' from the available organ.
5	What factors will help you to make a decision on this organ transplant?	The candidate can give a description of the factors involved as below: • Donor and recipient matching: not all organs can match all recipients. The process of ensuring a donated organ will not be rejected by the recipient's immune system requires specific testing, including blood group and human leukocyte antigen (HLA) matching. This would help in choosing an appropriate recipient.

Table 7.10.

Question themes	What is expected from the candidate?
	• Transplant waiting list: in the UK, living-related donors are rare for a liver transplant. Most of the donors are either donors after brain death or circulatory death. Despite the recent change in the organ donation law of presumed consent, donated organs are finite and patients often wait for many months. Once the patients have been identified for an organ transplant, they are allocated to a waiting list. Typically, the longest waiting person would get priority.
	• Comorbidities: coexisting illnesses and their severity, physiological reserve, functional status and frailty.
	• Quality Adjusted Life Years (QALY): this is simply a product of the perceived quality of life (0-1, 0 being poor health and 1 being perfect health) and the number of years expected to survive. This will determine how likely a proposed treatment would benefit the patient.

	• The pillars of medical ethics:
	  - beneficence: how likely is your treatment going to benefit the patient?
	  - non-maleficence: first do no harm;
	  - autonomy: giving the person freedom to choose, when they are able;
	  - justice: acting fairly.

	• Social circumstances: although this will not impact heavily on the decision-making process, it is worth highlighting social issues such as alcohol consumption and how these would impact the success of the transplantation and the risk of damage to the transplanted liver if habitual drinking continues.

Table 7.10.

Question themes	What is expected from the candidate?
6 The examiner will ask about individual patients and their suitability. It is prudent if the candidate can volunteer the order or reasons behind each scenario.	A 47-year-old man with alcoholism who is a father of two children: there is a high risk for going back to drinking after the transplant, but the patient could do well, as there is motivation to stop drinking due to his two children.
	A 73-year-old healthy, fit gentleman: even though considered fit, he will be a high-risk transplant recipient due to his age and the high risk of complications. The utility of the liver is not the same as for a young patient.
	A 32-year-old lady with well-controlled AIDS: high risk due to worsening AIDS with immunosuppression, but the patient is young, and there are better HIV medications available that could control the disease.
	A 6-year-old boy with genetic liver disease: a young boy but there might not be a genetic therapy available; this would depend on the prognosis of the condition and whether a liver transplant could improve his prognosis or life. A liver transplant could be the only option with which to lead a good quality of life; as he is young, he will do well in surgery. However, an assessment of other affected organs could change this scenario.
	A 34-year-old pregnant lady: probably acute/sub-acute liver failure, which could be due to HELPP syndrome, autoimmune issues or other common presentations in pregnancy. This patient will do well and probably will complete the pregnancy as well. Correcting the liver problem could save two lives.

Table 7.10.

	Question themes	What is expected from the candidate?
7	Triage order.	There is no right or wrong answer, but whatever order is mentioned, it is very important to give the reasoning behind this order.
		If the liver quality is good, there is a possibility that it could be resected and split into two recipients; if this is allowed, it could be split between the pregnant lady and the young boy with a genetic disease.
		If not, the order of priority could be (mention again, that there is no right or wrong answer, but the above reasoning is most important):
		1. A 34-year-old pregnant lady (saves two lives, top priority and correctable disease).
		2. A 6-year-old boy with genetic disease (longest utility of the organ if it is correctable).
		3. A 47-year-old father with alcoholism (modest benefit, provided he has proper counselling to avoid alcohol in future).
		4. A 32-year-old woman with AIDS (high risk of worsening of AIDS and liver condition, poor benefit, but this could be argued).
		5. A 73-year-old healthy man (lifespan of the transplanted liver: lowest utility, can be argued).
8	MDT decision.	The candidate concludes by saying that it is ultimately a multidisciplinary team (MDT) decision after reaching a consensus, and never an individual decision.
9	Four pillars of medical ethics.	The candidate has good awareness of the above-mentioned four pillars of medical ethics and quotes them whilst explaining the reasoning behind the triage order.
10	Conclusion.	The candidate concludes the station and thanks the examiner.

Discussion

This is a complex ethics question. It demands an order of priority to be given, but this should be justified based on sound ethical principles and reasoning used to order the patients.

Most candidates score less as they are worried about giving the right order or answer, but this is not possible in these scenarios. Always explain the reasoning and use sound judgement so that the examiner can understand that you have the aptitude and awareness of these problems.

Key Points

- Always introduce yourself/thank the examiner and appropriately close the session.
- Transplants are always an MDT team decision.
- There are multiple factors, but sound ethical and clinical principles decide the triage order.

References

1.   National Health Service blood and transplant. Organ donation and transplantation. Give the gift of life after your death. Available from: https://www.nhsbt.nhs.uk/what-we-do/transplantation-services/organ-donation-and-transplantation.

Section **8**

Data and mathematical calculations

Section editor: Thanthullu Vasu

Introduction to data and mathematical calculations

Some universities test candidates on mathematical calculations, statistics, research methods, data analysis, interpretation of graphs/charts and looking at other data. A basic knowledge of mathematics is essential in these stations. It might come as a shock to the candidates when they face a mathematical calculation question in the MMI, but please reassure yourself, understand that they are only checking the basics, break the question into smaller parts, start working from the basics and stay confident. Once the question is broken into smaller parts, it is easy to start at some point and start the calculations.

In mathematical calculations, it is important to understand how to change one unit to another; for example, converting milligrams (mg) to micrograms (μg). More complex is the calculation of a drug, which is available, for example in milligrams, to dilute it in liquid to a concentration in ml/hour (calculating concentrations, infusion flow rates, daily dose calculations, based on body weight calculations, etc.). We have suitable examples of such calculations in this book.

Interpretation of graphs and charts can look complex in the beginning, but if they are approached in a systematic way, they can be easily understood; the questions will be multiple and look at various aspects of the graph/chart.

Question 110

Comparing a graph of two painkillers

Prabhu Gandhimani

Question

The following is a graph showing the blood levels of two painkillers (short-acting and long-acting). In the next station, you will be asked questions based on the interpretation of these graphs.

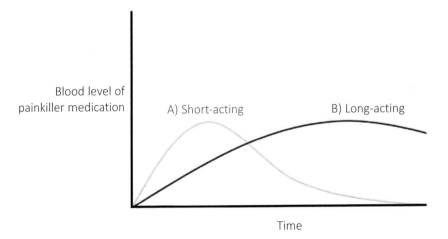

Themes for discussion (■ Table 8.1)

	Question themes	What is expected from the candidate?
1	Can you please explain what is shown in the graph?	The candidate starts with an introduction statement: this is a graph showing the relationship between the blood level of two different painkiller medications and time.
		The candidate voluntarily explains correctly what is in the x- and y-axes; the y-axis shows the blood level of the medication (units to be detailed if provided, e.g. mg/ml or µg/ml); the x-axis shows the time (units such as seconds or minutes to be detailed if provided).
		Summarise the graph and explain the graph. What happens to short-acting (blue) drugs with time and what happens to long-acting (red) drugs with time?
2	What do you think is happening with the blue curve (short-acting painkiller)?	The candidate answers that the blood level rises faster, reaches a peak and then falls down rapidly.
3	What do you think is happening with the red curve (long-acting painkiller)?	Blood levels are slow to rise, but the level is maintained for a longer period of time.
4	In what situations would the drug in graph A be used?	When a quick onset of action is needed and if the effect of the medicine does not need to last for long. The candidate gives an example of the need for medication in which a painkiller is needed immediately.
5	In what situations would the drug in graph B be used?	It can be used when the pain relief is intended for a longer duration; this gives stable levels for a longer duration.

Table 8.1.

Table 8.1.

Question themes	What is expected from the candidate?
6 What determines the blood concentration of the medicine?	This depends on various factors, the most important factor being the route of administration. When a medicine is given into a vein directly, the blood level will rise rapidly, whereas a medicine taken through the mouth needs to go to the stomach first, then it needs to be broken down by stomach juices and then absorbed by the intestines and then reach the bloodstream. There are slow-release preparations that release the medicine slowly into the bloodstream and so the effects of the medicine are prolonged.
7 What problems do you think the patient taking a medicine shown in the blue colour graph (short-acting) would have?	As the blood level of medicine rises rapidly, patients might experience immediate side effects from the medicine. An example is opioid painkillers: they act fast when given into a vein, but unfortunately a rapid rise in blood levels can cause side effects. In contrast, a slow-release preparation takes time to act but acts longer and the blood levels do not reach a high peak and, thereby, the chance of immediate side effects can be less.
8 Which drug will you use if you need immediate relief?	Short-acting (the one in the blue curve in the graph).
9 Conclusion.	The candidate thanks the examiner and concludes the station.

Discussion

It is important to describe the graph first, rather than jumping to an interpretation of the data. Just describe what you see:

- Is it a graph or table, or a chart?
- Describe what the title says.

- Describe the axes and units on each axis.
- Describe the trends in the graph.

You can score some points by just reading what is given in the question, and you would not want to miss those easy marks. Then you can start by analysing the graph and answering the questions thrown at you.

When a drug is administered, it needs to be absorbed by the body first, and the route of administration determines how much is absorbed, how fast it is absorbed, and how much reaches the systemic circulation. Drugs given into a vein or artery can enter the systemic circulation quickly and almost all of the drug you give goes to the bloodstream (100% bioavailability), whereas drugs given orally need to be broken down by stomach juices and enzymes, and need to be absorbed in the intestines before reaching the bloodstream. Only a portion of the drug is absorbed and, moreover, the absorbed medicine must go through the liver before reaching the systemic circulation.

In this example, when a patient is in severe pain, you need to do something that acts fast, and an intravenous route of short-acting drug administration is ideal. The blood concentration rapidly rises and, although this helps to reduce the pain, this can cause other undesirable side effects such as sleepiness, respiratory depression, vomiting, etc.

Oral drug administration can take 30-60 minutes to work, and the duration of action is generally longer than for intravenous preparations. The duration of action can be prolonged by slow-release preparations that are dissolved and absorbed slowly in the intestines. There are skin patches that release medication slowly for up to a week. The slow-release preparations are suited for someone who needs long-term pain control, such as someone suffering from long-term back pain.

Key Points

- The candidate should read the axes first and not jump to analysing the graph straight away.
- The candidate should mention the units if given in the chart whilst describing the x- and y-axes.
- The candidate should set out a good interpretation of the graph and use simple language to explain it clearly.
- Intravenous administration gives a rapid onset.
- Oral drug administration takes 30-60 minutes to work.

References

1. Argoff CE, Silvershein DI. A comparison of long-acting and short-acting opioids for the treatment of chronic non-cancer pain: tailoring therapy to meet patient needs. *Mayo Clin Proc* 2009; 84(7): 602-12.

2. Grogan S, Preuss CV. Pharmacokinetics. StarPearls. Available from: https://www.ncbi.nlm.nih.gov/books/NBK557744.

Question 111

A graph of COVID incidence

Thanthullu Vasu

Question

The following graph outlines the daily confirmed cases of coronavirus during the COVID pandemic in 2020-2021. (The source of data is from the Gov.uk dashboard.)

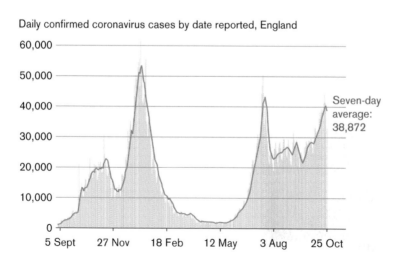

Daily confirmed coronavirus cases by date reported, England

Source: Gov.uk.

In the next station, the examiner will ask you questions based on how you interpret this graph.

Themes for discussion (■ Table 8.2)

Table 8.2.

Question themes	What is expected from the candidate?
1 Can you please explain what is shown in the graph?	The candidate starts with an introduction statement: this is a graph showing the relationship between the number of daily confirmed coronavirus cases and time.
2 Explain the graph with details.	The candidate voluntarily explains correctly what is in the x- and y-axes. The y-axis shows the number of coronavirus cases per day; the x-axis shows the chronological time from 5 September to 25 October of that year.
	The candidate summarises the graph and can explain the graph; they describe how the number of coronavirus cases increased and peaked around December and July and rose towards October.
3 Are these data reliable?	The data were sourced from the Gov.uk website, which is the website of the UK Government; it is very reliable.
	The candidate is aware enough to check the source of the data; this can be important if a research finding is reported.
4 Explain the reasons why there is a peak and trough.	The number of COVID positive cases went up in winter with a peak in December/January.
	The cases came down in early 2021, but later went up towards the summer of 2021.

Table 8.2.

	Question themes	What is expected from the candidate?
5	Why did the number of cases decrease between February and May 2021?	The candidate understands that the COVID vaccine was applied in late December/early January; the vaccine was successful in controlling the COVID pandemic.
6	What could be the reasons why the cases started increasing in August 2021?	The candidate thinks of various reasons such as: the mobility of people increased; social distancing was tapered off; there was increased contact between people; a return to a normal work schedule rather than home-working; the virulence of the virus increasing; the efficacy of the first dose of vaccine was waning; most people did not receive the second dose of vaccine. This question assesses whether the candidate can think logically and has good reasoning skills.
7	What do you think about the COVID vaccination scheme?	The COVID vaccination scheme was very successful, and the candidate is aware of how it has controlled the pandemic. The candidate has a positive approach towards the vaccination scheme.
8	What would have happened to the graph today?	The candidate is aware that there are COVID cases still reported, but these are very few and many go undiagnosed. The line would have come near to the x-axis, but not reached zero.
9	Conclusion.	The candidate interprets the graph clearly and has shown a good knowledge of COVID vaccination; they thank the examiner and conclude the station.

Discussion

It is important to describe the graph first, rather than jumping to an interpretation of the data.

Just describe what you see:

- Is it a graph or table or chart?
- Describe what the title says.
- Describe the axes and the units of both axes.
- Describe the trends in the graph.

It is expected for the candidate to be aware of the success of the COVID vaccination scheme and is positive in their approach towards the COVID vaccine.

Key Points

- The candidate should read the axes first and not jump to analysing the graph straight away.
- The candidate must state the units if given in the chart whilst describing the x- and y-axes.
- The candidate should interpret the graph well and use simple language to explain it clearly.

References

1. BBC News. COVID: are cases about to plummet without Plan B? Available from: https://www.bbc.co.uk/news/health-59039739; accessed 26 October 2021.

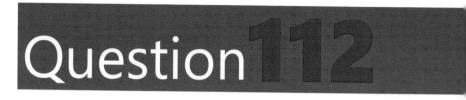

Question 112

A graph of COVID vaccination

Premkumar Sundaram

Question

The next station will be based on the interpretation of the graph shown below; the examiner will ask questions related to this graph.

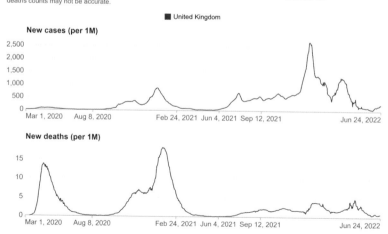

Daily new confirmed COVID-19 cases & deaths per million people
7-day rolling average. Limited testing and challenges in the attribution of cause of death means the cases and deaths counts may not be accurate.

■ United Kingdom

New cases (per 1M)

New deaths (per 1M)

Themes for discussion (■ Table 8.3)

	Question themes	What is expected from the candidate?
1	Can you please explain what is shown in the graph.	The candidate starts with an introductory statement: this is a graph showing the relationship between the number of COVID patients and the number of deaths due to COVID in the UK during the pandemic period, between March 2020 and June 2022.
2	Explain the graphs and compare them.	The candidate voluntarily explains what the two graphs show. They differentiate that the top graph is the number of new COVID-19 cases, and the bottom graph is the number of deaths due to COVID. The units are number per million people.
3	What is the trend in the graph?	The candidate summarises the graph and can explain the graph; they can detail each graph and then compare both.
4	Explain and compare both graphs.	The number of deaths was very high compared with the number of infected patients in March 2020. The number of deaths was very low compared with the number of infected patients in June 2022. Between February and June 2022, the number of cases were high.
5	What are the reasons that could explain the low infection rate but the higher death rate in April 2020?	The candidate understands the trend and could give reasons: • There was a lack of facilities for testing at the beginning of the pandemic. • Vaccination was not fully introduced, and this could have increased mortality. • The virulence of the virus was higher at the beginning of the pandemic.

Table 8.3.

Table 8.3.

	Question themes	What is expected from the candidate?
6	What could be the reasons that the death rate started to decline in August 2020?	The candidate thinks of various reasons such as: • Decreased transmission of viruses due to public health measures and education. • National lockdown measures. • Social distancing was strictly followed. • Wearing masks, handwashing, etc.
7	According to the graph, when did the second wave occur in the UK?	January to February 2021.
8	Explain the reasons for the high death rate during the second wave.	The candidate can think of a few reasons, including: • New variant (Delta variant) with a high virulence. • Most of the population was still not vaccinated.
9	What was the cause of the third wave in December 2021?	• New variants such as Omicron. • Relaxation of lockdown measures.
10	In the third wave, there is a low death rate despite the high infection case rate. Why?	• Most vulnerable people had been vaccinated.
11	Conclusion.	The candidate has interpreted the graph clearly and has shown a good knowledge of the COVID infection, trends, variants, and vaccination; they thank the examiner and conclude the station.

Discussion

It is important to describe the graph first, rather than jumping to an interpretation of the the data. Just describe what you see:

- Is it a graph or table or chart?
- Describe what the title says.
- Describe the axes and the units of both axes.
- Describe the trends in the graph.

It is expected that the candidate can read the trends in the graph; at the same time, they can think logically and give reasons why this could have happened. This also shows the awareness of the candidate about recent health topics.

Key Points

- The candidate should be able to analyse the graph by reading the x- and y- axes and their relationship.
- The candidate should interpret the graph well and use simple language to explain it clearly.
- They should also apply the knowledge of the graph to a practical situation.

References

1.   Our world in data. Coronavirus pandemic (COVID-19). Our world in data. Available from: http://www.ourworldindata.org/coronavirus.

Question 113

A graph of coronavirus deaths in varying deprived areas

Siva Thanthullu

Question

You are given a graph (see below) and the examiner will ask you questions based on this graph.

Coronavirus deaths per 100,000 people

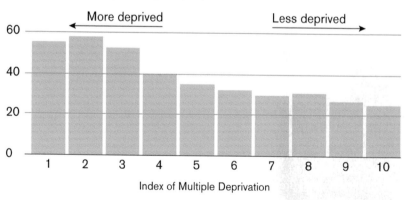

Source: ONS.

Themes for discussion (■ Table 8.4)

Table 8.4.	
Question themes	**What is expected from the candidate?**
1 What type of graph has been shown in this picture?	Bar diagram.
2 What does the x-axis represent?	Index of Multiple Deprivation; this is an index of poverty and is ranked from the most deprived communities (ranked low starting at 1) to the least deprived communities (higher rank up to 10).
3 What does the y-axis represent?	The number of deaths due to coronavirus per 100,000 people.
4 'A population of low-income people will have a higher Index of Multiple Deprivation'. Is this statement true or false?	False.

Low-income populations have a lower index of multiple deprivation. |
| 5 From where has this graph and data been sourced? Is the source reliable? | The candidate should check the reliability of any data or information.

These data were sourced from the Office for National Statistics (ONS); these data are reliable. |
| 6 According to this graph, who had higher death rates due to coronavirus: high-income or low-income people? | Low-income people had a higher death rate. |
| 7 Which rank of the Index of Multiple Deprivation group contains the highest number of deaths (from groups 1-10)? | Group 2. |

Table 8.4.

	Question themes	What is expected from the candidate?
8	What could be the reason for higher deaths in groups 1-3 on the Index of Multiple Deprivation?	The candidate can think logically and give a few reasons: • Poverty. • Less social distancing. • Poor education. • Less vaccination. • Poor nutrition.
9	What is the ratio of deaths in group 3 to deaths in group 9 of the Index of Multiple Deprivation in the given graph?	50/25 = 2.
10	If you wanted to reduce the deaths due to coronavirus, as per this graph, which group should you target? What would you advise for that group?	Low-income populations: groups 1-3. Encourage vaccination, education, social distancing, etc.

Discussion

At the outset, the graph might look complex, but if the questions are broken down and if there is a structured way of looking at the data, it can be made easier.

Graphs and data can come as a written question, or an examiner can ask the question.

Key Points

- The candidate should be able to analyse the graph by reading the x- and y- axes and their relationship.
- The candidate should interpret the graph well and use simple language to explain it clearly.
- They should also apply the knowledge of the graph to a practical situation.

References

1. BBC News. Coronavirus: higher death rate in poorer areas, ONS figures suggest. Available from: https://www.bbc.co.uk/news/uk-52506979; accessed 1 May 2020.

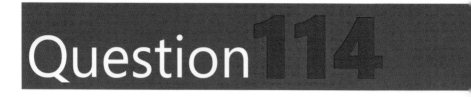

Question 114

Obesity versus calorie intake

Premkumar Sundaram

Question

You are given a graph (see below) and the examiner will ask you questions based on this graph.

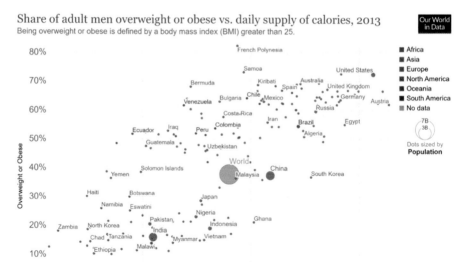

Share of adult men overweight or obese vs. daily supply of calories, 2013

Being overweight or obese is defined by a body mass index (BMI) greater than 25.

Themes for discussion (■ Table 8.5)

	Question themes	What is expected from the candidate?
	Table 8.5.	
1	What does this graph depict?	This is a graph comparing men who are overweight or obese with daily caloric supply in different countries.
2	What does the x-axis represent?	The x-axis represents the amount of daily calorie intake per person in 2013 in particular countries.
3	What does the y-axis represent?	The y-axis represents the percentage of people who were overweight or obese in particular countries in 2013. The term overweight or obese is defined as a body mass index (BMI) of more than 25 in this graph.
4	What is the body mass index (BMI)?	The body mass index is the weight in kilogrammes divided by the square of the height in metres. An index of more than 25 indicates overweight or obesity.
5	Which two continents have the lowest prevalence of overweight or obesity?	Africa and Asia.
6	Why are the dots representing countries different sizes in this graph?	In this graph, the dots are sized by population in that country. The countries with higher populations have bigger dots.
7	What is the relationship between overweight and daily caloric intake as per this graph?	There is a linear relationship between the incidence of being overweight and the daily caloric intake, showing a straight line between the x-axis and the y-axis. The more the caloric intake, the higher the incidence of overweight.

Figure: NCD Risk Factor Collaboration (NCD-RisC) and Food and Agriculture Organization of the United Nations (FAOstat). Published online at OurWorldInData.org (https://ourworldindata.org/grapher/share-of-adult-men-overweight-or-obese-vs-daily-supply-of-calories). (Creative Commons CC BY licence.)

Table 8.5.

	Question themes	What is expected from the candidate?
8	Explain the reason for the high prevalence of obesity in the USA.	The candidate can think logically and give a few reasons: • High intake of calories. • Eating calorie-dense food. • Easy access to fast food and sugar-containing drinks. • Sedentary lifestyle. • Decreased physical activity. • Increased use of screen time, restricting activities.
9	Which country has the highest rate of overweight or obesity as per this graph?	French Polynesia.
10	What are the long-term health effects of being overweight or obese?	The candidate gives a list of a few problems, such as: • Type 2 diabetes. • High blood pressure. • High cholesterol. • Coronary artery disease. • Stroke.

Discussion

At the outset, the graph might look complex, but if you break the questions down and if you have a structured way of looking at the data, it can be made easier.

Graphs and data can come as a written question, or an examiner can ask the question.

Sometimes, the graph can lead to some simple health- and lifestyle-related questions.

Key Points

- The candidate should be able to analyse the graph by reading the x- and y- axes and their relationship.
- The candidate should interpret the graph well and use simple language to explain it clearly.
- They should also apply the knowledge of the graph to a practical situation.
- Body mass index (BMI) is measured by dividing the weight in kilogrammes by the square of the height in metres.

References

1. Our World in Data. Share of adult men overweight or obese vs. daily supply of calories. Available from: https://ourworldindata.org/grapher/share-of-adult-men-overweight-or-obese-vs-daily-supply-of-calories.

Question 115

A graph of diurnal variation of hormones

Premkumar Sundaram

Question

You are given a graph (see below) and the examiner will ask you questions based on this graph.

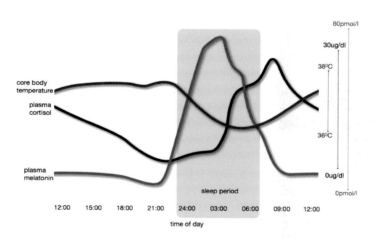

The normal synchronous relationships between sleep and daytime activity and cortisol, melatonin and body temperature. Hickie IB, Naismith SL, Robillard R, *et al*. Manipulating the sleep-wake cycle and circadian rhythms to improve clinical management of major depression. *BMC Med* 2013; 11: 79. (Creative Commons CC BY licence.)

Themes for discussion (■ Table 8.6)

Table 8.6.

Question themes	What is expected from the candidate?
1 What does this graph depict?	This is a graph showing the blood levels of melatonin and cortisol, as well as body temperature during different times of the day. It represents the variation in levels as per the time of the day.
2 What does the x-axis represent?	The x-axis shows the different times of the day, starting from 12 noon until the next 12 noon.
3 What does the y-axis represent?	The y-axis represents the plasma levels of melatonin and cortisol as well as body temperature. All these three parameters are shown in different coloured curves in this graph.

Melatonin is the sleep hormone and is measured in units of picomoles per litre in the blue graph. It is produced by the pineal gland in the brain, and controls the sleep-wake cycle.

Plasma cortisol is the steroid hormone measured in μg per dl (1dl=100ml) in the black-coloured graph. It is produced by the adrenal gland.

Core body temperature is measured at °C, shown as red on the graph. |
| 4 According to this graph, what time does melatonin reach its peak? | 3 a.m. in the morning. |
| 5 What is the effect of melatonin at this time with its peak level? | Peak levels of melatonin lead to deep sleep as per this graph. |

Table 8.6.

	Question themes	What is expected from the candidate?
6	What conditions can affect peak melatonin secretion and therefore deep sleep?	The candidate can think of logical reasons such as: • Late-night parties or being awake until late. • Night shift jobs. • Insomnia or sleep problems.
7	What time does the cortisol secretion increase to maximum?	7-8 a.m. in the morning.
8	What could be the function of cortisol, looking at the increase in the peak in the morning?	Increased cortisol happens at 7-8 a.m. in the morning and could help in preparing the body to wake up.
9	What happens to the core body temperature during deep sleep?	Core body temperature reduces by 1-2°C.
10	What could be the reasons for reduced body temperature during deep sleep?	The candidate gives a list of a few reasons, such as: • Inactivity, not being mobile. • Reduced metabolic activity. • Hormonal reasons, reduced cortisol and high melatonin. • Environmental, such as staying in the bedroom.

Discussion

At the outset, the graph might look complex; but if you break down the questions and if you have a structured way of looking at the data, this can be made easier.

Graphs and data can come as a written question, or an examiner can ask the question.

Sometimes, the graph can lead to some simple health- and lifestyle-related questions.

Key Points

- The candidate should be able to analyse the graph by reading the x- and y- axes and their relationship.
- The candidate should interpret the graph well and use simple language to explain it clearly.
- They should also apply the knowledge of the graph to a practical situation.

References

1.   Hickie IB, Naismith SL, Robillard R, Scott EM, Hermens DF. Manipulating the sleep-wake cycle and circadian rhythms to improve clinical management of major depression. *BMC Med* 2013; 11: 79.

Question 116

A pain chart and its interpretation

Prabhu Gandhimani

Question

In the next station, you will be given a figure and asked questions on how to interpret it and questions based on the science behind this tool.

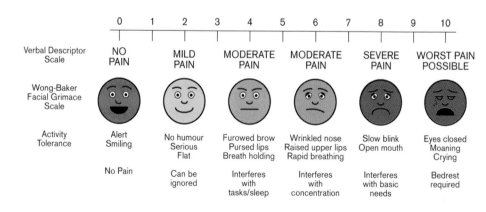

Themes for discussion (■ Table 8.7)

	Question themes	What is expected from the candidate?
Table 8.7.		
1	The candidate greets the examiner, has good body language and speaks coherently.	The candidate is presentable and uses good communication skills; always recommended in any station.
2	What do you think this is?	The candidate describes it broadly and says this is a pain scale/pain assessment chart and is used to quantify pain.
3	Why is the assessment of pain important?	Pain is the most important reason for a doctor's visit and to be free of pain is a fundamental human right. Pain is an important protective reflex and can draw one's attention to an injury and help to take remedial measures.
4	Can you think of some examples in which pain assessment is difficult?	If patients cannot communicate well, then pain assessment will be difficult. For example, in children and in adults with communication problems (e.g. confused adults, older patients, and people with learning difficulties).
5	How does pain assessment help?	Pain is a very subjective phenomenon, and the pain charts give some objectivity to it. Although a single measurement is important, multiple assessments give us a trend. Frequent pain assessment gives an indicator of whether the pain is getting better and is responding to treatment.
6	How is pain assessment done?	The patient is asked to describe how much their pain is, on a scale of 1-10, in which 0 will be no pain, 1 being minimal pain and 10 being the worst pain imaginable.

Table 8.7.

	Question themes	What is expected from the candidate?
7	Why are there faces on the pain scale?	It is difficult for children and people with communication problems to put a number to their pain, and it is easy for them to point at faces to quantify their pain. It is also easy for the assessor to document the patient's pain based on their facial expression.
8	How can you detect if an unconscious patient might be in pain?	When someone is in pain their heart rate and blood pressure increases and this is an indicator that they might be in pain. They might also have tears and we can tell by their facial expressions.
9	Conclusion.	The candidate has a clear flow of thoughts and concludes the session by saying 'thank you' to the examiner.

Discussion

The assessment of pain remains a challenge as it is very subjective, and everyone's pain perception is different. A survey found that acute pain is not well managed in 70% of hospitalised patients and untreated pain can affect the quality of life, prolong recovery from illness and impair mental well-being. Effective pain management is an important quality indicator of the care provided. To improve pain control, pain measurement has been included as the 'fifth vital sign' (in addition to pulse, blood pressure, respiratory rate and temperature) and pain scales are used to measure the pain being felt. A trend rather than a single measurement is important, as the same pain sensation can be felt as mild in someone and severe in another. Pain scales standardise the measurement of pain and make it easier to communicate the severity of pain within the medical multidisciplinary team and aids research.

The candidate might not know about pain scales and pain measurement in detail, but this station and question will test the candidate's broader knowledge about medicine and the importance of measurement, data and record-keeping in medicine.

Key Points

- The candidate should be able to describe the chart in detail.
- A pain chart standardises the measurement of pain and aids in communication.
- Assessment of pain is difficult in children and people with communication problems.

References

1. Dugashvili G, Van den Berghe LI, Menabde G, Janelidze M, Marks L. Use of the universal pain assessment tool for evaluating pain associated with TMD in youngsters with an intellectual disability. *Med Oral Patol Oral Cir Bucal* 2017; 22(1): e88-e94.

2. Lewis LM, Lasater LC, Brooks CB. Are emergency physicians too stingy with analgesics? *South Med J* 1994; 87(1): 7-9.

3. Todd KH, Ducharme J, Choiniere M, *et al*. Pain in the emergency department: results of the pain and emergency medicine initiative (PEMI) multicenter study. *J Pain* 2007; 8(6): 460-6.

4. Sinatra R. Causes and consequences of inadequate management of acute pain. *Pain Med* 2010; 11(12): 1859-71.

Question 117

Microgram versus milligram calculation

Premkumar Sundaram

Question

A 62-year-old gentleman is started on digoxin medication to treat his atrial fibrillation (abnormally fast heart rhythm). Digoxin is available on the market as 62.5μg (microgram) tablets.

The following questions will be based on the dosage for this patient.

Themes for discussion (■ Table 8.8)

Table 8.8.

	Question themes	What is expected from the candidate?
1	The candidate greets the examiner, has good body language and speaks coherently.	The candidate is presentable and uses good communication skills; always recommended in any station.

Table 8.8.

Question themes	What is expected from the candidate?
2 The loading dose (initial dose) of digoxin to treat atrial fibrillation is 0.75mg. What is the equivalent dose in µg?	1mg = 1000µg. 0.75mg = 0.75 x 1000 = 750µg.
3 In this patient mentioned, how many digoxin tablets should be prescribed for the initial loading dose?	Loading dose = 750µg. Each digoxin tablet is 62.5µg. Number of tablets needed = total loading dose/strength of each tablet = 750µg/62.5µg = 12 tablets.
4 Once the loading dose is given and atrial fibrillation is controlled, the patient needs a regular maintenance dose of 0.25mg per day. What is the equivalent dose in micrograms?	1mg = 1000µg. 0.25mg = 0.25 x 1000 = 250µg.
5 How many digoxin tablets are needed for a maintenance dose per day?	The dose needed for maintenance = 250µg per day. Each digoxin tablet is 62.5µg. Number of tablets needed = maintenance dose per day/strength of each tablet = 250µg/62.5µg = 4 tablets per day.
6 Conclusion.	The candidate concludes the session by saying 'thank you' to the examiner.

Discussion

It is important to know simple conversion equivalents of units. These could be commonly asked in mathematics stations:

- 1mg = 1000µg.
- 1µg = 0.001mg.
- 1g = 1000mg.
- 1mg = 0.001g.
- 1kg = 1000g.
- 1g = 0.001kg.
- 1µg = 10^{-6}g.
- 1ng = 10^{-9}g.
- 1l = 1000ml.
- 1l = 1000cc.
- 1 metre = 100 centimetres.
- 1 metre = 1000 millimetres.

Key Points

- The common conversion of units may be asked as they are used in medical practice.
- Read the question and think clearly as it will be a simple conversion.

Question 118

Calculation to ml/hour based on body weight

Siva Thanthullu

Question

The next question will test your ability to do mathematical calculations applied to medical practice; the examiner will assess your ability to calculate the concentration of a drug to be given to a patient.

Your consultant asks you to calculate the dose of lignocaine that is needed at a dose of 750µg per kg (microgram per kg) intravenously as an infusion over 1 hour. The patient weighs 80kg.

Your nurse colleague has loaded 0.25% lignocaine in a syringe pump ready for infusion. How many millilitres of this medicine should you administer per hour to achieve the calculated dose?

Themes for discussion (■ Table 8.9)

Table 8.9.	
Question themes	**What is expected from the candidate?**
1 The candidate greets the examiner, has good body language and speaks coherently.	The candidate is presentable and uses good communication skills; always recommended in any station.
2 Calculate the dose needed for this particular patient.	Dose needed is 750μg per kg. The patient weighs 80kg. Total dose needed is 750 x 80 = 60,000μg per hour.
3 Convert micrograms (μg) to milligrams (mg).	1000μg = 1mg. The total dose needed for this patient = 60,000μg per hour = 60,000/1000 = 60mg per hour.
4 Convert % preparation to mg/ml.	1% solution means 1g per 100ml, which is the same as 0.01g per ml, which is the same as 10mg per ml. If 1% is 10mg per ml, then: 0.25% (given in the question) is 2.5mg per ml.
5 Calculate the infusion rate needed for this patient.	The solution prepared by the nurse is 2.5mg per ml. Total dose needed for this patient = 60mg per hour. Infusion strength available = 2.5mg per ml. Infusion rate needed = 60mg divided by 2.5mg/ml = 24ml to be given per hour.
6 Conclusion.	The candidate concludes the session by saying 'thank you' to the examiner.

Discussion

It can be confusing when a candidate reads the question during stressful MMI time, but relax and break the question into smaller parts. In this question, use logical thinking:

- What is the dose needed for the patient?
- What is the strength of the solution available?
- What is the rate per hour needed for this strength?

Breaking complex questions into smaller chunks can help you to proceed.

In these mathematical questions, it will help to use the right units such as mg/ml or ml/hour.

Key Points

- Calculate the dose needed as per the body weight given. This involves multiplication.
- A 1% solution means 10mg/ml.
- The total dose (mg) divided by strength (mg/ml) gives the infusion rate (ml/h).
- Use the right units for each parameter.

Question 119

Drug dose calculations

Premkumar Sundaram

Question

The next question will test your ability to do mathematical calculations applied to medical practice; the examiner will assess your ability to calculate the concentration of drug to be given to a patient.

This question will assess the calculation of glucose infusion in a diabetic child who is hypoglycaemic (low blood sugar).

A 5-day-old baby born to a mother with type I diabetes presents with hypoglycaemia; the baby needs treatment with glucose solution given intravenously (given by vein into the blood). The protocol is to administer a 10% glucose infusion intravenously.

Themes for discussion (▧ Table 8.10)

Table 8.10.

	Question themes	What is expected from the candidate?
1	The candidate greets the examiner, has good body language and speaks coherently.	The candidate is presentable and uses good communication skills; always recommended in any station.
2	How much glucose is present in 1ml of 10% glucose?	10% means 10g per 100ml, which is the same as 0.1g per ml, which is the same as 100mg per ml.
3	How much glucose is present in 100ml of 10% glucose?	As per the previous calculation, 1ml contains 0.1g. 100ml will contain = 100 x 0.1 = 10g of glucose.
4	The baby weighs 4kg; the baby needs 5mg per kg per minute of a glucose infusion to correct the glucose levels to normal. How many mg of glucose does this baby need per hour?	Body weight = 4kg. The dose needed = 5mg per kg = 5 x 4 = 20mg per minute. 1 hour = 60 minutes. The dose needed per hour = 20 x 60 = 1200mg per hour.
5	How many ml of 10% glucose does this baby need in 1 hour?	Baby needs 1200mg per hour. Strength available = 10% glucose = 100mg per ml. Infusion rate needed = dose divided by strength of the drug = 1200mg per hour/100mg per ml = 12ml per hour. Baby needs 12ml per hour of 10% glucose.

Table 8.10.

	Question themes	What is expected from the candidate?
6	After 2 hours of treatment, the baby still has a low glucose. Your consultant advises you to increase the dose of glucose infusion to 10mg/kg/min. How many ml of 10% glucose does this baby need now?	Baby weight = 4kg. Dose needed = 4 x 10 = 40mg per min. = 40 x 60mg per hour = 2400mg per hour. Strength available = 10% = 100mg per ml. Infusion rate = 2400/100 = 24ml per hour. Baby now needs 24ml per hour of 10% glucose. (You can use the previous question to extrapolate this answer also. The dose needed is doubled, so the infusion rate will double.)
7	Conclusion.	The candidate concludes the session by saying 'thank you' to the examiner.

Discussion

It can be confusing when a candidate reads the question during stressful MMI time but relax and break the question into smaller parts. In this question, use logical thinking:

- What is the dose needed for the patient?
- What is the strength of the solution available?
- What is the rate per hour needed for this strength?

Breaking complex questions into smaller chunks can help you to proceed.

In these mathematical questions, it will help to use the right units such as mg/ml or ml/hour.

The MMI interview can end with a question asking what happens if the rate is doubled or halved or changed to a different proportion.

In many MMI interviews, these mathematical questions can be given as written stations where an invigilator hands you a paper to answer the question or mark in a tablet/ laptop, rather than orally asking the question.

Key Points

- Calculate the dose needed as per the body weight given. It involves multiplication.
- A 1% solution means 10mg/ml.
- The total dose (mg) divided by strength (mg/ml) gives the infusion rate (ml/h).
- Use the right units for each parameter.

Question 120

Calculation of an inhaler dose

Thanthullu Vasu

Question

A mother has questions about her daughter's inhaler prescription. She is using a medical device called a BreathSmooth Inhaler (which comes in two different strengths), and which is used to treat asthma. Her daughter usually takes two puffs from a BreathSmooth A Inhaler (which contains 50μg per puff of BreathSmooth medicine) twice a day. Today, her prescription was changed to BreathSmooth B, which contains 100μg per puff.

Both BreathSmooth A and BreathSmooth B contain the same chemical BreathSmooth, but in different concentrations.

In the next scenario, you will be asked questions and asked to do some mathematical calculations in the various settings.

Themes for discussion (▦ Table 8.11)

<table>
<tr><td colspan="3">Table 8.11.</td></tr>
<tr><td></td><td>Question themes</td><td>What is expected from the candidate?</td></tr>
<tr><td>1</td><td>What was the original total daily dose of BreathSmooth A in micrograms that the patient was taking until yesterday?</td><td>She used BreathSmooth A, which contained 50µg per puff.
She used 2 puffs twice a day.
Total dose = 4 puffs per day
= 4 x 50 = 200µg per day.</td></tr>
<tr><td>2</td><td>If you want the child to use the same dose of BreathSmooth B, how many puffs should she use?</td><td>Until yesterday, the child used BreathSmooth A that gave 100µg BreathSmooth twice a day (making a total dose of 200µg).

BreathSmooth B is stronger and contains 100µg per puff. To have the child achieve 100µg twice a day (the same as the old dose), she will need 1 puff of BreathSmooth twice a day.</td></tr>
<tr><td>3</td><td>How many micrograms make a milligram?
How many micrograms make a gram?</td><td>1mg = 1000µg (10^3µg).
1g = 1000mg.
1g = 1,000,000µg (10^6µg).</td></tr>
<tr><td>4</td><td>In the case of worsening asthma, she can use 400µg of BreathSmooth with a half-hour gap in between additional doses, on top of her routine use.
If so, how many puffs of BreathSmooth A can she use if her asthma worsens in addition to her routine dose (if she was on BreathSmooth A)?</td><td>BreathSmooth A contains 50µg per puff.
In the case of worsening asthma, she needs 400µg, which is equivalent to 400/50 = 8 puffs.</td></tr>
</table>

Table 8.11.

	Question themes	What is expected from the candidate?
5	If her asthma worsens, how many puffs of BreathSmooth B could be used (if she was on BreathSmooth B regularly)?	BreathSmooth B contains 100µg per puff. In the case of worsening asthma, she needs 400µg, which is 4 puffs.
6	In the case of a flare-up of asthma that lasts for 45 minutes, what is the maximum dose of BreathSmooth in micrograms that this patient can use (in addition to her regular dose)?	In the case of worsening asthma, she could use 400µg with a 30-minute gap in between repeat uses (in addition to her regular doses). This means that she could use two doses of 400µg with a half-hour gap in between, making a total of 800µg.
7	Which drug is more potent: BreathSmooth A or BreathSmooth B?	A more potent drug has a stronger concentration. BreathSmooth B is more potent.
8	How will you make sure that the mother and child understood what you have explained?	The candidate gives reasonable explanations such as: • Explain clearly in simple language, using puffs as the measure. • Ask the mother/child to repeat the instructions to make sure that she has understood. • It can be written down and given in addition to verbal instructions.
9	If the inhaler BreathSmooth B contains enough drug for 100 puffs, and assuming there is no flare-up or worsening, how long will a single inhaler last for this patient?	The patient uses 2 puffs per day of BreathSmooth B. If there are 100 puffs, this inhaler should last for 50 days.

Table 8.11.

Question themes	What is expected from the candidate?
10 If you want to give a prescription of BreathSmooth B for 10 weeks, assuming that there is no flare-up, how many inhalers do you need to prescribe (assuming one inhaler of BreathSmooth B contains 100 puffs)?	10 weeks = 10 x 7 = 70 days. Each day, the child needs 2 puffs. Total dose needed = 70 x 2 = 140 puffs. Each inhaler contains the dose of 100 puffs. We need to prescribe two inhalers.

Discussion

At the outset, the question can look very complex as an A-level student may not be familiar with specific drugs. This is an imaginary drug and the question assesses how the candidate can tackle drug doses and can make simple calculations.

The candidate should relax, read the question properly, think and make simple baseline calculations. Then, when the specific question comes up, these baseline calculations form part of further calculations.

If you do not know the specific drug or details of the medical condition, please do not worry; you need to stay calm and let yourself do some simple calculations.

Key Points

- Stay calm, read the question properly and make baseline calculations from the question.
- In further questions, it will be simple calculations.
- Make sure you write down the units, as it will be a simple change of units that can cause confusion.

Question 121

Calculation of calories needed

Thanthullu Vasu

Question

A dietician is creating a meal for a patient admitted to an intensive care unit. She needs to create a meal of 300kcal for this patient.

The standard measurements are given below for the food ingredients that she is using:

- Chicken = 1.25kcal per g.
- Potato = 0.75kcal per g.
- Peas = 0.75kcal per g.
- Gravy = 0.25kcal per g.

Using these data, you will be asked to do calculations in this next question.

Themes for discussion (■ Table 8.12)

Table 8.12.

Question themes	What is expected from the candidate?
1 If the dietician uses 70g of chicken, 80g of peas, and 100g of gravy, what is the amount of calories in this food?	1g chicken contains 1.25kcal. 70g chicken = 70 x 1.25 = 87.5kcal. 1g peas contains 0.75kcal. 80g peas = 80 x 0.75 = 60kcal. 1g gravy contains 0.25kcal. 100g gravy = 100 x 0.25 = 25kcal. Total = 87.5 + 60 + 25 = 172.5kcal.
2 As mentioned in this question, the patient needs 300kcal in the meal. How many more calories can the dietician add?	300 − 172.5 = 127.5kcal. The dietician can add 127.5kcal more to this food preparation.
3 The dietician decides to use potatoes to make up the extra needed calories. How many grams of potato can she use?	1g potato contains 0.75kcal. The dietician needs 127.5kcal from potato. Amount of potato needed = 127.5/0.75 = 170g. The dietician can add 170g of potato to make it in total a 300kcal meal.

Discussion

At the outset, the question can look very complex, as an A-level student may not be familiar with dietary needs and kilocalories. The question only tests basic mathematical calculations and the ability to think. It is essential to stay calm, understand the basics of the question and then think logically.

It would be prudent for the candidate to practise more mathematical questions. Some universities have stopped asking mathematical questions, whilst others give a mathematics paper as part of the interview or include a station in their MMI.

Key Points

- Stay calm, read the question properly and make baseline calculations from the question.
- In further questions, there will be simple calculations.
- Make sure you remember to check the units after the answers and calculations.

Question 122

Mean, median and standard deviation

Siva Thanthullu

Question

Given below are the haemoglobin levels of 10 different patients (in g/L):

132, 136, 148, 131, 132, 143, 132, 151, 128, 144.

In the next station, questions will be based on mathematical/statistical calculations based on these values.

Themes for discussion (■ Table 8.13)

Table 8.13.

	Question themes	What is expected from the candidate?
1	What is the mean of the haemoglobin values of these 10 patients?	Mean = sum of all variables/number of variables = (132+136+148+131+132+143+132+151+128+144)/10 = 1377/10 = 137.7g/L.

Table 8.13.

Question themes	What is expected from the candidate?
2 What is the median value of haemoglobin in this set of patients?	First, the values are written in ascending order as below: 128, 131, 132, 132, 132, 136, 143, 144, 148, 151. Given that this is an even set of numbers (total of 10 variables), the middle two values are 132 and 136. The average of these two numbers is the median: median = (132+136)/2 = 268/2 = 134g/L. If there were 11 numbers or variables, there is no need to find the average and the sixth variable would be automatically the median (after writing the values in ascending or descending order).
3 What is the mode of this set of variables given?	Mode = most frequently occurring data set = 132g/L.
4 What does the standard deviation value denote for a healthcare professional?	The standard deviation describes how far a value lies from the mean, in a normal distribution. If the value of the standard deviation is high, that means that values are generally far from the mean/average; a low standard deviation means that values are clustered near the mean.
5 What is a randomised controlled trial (RCT)?	A trial that is controlled by randomising the allocation of patients into two or more research groups is called an RCT. If patients are not randomised, there is a bias that patients are not balanced in these two groups, and this could lead to errors in the interpretation of the research. The RCT is the gold standard in clinical research.

Table 8.13.

Question themes	What is expected from the candidate?
6 Apart from this example, can you give some examples of how statistics can help healthcare professionals?	The candidate has good knowledge and can give a few answers or examples: • To plan a service: identify the need and demand. • Research and analyse the evidence. • Allocate resources appropriately (e.g. vaccine need and population). • Bed utilisation, waiting times, etc. • Identify mortality and morbidity data. • To find the relationship between cause and effect (e.g. disease and pathogens). • To assess risk for various health conditions.

Discussion

Having a basic knowledge of statistical calculations is important for a healthcare professional. When they are faced with huge amounts of data, it is vital to know how to interpret these data for the benefit of their patients. The analysis of data and how to interpret it quickly, helps in the interpretation of the scientific evidence.

The mean (or average) is the average of the set of data available. It is calculated by dividing the sum of all variables by the number of variables:

Mean = $(X_1 + X_2 + X_3 + ... + X_n)/n$

where X_1, X_2, X_3, ... X_n are the variables, and n is the total number of variables given.

The median is the middle value of the set of numbers, when they are written in ascending or descending order. If there is an even set of numbers, the middle two numbers are added and divided by two to get the average median value. If the distribution of the variables in the set of values are skewed, then the median gives a better understanding of the set of variables than the mean. In healthcare statistics, the median is often used to measure a central tendency when the distribution is skewed.

The mode is the variable or data set that is most frequently repeated. It has the highest frequency in that data set.

Key Points

- The mean is the average of all values; add the variables and divide by the number of variables to get the mean.
- The median is the middle value if written in ascending or descending order; if there are two middle numbers, the average of these two is the median.
- The mode is the most frequently occurring variable.
- RCTs are the gold standard in research.

Question 123

Insulin calculation

Thanthullu Vasu

Question

A patient in the intensive care unit needs an intravenous insulin infusion. The standard practice in the unit is to dilute 50 units (1ml) of Actrapid® insulin with 49ml of normal saline solution.

Below is the sliding scale of the insulin in this unit (■ Table 8.14).

Table 8.14.

Blood sugar (mmol/L)	Insulin infusion (units per hour)
0 to 4mmol/L.	0; call the doctor ASAP as the patient needs a glucose infusion.
4.1 to 8mmol/L.	1 unit per hour.
8.1 to 12mmol/L.	2 units per hour.
12.1 to 16mmol/L.	4 units per hour.
More than 16mmol/L.	4 units per hour and call the doctor ASAP.

In this section, questions will be based on the calculation of a dose of insulin based on the sliding scale given above.

Themes for discussion (■ Table 8.15)

Table 8.15.

Question themes	What is expected from the candidate?
1 As per standard practice, how much insulin is present in one ml of the diluted solution?	50 units of insulin is diluted with 49ml saline making a total of 50ml. 50 units in 50ml. 1 unit insulin in 1ml.
2 A patient has a blood sugar of 13.1mmol/L. What will be the rate of insulin needed for this patient in ml/h?	4 units per hour. 4ml per hour of the solution.
3 If the blood sugar changes to 19.4mmol/L in the next hour, what will you do?	Continue the infusion at 4 units per hour and call the doctor as the patient will need more insulin or investigate for the cause of high sugar levels.
4 After a period of 4 hours, the blood sugar drops to 2.3mmol/L. What will you do now?	Stop the infusion and call the senior doctor; this patient will need a glucose infusion and constant monitoring of blood sugar levels.
5 Insulin prescription errors are one of the most common errors in hospitals. How will you prevent such errors?	• Follow standard procedures on the ward or unit as per the protocols. • Different insulin preparations have different strengths and dilutions; being aware of these is essential.

Table 8.15.

Question themes	What is expected from the candidate?
	• Prescriptions should be clearly written and checked as units and ml can be confused easily. • Education of the staff and team, good communication, and cross-checking the prescription are vital.
6 Conclusion	The candidate concludes the session by saying thank you to the examiner.

Discussion

Prescription errors are to be avoided by constant education and working together as a team. Following standard protocols specific to the unit will help to achieve the same practice and can avoid errors. Rechecking and cross-checking to make sure that what is given to the patient is the same as what is prescribed is essential.

Errors can happen due to dispensing an incorrect medication, giving the wrong dose strength or form, or a failure to identify an allergy or contraindication. With regards to insulin-related errors, it is common for the miscalculation of units to contribute to problems.

Key Points

- Check the dilution of insulin as units (units/h) can be different from the dilution (ml/h).
- Education of the team is essential to avoid errors; following the same protocols across the ward or unit is vital.
- Clinical governance methods employ education via errors to prevent them happening in future.

References

1. Getting it right first time (GIRFT). GIRFT videos highlight measures to improve insulin safety for inpatients with diabetes. Available from: https://gettingitrightfirsttime.co.uk/girft-videos-highlight-measures-to-improve-insulin-safety-for-inpatients-with-diabetes.

Question 124

Calculation based on a Venn diagram

Siva Thanthullu

Question

From the diagram below, the examiner will ask questions in the next station. Please analyse this diagram and the data below the figure for the next 2 minutes. You have a rough sheet to write on if you need.

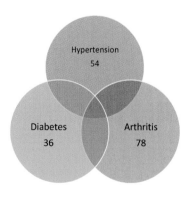

In a GP surgery cohort of 300 patients:

- 54 patients have hypertension.
- 36 patients have diabetes.
- 78 patients have arthritis.

Further, in the same cohort:

- 27 patients have both hypertension and arthritis.
- 12 patients have both hypertension and diabetes.
- 19 patients have both arthritis and diabetes.
- 7 patients have all three conditions: hypertension, diabetes and arthritis.

Themes for discussion (■ Table 8.16)

Table 8.16.

Question themes	What is expected from the candidate?
1 In this cohort of patients, how many of them have any one of the diseases mentioned (hypertension, diabetes or arthritis)?	54 + 36 + 78 = 168 patients.
2 In this cohort of patients, how many patients do not have any one of the diseases mentioned (hypertension, diabetes and arthritis)?	300 − (54 + 36 + 78) = 300 − 168 = 132 patients.
3 How many patients in this group suffer from hypertension and diabetes, but do not suffer from arthritis?	12 − 7 = 5 patients. See the calculated Venn diagram below in the discussion section.

Table 8.16.

	Question themes	What is expected from the candidate?
4	How many patients suffer from diabetes and arthritis, but not from hypertension?	19 – 7 = 12 patients.
5	How many patients suffer from hypertension and arthritis, but not from diabetes?	27 – 7 = 20 patients.
6	What percentage of the cohort population has any one of the diseases mentioned: hypertension, diabetes or arthritis?	(168/300) x 100 = 56%.
7	What percentage of the cohort population has arthritis alone?	(78/300) x 100 = 26%.
8	How many patients have diabetes alone, but do not have either hypertension or arthritis?	36 – (5 + 7 + 12) = 36 – 24 = 12 patients. See the calculated Venn diagram below for details (in the discussion section).
9	Which two diseases have the highest prevalence in this cohort of the study?	Arthritis and hypertension (78 and 54 patients).
10	What is the likelihood of the ratio of a patient to have diabetes compared with one without any disease in this cohort?	36:132 = 18:66 = 9:33 (36 patients have diabetes, and 132 patients have no diseases mentioned: see calculation in question 2).

Discussion

If you are given a question based on a Venn diagram, try to be calm even if it is an obscure diagram; try to break it into smaller parts and analyse the data given. Use a systematic approach:

- What data or information are given in the picture?
- Break down the information into smaller chunks.
- If there is any missing information, try to fill in and find those numbers.
- Try to find what conclusions could be arrived at based on the information that you have streamlined.
- Read the question again and check that you have the answer.

You could re-write the Venn diagram with the values given below, which will help to answer the specific questions.

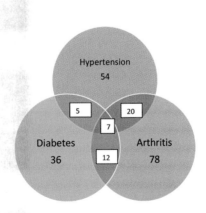

Key Points

- Read the question and try to work out separate parts of the Venn diagram.
- If a percentage is asked for, work out the numerator and denominator and multiply by 100.
- If a ratio is asked for, the answer will be in the format x:y.

Section 9

Other topics

Section editor: Thanthullu Vasu

Introduction to other topics

MMI stations can throw up surprising vague questions for the candidate; the aim is to see how the candidate can cope with these scenarios and answer them. Doctors have to cope with unplanned scenarios; keeping calm and tackling problems in a systematic way are essential in these scenarios. These non-clinical situations can assess the candidate's ability to deal with unplanned difficult times, and this could be extrapolated to their ability to deal with clinical situations. We have discussed a few odd questions that have appeared in MMI interviews in the past and have given brief ideas on answers, as these are not common questions.

Question 125

Conflict with superiors and how to deal with it

Jatin Naidu

Question

Have you ever experienced a conflict with your superiors and how did you deal with it at the time?

Discussion

The current scenario has been designed to manage a situation of conflict with senior colleagues and to still maintain a good rapport for ongoing working harmony. Give an appropriate example from your past experience. It could vary from simple school/college life to your work experience. One such example is described below:

In my A-level Extended Project Qualification, I had a supervisor in the college to oversee my project work. I was asked to draft a write-up on an experimental work that I was involved in for a few months. I had a deadline, but due to my ill health from COVID and end-of-year assessments, I could not correspond with my supervisor in a timely way and could not complete the task. My supervisor was annoyed and arranged a meeting with me.

This can be structured in the following way (RUES):

- R: maintain **R**apport:
  - thank him for giving you an opportunity to take part in the research and for ongoing support during the research.
- U: **U**nderstand their position:
  - I fully understand your position and there was a timeline and a deadline for this project that is important to meet to accomplish the task;
  - I am aware that you have other projects with tight timelines and these things will cause delays to other projects.
- E: **E**xplain your situation:
  - my situation happened a few weeks ago; I had COVID with a prolonged recovery. This left me with malaise and weakness that lasted longer than I expected. During this time, I was unable to attend my lectures and I had to catch up with the recorded lectures later on;
  - my end-of-year exams were closing in which also took priority and I could not put in the required effort into the writing up. I apologise as I could not explain my situation.
- S: provide a **S**olution:
  - my exams will finish next week and following that I can just concentrate on this task and will be expected to finish in the next couple of weeks;
  - I will make an appointment following that. We have some great results and are very close to publishing these in some good journals.

Key Points

- Have a structure to answer the question.
- Use good real-life examples, if possible, from your work experience or voluntary work.

Question 126

Writing a letter to yourself when you were 12 years old

Swetha Sridhar

Question

In the next station, you will be given paper and a pad; you have to write a letter to yourself when you were 12 years old. If you get an opportunity to talk to yourself about when you were 12 years old, what would you say or write? The paper will be marked by an examiner at the end of the session. You have 6 minutes for this station.

Discussion

This is a difficult question; especially when faced with an MMI interview scenario and in the restricted time limit. Do not complicate the question; keep it simple and informative.

You could think of various themes as below:

- The candidate may wish to write things that they achieved that they are proud of.
- The candidate can mention things they achieved that they did not think were possible before.

- The candidate can write any regrets that they have.
- The candidate can mention anything that they are looking forward to.
- The candidate may write down their current dreams and aspirations.

There is no right or wrong way of writing this letter, but it is prudent to think in a simple and logical manner. The examiner will assess how you can tackle and cope with difficult circumstances in this station by your answer in this short time.

Key Points

- Keep it simple and informative.
- Think of what you achieved that you are proud of, or any regrets that you have.
- This question assesses how you tackle difficult circumstances.

Question 127

Knowing about the university, curriculum and city

Thanthullu Vasu

Question

Do you know about the curriculum and the teaching methods used at our university?

Discussion

The medical school expects that the candidate has done enough research about the school and university before applying and coming for the interview. It is prudent that the candidate visits the school/university website and has enough knowledge about the history of the university, its facilities, curriculum, teaching methods, and the course itself.

Some universities use problem-based teaching, whilst others use traditional methods or integrated teaching. It is vital that the candidate knows what methods are followed in their chosen university.

It is also wise to find out whether they have cadaver-based teaching, what sort of research activities are available, what integrated courses are available, and what other opportunities are available. Some universities have links with foreign universities and there are opportunities for studying in these countries, and the candidate should be aware of these.

It is also wise for the candidate to do some research about the city where the university is based. Students also have to live a life in this city for 5-6 years and it is important that they are positive about the city.

Finally, it is important to find out about the extracurricular opportunities available such as sports and hobbies. Universities have lots of societies or cultural groups and it might be worth looking into these to have a good social life.

Open days in the universities help a lot in this regard, but if you have missed them, you can go to the university website to have a look at recorded videos, or YouTube videos; the website will have lots of details about the above-mentioned aspects and we strongly recommend that candidates do extensive research before the interview.

Key Points

- You should know about the curriculum of the university that you have applied to.
- Think about how this curriculum would suit you and your learning style.
- Analyse what you observed during the open day; research the university website regarding the curriculum.

Question 128

Stuck on an island

Subramanian Ganesan

Question

You will be stuck on an island for a few months; you can take only three things with you. What three things would you prefer and why?

Discussion

This is a difficult question that calls on your imagination skills and how you respond to a situation. There is no right or wrong answer, but we will discuss some broad aspects of how to answer this question.

The question does not specify what type of island and where (weather, wildlife and natural resources), and whether you could bring your loved one(s), so just assume it is a tropical island with lush vegetation and no violent inhabitants, and that you will be there for a few months. However, treat this island scenario as a survival scene instead of a leisurely vacation. That means that you do not sit around waiting for someone to arrive and save you. You need to get moving and think about how you are going to survive. But take it easy and enjoy your time. Make sure you are choosing at least one of the items from the things that help us to survive.

In any of these island scenarios, the five pillars of survival are: shelter, water, fire, food, and a positive attitude and mindset. You can add clothing and medicines to this list.

You can mention any of the items listed here based on the scenario whether you are stuck but assuming it's safe to stay there or you are struck and your safety is compromised, etc. Whatever you choose, it needs an explanation or reason why you have selected them. Adaptability according to the situation is the key here.

In general, you can categorise the three things from various themes mentioned below, assuming that you are there for a few months and it is a safe place to live and return home after a few months. If you are stuck and have no rescue plan in place, then you should choose three essential things from these!

Things to help us survive

- An endless supply of safe drinking water as it is essential for survival, especially if it is a desert where water is scarce. You need to stay hydrated to stay alive.
- A cooking vessel to boil and purify water.
- A magnifying glass or a mirror to start a fire, to feel warm and be able to cook.
- A giant box of matches. If you want to avoid spending hours trying to start a fire!
- A Swiss army knife to prepare food and for hunting, protecting ourselves, and building a shelter. A good knife is essentially vital in survival situations.
- Paracord: this is a very strong nylon rope originally designed for use in parachuting. It is versatile in survival situations and can be used for many purposes. Uses may include creating fishing lines and netting, bow drills to create fire, or even twine to bind a shelter together. It can be used to create splints in case of injuries. You can use this to tie logs together as needed to create a raft. You may also choose to work on your archery skills and build yourself a bow to shoot arrows useful for hunting! You may even weave yourself a comfortable

hammock to rest upon. You have got enough time on your hands to keep yourself occupied!

- Fishing net: fish are a very healthy protein choice, and having a net will ensure that fish are caught more easily.
- A solar-powered torch to be able to see at night, so you do not need batteries.
- A first aid kit with essential medicines in case of injuries and illness.
- A spear: this item would also come in handy for spear-fishing and for hunting.
- Rescue items: to create a rescue plan in case of dangerous situations such as signal fires, giant SOSs on the beach, and signal flags created from washed-up flotsam and jetsam to catch the eye of passing boats and overhead seaplanes.
- Map and compass.

Things to keep us updated/communication

- Satellite phones with solar batteries. It is great to start the morning by reading newspapers or magazines, or by checking newsfeeds on Facebook and Twitter. These will occupy your time from listening to music to watching your favourite films.
- Reading books. To kill the time.
- Take a friend.

Things to help us feel comfortable

- A hammock — many deserted islands are filled with trees, and a hammock would provide a comfortable place to sleep and be away from any nocturnal creatures.
- A can of bug spray — you know how useful it is to have bug spray if you have ever spent some time in the tropics.
- A bottle of sunblock. Sunscreen is one item that should not be left out of your deserted-island packing list to avoid sunburn leading to infections.

An inflatable raft with rows

- Row your boat to look at the scenic beauty of the sea; also useful for fishing in the sea.

Others

- A comfortable reclining chair for sleeping and relaxing.
- Sleeping bag.
- Fancy ideas such as your favourite pair of shoes, a guitar so that you can play watching the stars at night. Life is for enjoying anyway.

This question can throw up various opportunities to answer, but the main key is to stay positive and enjoy the answering process. The examiner is assessing your attitude rather than the correct answers.

Key Points

- Stations like this will assess your imagination skills and response to difficult situations.
- Have a logical way of answering these questions; keep it simple and informative.

Question 129

Creative thinking: why are schools needed for children?

Swetha Sridhar

Question

In the next station, the examiner will ask you why you think it is important for children to attend school.

Discussion

- School can be a good way to develop knowledge in a variety of subjects and can be beneficial for the development of life skills.
- The candidate may also mention that intelligence is not determined by whether or not a child attends school.
- Going to school involves conversing with other children their age and so is good for socialising and developing confidence.
- Schools are not solely academically based, as there are expressive art subjects, as well as cooking lessons, that are usually available.
- Children also have the opportunity to take part in extracurricular activities and may find interests outside the academic subjects that they enjoy.

Key Points

- Even though the question is based in favour of children attending school, make sure to acknowledge both sides.
- Make sure the language used is appropriate and does not belittle anyone.
- Keep your answer clear and succinct.

Question 130

Desert island: one person that can join you

Swetha Sridhar

Question

You can take one famous personality with you to a desert island. Who would you choose?

Discussion

This is a vague question, but the examiner is assessing whether the candidate can respond to difficult scenarios and can think coherently. It is prudent to keep the right attitude, stay focused and be positive:

- The candidate says who they would want to join them, with a reasonable explanation.
- The candidate could describe the celebrity's personality and qualities to justify why they chose that person.
- The candidate could also mention why they would be interested in going to a desert island.
- Think of someone with skills who would prove useful on a desert island.

Key Points

- This questions assesses your imagination skills and how you would respond to a difficult situation.
- Keep it simple and interesting.

Question 131

Asking 20 questions with a yes or no answer

Thanthullu Vasu

Question

The examiner thinks of a thing in his mind; you can ask 20 questions that have a yes or no answer only. You have to try to guess the thing that the examiner has thought of. All questions should have only a yes or no answer.

Discussion

Most candidates fail this station as they are under pressure to guess the right thing; rather, the examiner is assessing the way the candidate thinks and structures their questioning. This is a specific skill and can be practised before. Have a systematic approach rather than asking random questions.

Do not waste your limited supply of questions; any question that you ask should have the purpose of eliminating a group and focusing on another group.

Start the questions broad and then gradually go to more specific questions. Do not become frustrated in the middle and be focused. A doctor's career can be frustrating sometimes with puzzles in a medical conundrum, and those who stay focused are the ones who can help their patients.

There are a few examples below on how to do it and the candidate should practise them. It is wise to narrow it down to whether it is a person, place, object, animal, real or fictional and then proceed to specifics.

If it is an animal, the questions could be as below:

- Is it a living thing?
- If living: is it an animal?
- Does it live on land?
- Is it bigger than a car?
- Is it a pet animal?
- Does it have four legs?
- Is it a bird?

and so on.

If it is a personality rather than an animal, questions can go on as below:

- Is it a real person?
- Are they alive?
- Have I met them?
- Is it a male?
- Is it a movie star or politician or athlete?

and so on.

Categorising a movie star, a politician and a athlete together eliminates all three groups. If they say yes, then it is one of the three groups and then go to specifics.

If it is an edible thing, the questions go on as below:

- Is it eaten raw?
- Is it a fruit or vegetable?
- Is it sweet?
- Have I eaten it before?

and so on.

If it is a place, then questions can be:

- Is it in the UK?
- Do I need to take a plane to reach it?
- Is it a hot place?
- Is it a crowded place?

and so on.

If it is an object, then you can ask:

- Is it in this room?
- Is it light enough to pick up?
- Is it expensive?
- Is it used for fun?

and so on.

As mentioned before, the examiner assesses your structure and systematic way of working things out rather than arriving at the answer. Stay focused, be positive and do not get frustrated. If you cannot find the answer, convey apologies, smile and show your enthusiasm to find the answer.

Key Points

- The examiner will assess whether you have a structure for finding the answer.
- The key is in the structure rather than finding the answer.
- Stay calm and focus on a systematic approach.

Question 132

If you could have a superpower

Subramanian Ganesan

Question

If you could have one superpower, what would it be? Why?

Discussion

This type of question is asked to see how well you think outside of the box and see whether you are imaginative/creative. These kinds of questions are also used to see if a candidate has a good sense of humour, a very desirable trait when you are faced with a complex medical career. You should use this opportunity to showcase your personality and make yourself stand out from the other candidates. There must have been a time in your personal life when you put some thought into what superpower you would like to have.

Superpowers generally show the powers of speed, agility, power to influence, extraordinary strength/stamina/endurance, creativity/imagination, resilience, in-depth observation, time management, and the ability to prioritise.

Some examples you could choose from the following powers are shown below; this list is not exhaustive:

- Mind reading.
- Money pot.
- Predicting the future.
- Superhero.
- X-ray vision getting in-depth detail (observation).
- Time travel.
- Shape shifting.

If the topic of superhero powers comes up, feel free to have some fun with your response:

- It does not really matter what specific power you mention.
- Relate the power you want, and how it would apply to you doing your role.
- Relate the power to your personality.
- Try to be unique.

You should draft a story/scenario about choosing a superpower using the STARR framework:

- Situation: what is the challenging situation?
- Task: your role to help/solve the situation.
- Action: what did you do to resolve the situation?
- Result: achievement.
- Reflection: how to do better next time.

There are three important components for this scenario:

- Choose a suitable power that best represents you.
- Explain how it relates to you.
- Explain how things can be changed using your superpower.

Below are some sample answers to give you an idea:

Example 1: I have done volunteering work in a tribal area in India where access to the healthcare system is very remote. The nearest hospital with secondary care services is 50 kilometres away and it takes 3 hours to reach it by the hilly route. I have seen a mother in difficult labour, ending in the death of the baby due to a delay in getting to the hospital. This affected me significantly. If I had the chance, I would want to become a superhero with flying powers, so that I can take these patients with difficult medical illnesses to secondary care facilities in time to receive appropriate treatment. The satisfaction of averting an avoidable death is beyond description.

Example 2: my superpower would have to be supersonic speed, such as lightning. In the NHS there is a huge waiting list for elective surgeries that has been further worsened due to the COVID pandemic. This has compromised patient safety and care. I would like to use my superpower to perform surgery at a lightning pace that enables me to work more productively. This will enable me to finish the given task quicker, making it possible to increase the throughput.

You can tell different stories, but always explain why you chose that superpower in a simple logical way.

Mistakes you should avoid

There is not necessarily a wrong answer to give with this question, so make sure you do not make any of these easily avoidable mistakes:

- Do not say a superpower without giving a reason why you want it.
- Avoid saying you cannot think of one.
- Do not act like the question is silly.
- Do not spend too much time thinking about it.

Key Points

- Think of similar imaginative questions and practise before the interview.
- Choose a power that actually suits your strengths.
- Explain how this superpower will benefit you to help others or make a change.
- Remember you are attending a medical interview; your answers should be relevant to health and humanity!

Question 133

Explaining to a 6-year-old boy how an aeroplane flies

Swetha Sridhar

Question

Your 6-year-old nephew has taken an interest in aeroplanes and asks you whether you know how aeroplanes can fly. How would you explain to him how aeroplanes fly?

Themes for discussion (■ Table 9.1)

Table 9.1.

	Question themes	What is expected from the candidate?
1	The candidate greets the examiner acting as their nephew.	The candidate says hello, introduces themselves, and talks in a friendly manner. It is important that you are talking to a 6-year-old person and keep the language simple and clear.

Table 9.1.

Question themes	What is expected from the candidate?
2 The examiner mentions how he has been watching a TV show with cartoon aeroplanes and is wondering how aeroplanes fly.	The candidate appreciates the nephew's interest and curiosity towards aeroplanes. The candidate then proceeds to explain the process of flight of an aeroplane, using language tailored to the age of their nephew: • The aeroplane is driven by the pilot and his team; it has a powerful engine that gives the energy to fly. • The pilot starts the engine and pulls a lever that allows the aeroplane to take off from the ground, into the sky. This is called a take-off. The plane has to go at high speed and then the pilot pulls the lever to take it off the ground to the sky. • The aeroplane has wings that help it move across the sky. • When landing the aeroplane, the pilot moves the lever, so that the front of the aeroplane faces the ground and the plane can land at its destination. The candidate asks if their nephew understood. The candidate can volunteer to show a paper model and explain the science behind flight
3 The examiner apologises and says they do not understand and asks whether you can repeat a part of your explanation.	The candidate shows compassion and reassures the nephew that it is OK that they did not understand. The candidate then proceeds to repeat what their nephew did not understand, in a way that is easier to understand.
4 The examiner expresses interest in your explanation and thanks you for explaining.	The candidate asks if they have any more questions.
5 Conclusion.	The candidate says 'thank you' to the examiner.

Discussion

It is important to be patient and compassionate. Your nephew, in this instance, may not understand what you have said, so be prepared to repeat what you have said, and perhaps simplify your description of how aeroplanes fly, if necessary.

Make sure to explain how aeroplanes fly in non-technical terms so that it is interesting and easy to understand for your nephew.

Key Points

- Tailor your words and expression to the person you are talking to.
- Take your time explaining and showing that you are interested when your nephew is talking to you.
- Take the initiative and ask if your nephew understands what you have said.
- Make sure to keep the explanation short, concise and engaging, so that you answer your nephew's question, but do not overcomplicate it.

RISE Foundation Leicestershire

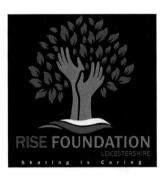

Registered Charity Number 1190740

www.risefoundationuk.com

Sharing is Caring

The RISE Foundation Leicestershire is a charity that aims to advance community education and promote health and wellbeing. Our vision is 'Sharing is Caring'. We are a group of like-minded friends living in Leicestershire who have come together to make small changes in the local community and abroad where there is a need. We host events and seminars regularly to further our objective; all the money raised has been donated for needed causes. All our trustees and committee members are busy professionals who have volunteered their time and effort to bring a cohesiveness to the community.

We have huge expertise in running popular MMI courses in Leicester that have been attended by hundreds of candidates who have benefited immensely; the money raised from these courses has gone to charitable causes through the Foundation. Our courses have been successful with excellent outcomes and feedback. We have pooled our expertise to produce this easy-to-read textbook which should help budding doctors who are preparing for their interviews. We wish them all the best in their interviews, career and future.

We thank you for buying this book and supporting our charity. All author royalties from the sales of this book will be donated to worthy causes through the RISE Foundation Leicestershire charity.